T0263106

Liver Transplantation and Transplantation Oncology

Editor

SHIMUL A. SHAH

SURGICAL CLINICS
OF NORTH AMERICA

www.surgical.theclinics.com

Consulting Editor
RONALD F. MARTIN

February 2024 • Volume 104 • Number 1

ELSEVIER

1600 John F. Kennedy Boulevard • Suite 1800 • Philadelphia, Pennsylvania, 19103-2899

http://www.surgical.theclinics.com

SURGICAL CLINICS OF NORTH AMERICA Volume 104, Number 1
February 2024 ISSN 0039–6109, ISBN-13: 978-0-443-12987-2

Editor: John Vassallo (j.vassallo@elsevier.com)

Developmental Editor: Anita Chamoli

© **2024 Elsevier Inc. All rights reserved.**

This periodical and the individual contributions contained in it are protected under copyright by Elsevier, and the following terms and conditions apply to their use:

Photocopying

Single photocopies of single articles may be made for personal use as allowed by national copyright laws. Permission of the Publisher and payment of a fee is required for all other photocopying, including multiple or systematic copying, copying for advertising or promotional purposes, resale, and all forms of document delivery. Special rates are available for educational institutions that wish to make photocopies for non-profit educational classroom use. For information on how to seek permission visit www.elsevier.com/permissions or call: (+44) 1865 843830 (UK)/(+1) 215 239 3804 (USA).

Derivative Works

Subscribers may reproduce tables of contents or prepare lists of articles including abstracts for internal circulation within their institutions. Permission of the Publisher is required for resale or distribution outside the institution. Permission of the Publisher is required for all other derivative works, including compilations and translations (please consult www.elsevier.com/permissions).

Electronic Storage or Usage

Permission of the Publisher is required to store or use electronically any material contained in this periodical, including any article or part of an article (please consult www.elsevier.com/permissions). Except as outlined above, no part of this publication may be reproduced, stored in a retrieval system or transmitted in any form or by any means, electronic, mechanical, photocopying, recording or otherwise, without prior written permission of the Publisher.

Notice

No responsibility is assumed by the Publisher for any injury and/or damage to persons or property as a matter of products liability, negligence or otherwise, or from any use or operation of any methods, products, instructions or ideas contained in the material herein. Because of rapid advances in the medical sciences, in particular, independent verification of diagnoses and drug dosages should be made.

Although all advertising material is expected to conform to ethical (medical) standards, inclusion in this publication does not constitute a guarantee or endorsement of the quality or value of such product or of the claims made of it by its manufacturer.

Surgical Clinics of North America (ISSN 0039–6109) is published bimonthly by Elsevier Inc., 360 Park Avenue South, New York, NY 10010-1710. Months of publication are February, April, June, August, October, and December. Business and Editorial Offices: 1600 John F. Kennedy Blvd., Suite 1800, Philadelphia, PA 19103-2899. Periodicals postage paid at New York, NY and additional mailing offices. Subscription prices are $503.00 per year for US individuals, $100.00 per year for US & Canadian students and residents, $592.00 per year for Canadian individuals, $597.00 for international individuals, and $250.00 per year for foreign students/residents. For institutional access pricing please contact Customer Service via the contact information below. To receive student/resident rate, orders must be accompanied by name of affiliated institution, date of term, and the *signature* of program/residency coordinator on institution letterhead. Orders will be billed at individual rate until proof of status is received. Foreign air speed delivery is included in all *Clinics* subscription prices. All prices are subject to change without notice. POSTMASTER: Send address changes to *Surgical Clinics*, Elsevier Health Sciences Division, Subscription Customer Service, 3251 Riverport Lane, Maryland Heights, MO 63043. **Customer Service (orders, claims, online, change of address): Telephone: 1-800-654-2452 (U.S. and Canada); 314-447-8871 (outside U.S. and Canada). Fax: 314-447-8029. E-mail: journalscustomerservice-usa@elsevier.com (for print support); journalsonlinesupport-usa@ elsevier.com (for online support).**

Reprints. For copies of 100 or more, of articles in this publication, please contact the Commercial Reprints Department, Elsevier Inc., 360 Park Avenue South, New York, New York 10010-1710. Tel. 212-633-3874, Fax: 212-633-3820, E-mail: reprints@elsevier.com.

Surgical Clinics of North America is also published in Spanish by McGraw-Hill Interamericana Editores S.A., P.O. Box 5-237 06500 Mexico D.F. Mexico; and in Portuguese by Interlivros Edicoes Ltda., Rua Comandante Coelho 1085, CEP 21250, Rio de Janeiro, Brazil; and in Greek by Paschalidis Medical Publications, Athens Greece.

Surgical Clinics of North America is covered in *MEDLINE/PubMed (Index Medicus)*, *EMBASE/Excerpta Medica*, *Current Contents/Clinical Medicine*, *Current Contents/Life Sciences*, *Science Citation Index*, and *ISI/BIOMED*.

Contributors

CONSULTING EDITOR

RONALD F. MARTIN, MD, FACS
Colonel (Retired), United States Army Reserve, Department of General Surgery, Pullman Regional Hospital and Clinic Network, Pullman, Washington

EDITOR

SHIMUL A. SHAH, MD, MHCM
The James and Catherine Orr Endowed Chair in Liver Transplantation, Chief, Solid Organ Transplantation, Vice-Chair, Health Services Research, Professor of Surgery, Division Chief of Transplantation, Professor of Clinical Surgery, Division of Transplantation, Department of Surgery, Cincinnati Research in Outcomes and Safety in Surgery (CROSS) Research Group, University of Cincinnati College of Medicine, Cincinnati, Ohio

AUTHORS

MICHIE ADJEI, MD
Department of Surgery, Cedars-Sinai Medical Center, Los Angeles, California

SANDRA ARIAS, MD
General Surgery Resident, Division of Transplant Surgery, Department of Surgery, Mayo Clinic, Phoenix, Arizona

HASSAN AZIZ, MD
Assistant Professor, Division of Transplant and Hepatobiliary Surgery, Department of Surgery, University of Iowa Hospital and Clinics, Iowa City, Iowa

ANDREW M. CAMERON, MD, PhD
Director and Chief, Professor of Surgery, Department of Surgery, Johns Hopkins Medicine, Baltimore, Maryland

WILLIAM CHAPMAN, MD, FACS
Professor and Chief, Section of Transplantation, Chief, Division of General Surgery, Washington University School of Medicine, St Louis, Missouri

KENDRA D. CONZEN, MD
Associate Professor of Surgery, Colorado Center for Transplantation Care, Research and Education (CCTCARE), University of Colorado Anschutz Medical Campus, Aurora, Colorado

J. MICHAEL CULLEN, MD
Fellow, Colorado Center for Transplantation Care, Research and Education (CCTCARE), University of Colorado Anschutz Medical Campus, Aurora, Colorado

NEHA DEBNATH, MD
Biostatistician, Division of Nephrology, Department of Medicine, Liver Transplant
and Hepatobiliary Surgery, Recanati/Miller Transplantation Institute, Icahn School of
Medicine at Mount Sinai, New York, New York

MARIA BERNADETTE MAJELLA DOYLE, MD, MBA, FACS
Professor, Division of Abdominal Organ Transplantation, Department of Surgery,
Washington University School of Medicine, St Louis, Missouri

OLANREWAJU A. ELETTA, MBBS
Department of Surgery, Rutgers Robert Wood Johnson Medical School, New Brunswick,
New Jersey

ZHI VEN FONG, MD, MPH, DrPH
Assistant Professor, Division of Surgical Oncology and Endocrine Surgery, Department of
Surgery, Mayo Clinic, Phoenix, Arizona

ANA L. GLEISNER, MD, PhD
Associate Professor, Department of Surgery, University of Colorado Anschutz Medical
Campus, Aurora, Colorado

STEPHEN J. HARTMAN, MD
Resident Physician, Department of Surgery, University of Cincinnati College of Medicine,
Cincinnati, Ohio

ANGELA HILL, MD, MPHS
Research Fellow, Department of Surgery, Washington University School of Medicine, St
Louis, Missouri, USA

NITIN N. KATARIYA, MD
Transplant and Hepato-Pancreato-Biliary Surgeon, Division of Transplant Surgery,
Department of Surgery, Mayo Clinic, Phoenix, Arizona

IRENE KIM, MD
Professor of Surgery, Director, Comprehensive Transplant Center, Cedars-Sinai Medical
Center, Los Angeles, California

KAYLA KUMM, MD
Transplant Surgeon, Division of Transplant Surgery, Department of Surgery, Mayo Clinic,
Phoenix, Arizona

KRISTINA LEMON, MD
Assistant Professor, Department of Surgery, University of Cincinnati College of Medicine,
Cincinnati, Ohio

JESSICA LINDEMANN, MD, PhD
Abdominal Transplant Surgery Fellow, Division of Abdominal Organ Transplantation,
Department of Surgery, Washington University School of Medicine, St Louis, Missouri

ALBAN LONGCHAMP, MD, PhD
Transplant Surgery Fellow, Department of Surgery, Center for Engineering in
Medicine, Massachusetts General Hospital, Harvard Medical School, Boston,
Massachusetts

KERI E. LUNSFORD, MD, PhD, FACS
Liver Transplant and Hepatobiliary Surgeon and Translational Transplant Immunologist, Department of Surgery, Rutgers New Jersey Medical School, Newark, New Jersey

JAMES F. MARKMANN, MD, PhD
Chief, Division of Transplant Surgery, Department of Surgery, Center for Engineering in Medicine, Harvard Medical School, Massachusetts General Hospital, Mass General Brigham, Boston, Massachusetts

THOMAS MARRON, MD, PhD
Associate professor of Medicine, Liver Transplant and Hepatobiliary Surgery, Recanati/Miller Transplantation Institute, Icahn School of Medicine at Mount Sinai, New York, New York

LAUREN MATEVISH, MD
Division of Surgical Transplantation, Department of Surgery, The University of Texas Southwestern Medical Center, Dallas, Texas

AMIT K. MATHUR, MD, MS, FACS
Transplant Surgeon and Professor, Division of Transplant Surgery, Department of Surgery, Mayo Clinic, Phoenix, Arizona

DAVID C. MULLIGAN, MD, FACS, FAASLD, FAST
Professor and Past Chair, Division of Transplantation and Immunology, Director, Transplant Innovation and Technology, Department of Surgery, Past President, UNOS/OPTN, Yale New Haven Health Transplantation Center, Yale School of Medicine, New Haven, Connecticut

BRYAN MYERS, MD
Liver Transplant and Hepatobiliary Surgery, Recanati/Miller Transplantation Institute, Icahn School of Medicine at Mount Sinai, New York, New York

TSUKASA NAKAMURA, MD, PhD
Clinical Fellowship, Division of Transplant Surgery, Department of Surgery, Massachusetts General Hospital, Harvard Medical School, Boston, Massachusetts

PARAMITA NAYAK, BSc
Division of Transplant and Hepatobiliary Surgery, University of Iowa Hospital and Clinics, Iowa City, Iowa

FRANKLIN OLUMBA, MD, MPHS
Research Fellow, Division of General Surgery, Department of Surgery, Washington University School of Medicine, St Louis, Missouri

GUERGANA G. PANAYOTOVA, MD
Division of Transplant and Hepatobiliary Surgery, Department of Surgery, Rutgers New Jersey Medical School, Newark, New Jersey

MADHUKAR S. PATEL, MD, MBA, SCM
Assistant Professor, Division of Surgical Transplantation, Department of Surgery, The University of Texas Southwestern Medical Center, Dallas, Texas

ELIZABETH A. POMFRET, MD, PhD, FACS
Professor of Surgery, Chief, Division of Transplant Surgery, Igal Kam, MD Endowed Chair in Transplantation Surgery, Executive Director, Colorado Center for Transplantation Care, Research and Education (CCTCARE), University of Colorado Anschutz Medical Campus, Aurora, Colorado

CATHERINE G. PRATT, MD
Research Fellow, General Surgery Resident, Cincinnati Research in Outcomes and Safety in Surgery (CROSS) Research Group, Department of Surgery, University of Cincinnati College of Medicine, Cincinnati, Ohio

RALPH C. QUILLIN III, MD
Associate Professor, Division of Transplantation, Department of Surgery, University of Cincinnati College of Medicine, Cincinnati, Ohio

BRIANNA RUCH, MD
Transplant Surgeon, Division of Transplant Surgery, Department of Surgery, Mayo Clinic, Phoenix, Arizona

EMILY J. SCHEPERS, MD
Fellow/Resident, Division of Transplantation, Department of Surgery, University of Cincinnati College of Medicine, Cincinnati, Ohio

SHIMUL A. SHAH, MD, MHCM
The James and Catherine Orr Endowed Chair in Liver Transplantation, Chief, Solid Organ Transplantation, Vice-Chair, Health Services Research, Professor of Surgery, Division Chief of Transplantation, Professor of Clinical Surgery, Division of Transplantation, Department of Surgery, Cincinnati Research in Outcomes and Safety in Surgery (CROSS) Research Group, University of Cincinnati College of Medicine, Cincinnati, Ohio

CHRISTOPHER J. SONNENDAY, MD, MHS
The Darrell A. Campbell, Jr, MD Collegiate Professor of Transplant Surgery Transplant Center Director, University of Michigan Health, Ann Arbor, Michigan

PARISSA TABRIZIAN, MD, MSc, FACS
Associate Professor of Surgery, Liver Transplant and Hepatobiliary Surgery, Recanati/Miller Transplantation Institute, Icahn School of Medicine at Mount Sinai, New York, New York

FRANCIS J. TINNEY, Jr, MD
Instructor in Surgery, Abdominal Transplant Surgery Fellow, Division of Transplant Surgery, Department of Surgery, Johns Hopkins Medicine, Baltimore, Maryland

KIARA A. TULLA, MD
Instructor in Surgery, Abdominal Transplant Surgery Fellow, Division of Transplant Surgery, Department of Surgery, Johns Hopkins Medicine, Baltimore, Maryland

KORKUT UYGUN, PhD
Associate Professor, Division of Transplant Surgery, Department of Surgery, Center for Engineering in Medicine, Massachusetts General Hospital, Harvard Medical School, Boston, Massachusetts

PARSIA A. VAGEFI, MD
Professor & Division Chief, Division of Surgical Transplantation, Department of Surgery, The University of Texas Southwestern Medical Center, Dallas, Texas

JENNA N. WHITROCK, MD
Research Fellow, General Surgery Resident, Cincinnati Research in Outcomes and Safety in Surgery (CROSS) Research Group, Division of Transplantation, Department of Surgery, University of Cincinnati College of Medicine, Cincinnati, Ohio

ALLEN YU, MD, PhD
Resident Physician, Liver Transplant and Hepatobiliary Surgery, Recanati/Miller Transplantation Institute, Icahn School of Medicine at Mount Sinai, New York, New York

SARA-CATHERINE WHITNEY ZINGG, MD
Clinical Instructor, Chief Resident, Department of Surgery, University of Cincinnati College of Medicine, Cincinnati, Ohio

IOANNIS A. ZIOGAS, MD, MPH
General Surgery Resident, Department of Surgery, University of Colorado Anschutz Medical Campus, Aurora, Colorado

Contents

setting, although more research is needed to delineate its role in current treatment paradigms.

transplantation being formally contraindicated for patients with iCCA; however, recent advances in patient selection and neoadjuvant therapy have resulted in a paradigm shift in liver transplant oncology. As a result, the feasibility of liver transplantation for iCCA is being reevaluated by several centers as a therapeutic alternative for select patients with locally advanced unresectable disease.

Liver Transplantation for Colorectal Liver Metastases

Emily J. Schepers, Stephen J. Hartman, Jenna N. Whitrock, and Ralph C. Quillin III

Colorectal cancer is one of the most common malignancies worldwide. Approximately half of the patients diagnosed will develop colorectal liver metastases (CRLM). Liver resection has a 50% 5-year survival; however, only a fourth of cases are resectable. Unresectable CRLM has poor prognosis despite improved systemic and local ablative treatments. Liver transplantation (LT) has demonstrated a survival benefit in initial prospective clinical trials. Current use of LT for CRLM is limited to several randomized trials and high-performing centers. Improving patient selection criteria and perioperative management, LT will likely become an important part of the multidisciplinary approach to managing the metastatic disease.

SURGICAL CLINICS
OF NORTH AMERICA

SERIES OF RELATED INTEREST

Advances in Surgery
https://www.advancessurgery.com/
Surgical Oncology Clinics
https://www.surgonc.theclinics.com/
Thoracic Surgery Clinics
https://www.thoracic.theclinics.com/

THE CLINICS ARE AVAILABLE ONLINE!
Access your subscription at:
www.theclinics.com

Foreword

Liver Transplantation and Transplantation Oncology

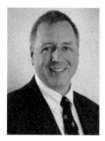

Ronald F. Martin, MD, FACS
Editor

The liver is an organ that has been shrouded in mystery and fascination since antiquity. As the Greek myths taught us, Zeus ordered Prometheus chained to a rock while his liver was pecked at daily by eagles (or vultures, depending on the translation). His liver regenerated after these insults, and the whole process began anew. His alleged crime against the gods was giving the forbidden knowledge of fire to humans. The concept of the liver being renewable yet somehow foreboding lies deep at the center of the human psyche. Most of us who have practiced for a while have learned that a patient can have almost any organ falter due to injury or infection and said organ, and the patient, will recover—with the notable exception of liver failure (and of course, major CNS failure). Or at least that is the way it was. Our ability to rescue the patient with a faltering liver has been completely redefined within a few short decades.

The above notwithstanding, at present one does very much need a liver. How much is debatable. Whose liver is debatable. But for the moment, a biologically active liver is a requirement. As with other aspects of liver care, that may be evolving as well. Perhaps when we cycle back to this topic in half a dozen years or so, other forms of "liver capability" will exist.

Early in my career, we focused on how much liver one could remove. Which segments could go with which. Largely the focus was on technical issues that ended in, "But you can't do that because…" Over a fairly short period of time, we progressed to: how much liver do we have to preserve? We decided to not bog ourselves down with technical details of lobes and segments but rather focus on how much functioning (and bile draining) hepatocellular mass we could maintain. Many bright and talented people literally rewrote the textbooks on how we approach operations to remove liver tissue that was misbehaving in some manner.

Surg Clin N Am 104 (2024) xv–xvi
https://doi.org/10.1016/j.suc.2023.09.011
0039-6109/24/© 2023 Published by Elsevier Inc.

Despite all those advances, there remained plenty of scenarios in which there would not be enough functional hepatic reserve to maintain viability. More liver would be required. As if on cue, significant developments in transplantation biology and practice had been developing that would open a new door. For some time, most of the partial hepatic resections fell to one type of specialist (hepatopancreatobiliary surgeons or surgical oncologists), while the allograft work fell to the transplanters. There was never a compelling reason for it to be that way—it just mostly was. Of course, there were always groups that did much of both; they were relatively rare by comparison. There were far more hospitals that were rigged to perform metastasectomies and resections for primary liver tumors than perform solid organ transplants.

Now, we have developed far more sophisticated pathways to remove liver that is malfunctioning or life-threatening and replace it with allograft. Dr Shah and his colleagues have provided us with a comprehensive resource to guide us through not only how we determine what to resect and how to replace it, when necessary, but also how to maximize the efficacy of a scarce resource. As with any other solid organ for transplantation, there are challenges acquiring donor tissue. Many of the advances in other medical branches and advances in overall safety have reduced the donor supply among the recently deceased. However, advances in using living donor material and methods for preserving and allocation of donor material are somewhat of an offset against the overall shortage. I can think of no other concise compendium such as has been collected to help any of us understand this complicated subset of issues.

The issue of competing immunologic paradigms for preventing rejection of allograft while maintaining competent immune surveillance in the setting of malignancy remains challenging as well. As "precision" medicine becomes more precise for preventing rejection and/or for tumoricidal effect, this hurdle may lessen as well.

Not all of us surgeons perform liver operations. Even fewer of us surgeons perform liver transplantations. That stated, nearly all of us general surgeons do or will take care of someone who has or will develop liver metastases. All of us need to be aware of what options are available and feasible for our patients who develop these concerns. And all of us of need to know how those who are already in this treatment group will present with other problems that may be in our wheelhouse.

Unlike the gods of the Greek myths, we surgeons should not guard our developments jealously. We share what we know when we know it in the hopes of serving the collective good. We at the *Surgical Clinics* are committed to providing a platform for those with extensive knowledge and opportunity to disseminate their hard-earned wisdom to all who care to partake. I encourage you to read this material and share it with your colleagues and trainees without fear of being chained to a rock or being assaulted by birds.

Ronald F. Martin, MD, FACS
Colonel (Retired), United States Army Reserve

Department of General Surgery
Pullman Surgical Associates
Pullman Regional Hospital and Clinic Network
825 Southeast Bishop Boulevard, Suite 130
Pullman, WA 99163, USA

E-mail address:
rfmcescna@gmail.com

Preface

Changing Paradigm of Liver Transplantation and Transplant Oncology

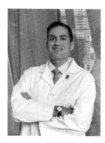

Shimul A. Shah, MD, MHCM
Editor

The landscape of liver transplantation is changing rapidly. The indications, needs, and access to organs are evolving, and our community needs to be kept abreast of the latest developments and emerging concepts in the field. This issue of *Surgical Clinics* provides the reader with the latest data and trends in liver transplantation in general and then focuses on a new concept of transplant oncology. Transplant oncology is an emerging concept with growing interest in our community, and the newest and emerging findings, protocols, and trends are discussed in this issue.

Shimul A. Shah, MD, MHCM
Solid Organ Transplantation
Health Services Research
University of Cincinnati College of Medicine
231 Albert Sabin Way, MSB 1555B
Cincinnati, OH 45257, USA

E-mail address:
shimul.shah@uc.edu

Twitter: @shimulshah73 (S.A. Shah)

Conflict of interest/disclosures: Organ Recovery Systems, grant funding; CareDx, grant funding; Genentech, medical advisory board.

surgical.theclinics.com

Current Status of Liver Transplantation in North America

Hassan Aziz, MD[a], Paramita Nayak, BSc[a], David C. Mulligan, MD[b],*

KEYWORDS

- Liver transplantation • Machine perfusion • Transplant oncology

KEY POINTS

- The rise of transplant oncology brings higher survival rates in patients.
- Donors are becoming older/more obese/having more comorbidities.
- Liver transplant complications are rising.
- The organ shortage is impacting liver recipients and giving way to the rise of living donors.
- Machine perfusion is allowing organs to be salvaged for longer, therefore, improving lifespan.

INTRODUCTION

Liver transplantation has made tremendous progress over the past 2 decades. The deceased donor pool has been significantly increased over the past decade. As a result of the effort in this area, liver allografts from donors after cardiac death (DCD), marginal donors, and those with extended criteria have been used more frequently. In addition, developing mechanical perfusion strategies has been made possible due to an improved understanding of the pathophysiology of liver allografts procured following circulatory arrest. Early findings showing hypothermic and normothermic perfusion's clinical relevance and their potential to enhance allograft function and patient survival have generated a great deal of interest.

Despite progress, some challenges remain: one is organ shortage, which accounts for a large portion of waitlist mortality. The number of liver transplants has increased in Asian countries through living donation but has stagnated in Western countries.

[a] Division of Transplant and Hepatobiliary Surgery, University of Iowa Hospital and Clinics, Iowa City, IA, USA; [b] Division of Transplantation and Immunology, Transplant Innovation and Technology, Department of Surgery, UNOS/OPTN, Yale-New Haven Health Transplantation Center, Yale University School of Medicine, 333 Cedar Street, Farnum Medical Building Room 121, New Haven, CT 06520, USA
* Corresponding author.
E-mail address: david.mulligan@yale.edu

Surg Clin N Am 104 (2024) 1–9
https://doi.org/10.1016/j.suc.2023.08.002
0039-6109/24/© 2023 Elsevier Inc. All rights reserved.
surgical.theclinics.com

Finally, long-term outcomes for liver transplant recipients have not improved significantly, as they continue to suffer from infection, malignancy, and renal failure. This study discusses the current status of liver transplantation in North America and its potential challenges.

DONOR CHARACTERISTICS
Age

The age of the donors being utilized continues to rise. The United Network for Organ Sharing reported that 2.4% of liver donors were above 50 years in age in 1989, but that rate increased to 29% in 1999 and 33% in 2013, indicating that the average liver donor's age is increasing.[1] The transplantation of older donors has been associated with a higher risk of delayed graft function and primary nonfunction and therefore requires a careful selection of recipients who have lower medical acuity for these livers. Therefore, despite the early growth in liver transplants from older donors between 1990 and 2009, usage of older donor livers has plateaued.

Opioid Crisis

Recent studies have shown an increase in deceased donors due to the opioid crisis. Drug-related donor deaths increased by 48%, and national drug-related deaths increased by 102% within the past decade. It is hypothesized that the same phenomena are in play when observing the significant increase in donor deaths due to anoxic brain injury within the 18 to 34 years age group.[2] The Centers for Disease Control also noted that these donors are more likely to have diseases like hepatitis B virus (HBV), hepatitis C virus (HCV), and human immunodeficiency virus due to the opioid crisis.[3,4]

Hep C Donors

Increasingly, livers from HCV-positive donors are being utilized for transplantation in the United States following the introduction of direct-acting antivirals (DAAs), with sustained viral response rates approaching 100%. Several centers have accepted livers from HCV-viremic (HCV-RNA+) and HCV Ab+ donors for HCV-negative recipients thanks to the efficacy and low side effect profile of DAAs. There is no significant difference in early graft and patient outcome between recipients of HCV-positive and HCV-negative grafts in the post-DAA era.

Obese Donors

Obesity is rising within the donor population as well. As a result, there has been an increase in the use of obese donors and livers with micro and macrovascular steatosis. The incidence of primary graft nonfunction and biliary complications are higher in steatotic grafts. Therefore, patient selection continues to be the key to using these donors.

LIVER RECIPIENTS CHARACTERISTICS

The United States continues to see a growth in the number of waitlist registrants and transplants performed. The number of registrations and transplants for HCV-related indications has decreased significantly, while alcoholic liver disease and nonalcoholic steatohepatitis (NASH) have increased. Similarly, there has been an increase in elderly patients undergoing liver transplant (LT) (**Fig. 1**).[5] It is suspected that alcoholic liver disease will surpass HCV in the coming year as an indication for LT. As a result of a lack of awareness and knowledge about transplant as a curative option, most patients with alcoholic liver disease seen in the community or rural areas do not get referred for LT.[6] According to population studies, alcohol-related liver disease death rates have

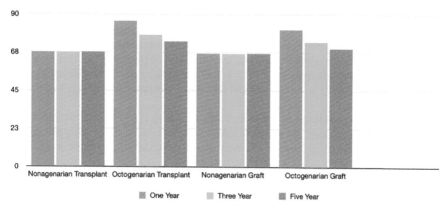

Fig. 1. Octogenarian and nonagenarian transplant and graft survival rates.

been increasing and most recently was found to have the highest mortality rate among gastrointestinal diseases (6.8 per 10,000). Recent studies have shown that acute alcoholic hepatitis (AAH) is a new and rising indication for LT. In cases such as these, LT is indicated for specific reasons.[7] This has been made possible by a consensus statement that has defined many parameters. In the setting of AAH, patients must have the following[1]: patients with AAH presenting for the first time with decompensated liver disease that cannot be treated with medical therapy without severe medical or psychiatric comorbidities,[2] no fixed period of abstinence before transplantation, and[3] psychosocial assessment by a multidisciplinary team. Lack of repeated unsuccessful attempts at addiction rehabilitation, no other substance use/dependency, acceptance of diagnosis with a commitment to sobriety, and formal agreement to adhere to total alcohol abstinence were all supportive factors. When patients with AH are likely to recover spontaneously, LT should be avoided.[8] Long-term and short-term survival must be comparable to other indications for LT. The treatment of alcohol-use disorders should be incorporated into pre- and post-LT care. This lifesaving indication had shown excellent results when appropriately indicated, with comparable survival and similar recidivism rates.

There is an increasing incidence of nonalcoholic fatty liver disease (NAFLD) in the Western world, particularly in North America, and this trend is predicted to continue for another 10 to 15 years. In parallel with obesity, diabetes, and other lifestyle-related diseases, NAFLD will rise, such as nonalcoholic steatohepatitis, liver fibrosis, liver cirrhosis, liver-related morbidity, and mortality. As a result of its widespread prevalence and associated economic burden, it has attracted significant attention and research. There is no targeted treatment for this condition, so prevention has been the focus.[9,10] As with alcoholic liver disease, its incidence and indication are rising. NASH accounts for 30% of liver transplant indications in many centers. Cardiovascular comorbidities and complications of diabetes are prevalent in this subpopulation of patients, posing unique challenges for transplant physicians and surgeons. A record of 51.4 deceased donor transplants per 100 waitlist years has been recorded due to the increase in deceased donors, while waitlist mortality has decreased across demographic groups, including gender, race, diagnosis, and urgency. Twenty-two percent of patients were older than 65 years in 2017, almost double the number 10 years ago. Waitlist mortality varies by geography and does not reflect organ availability, suggesting that center behavior, referral practices, and waitlist management vary across the country.[5]

It has been shown that recipients of rHCV-positive livers have a higher 3 year and 5 year mortality rates than recipients of a non-HCV liver donor. Between 2016 and 2019, there was an increase in the amount of HCV-/R+ liver transplants; within the first 3 months of 2020, there were 73 transplants of this nature performed.[11] The data indicate a 35x increase in the amount of HCV + liver transplants performed within 4 years; in 2016, there were only 8 transplants performed of this nature; by 2019, there were 300 (**Fig. 2**).

Obesity is a rising epidemic in the United States as well. It has been shown that liver recipients have rising body mass index (BMI); around 17% of liver transplant candidates have a BMI above 35 kg/m^2.[6] Morbidly obese candidates, described as patients with a BMI of over 40 kg/m2, are observed to have higher waitlist mortality rates alongside a higher risk factor for acute-on-chronic liver failure. In addition, it was shown that obese patients had significantly reduced 5 year grafts and survival rates compared with nonobese patients, going from 75.8% to 49% and 78.8% and 51.3%, respectively.[12]

Waitlist times are increasing due to organ shortages, leading to higher complication and death rates. It is shown that the longer the wait period proceeds, the higher the likelihood of complications and death becomes. It was shown that at the 3, 6, and 12 month marks, the survival rates of people on the waitlist were 92%, 80%, and 69%, respectively.[7]

Waiting List Registration

Owing to a steady increase in transplants over the past decade, the waitlist has reduced, albeit slightly, with 11,772 candidates still waiting on December 31, 2020. In addition, an increasing proportion of older (aged >65 years) candidates were on the adult waiting list in 2020, representing 21.7%, compared with 9.4% in 2010. There is relatively little change in the gender and racial composition of the waiting list: 61.6% male, 38.4% female, 68.7% White, 7.0% Black, 17.9% Hispanic, and 4.8% Asian.

Alcohol-associated liver disease and other/unknown diagnoses (often representing liver disease due to nonalcoholic steatohepatitis) are currently the leading indications for liver transplant listing, while acute liver failure, cholestatic liver disease, and, especially, HCV have decreased. Hepatocellular carcinoma (HCC) accounts for 10.9% of new waiting list registrations, nearly doubling in the past decade.

Based on the first active laboratory model for end-stage liver disease (MELD) during the calendar year, the severity of liver disease has increased, with a greater proportion of listings with MELD 25 to 34 (12.0%), MELD 35 to 40 (3.4%), and MELD 40+ (3.0%). Among the candidates on the waiting list, 17.8% had a BMI of 35 kg/m^2, the only category with a steadily increasing trend. In 2020, 3.2% of candidates had a history of liver transplants.

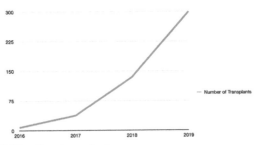

Fig. 2. Number of HCV + liver transplants per year.

Over the past 5 years, there was a distinct shift in attitudes as DAA therapy became available, resulting in a nearly threefold increase in liver candidates willing to accept HCV-positive donors.

WAITING LIST OUTCOMES

The overall deceased donor transplant rate among adult waiting list candidates rose to 65.2 per 100 waiting list years in 2020 from 35.7 per 100 in 2009. There was an increase in all age groups, major racial/ethnic groups, blood types, and places of residence. Regarding deceased donor transplants, women continue to experience a lower rate than men (59.9 vs 68.6). There has been a narrowing gap between candidates with and without HCC exception points (79.0 vs 63.7 per 100 waiting list years), reflecting the May 2020 policy that will lower waitlist priority for exceptional cases.

In 2020, the pretransplant mortality rate was 12.2 per 100 waiting list years, an all-time low. Pretransplant mortality rates were higher among women (13.1 vs 11.6 deaths per 100 waiting list years). Among those with acute liver failure, pretransplant mortality was highest (19.0 deaths per 100 waiting list years) and lowest (9.1 deaths per 100 waiting list years for both HCV and HCC). Despite improvements in the higher MELD categories (ie, MELD 25 or higher), pretransplant mortality was still high for those with MELD 35 to 40 or 40+ (167 and 124 deaths per 100 waiting list years, respectively).

Donation

The number of deceased liver donors increased to 9211 in 2020, despite fewer pediatric donors (age 18 years) (Figure LI 36, Figure LI 39). A total of 61.4% of donors are male, 38.6% female, 63.3% white, 17.8% black, 15.1% Hispanic, and 2.8% Asian. Among the deceased donor livers recovered in 2020, 9.7% were HCV-positive.

Overall, 9.5% of livers recovered were not transplanted; livers from older donors were less likely to be transplanted. Positive hepatitis C antibodies and those at an increased risk of disease transmission were not more likely to be discarded. Donors' livers recovered after circulatory death (DCD) were discarded at a lower rate than in previous years. Still, they remained much more likely not to be transplanted than livers recovered after brain death (26.6% vs 7.1%). Amid the ongoing opioid epidemic in the United States, anoxic brain injuries continue to be the leading cause of death among deceased donors.

Compared with the year before (n = 516), 485 living donor liver transplants were performed in 2020, a 6% decrease. With a small but growing proportion of nondirected living donations (12.0%) and paired donations (2.9%), most donors were related to or directed to the recipient. Most living donors were between 18 and 54 years, with a minority over 55 years (5.5%). Female (58.0%) and white donors (79.5%) were more likely to be living donors. Over the past decade, the right liver lobe has been used in most cases (76.2%). For living liver donors (2015–2019), the readmission rate was 9.0% at 6 months and 11.0% at 12 months. Biliary complications (2.6%), vascular complications (0.8%), reoperations (2.1%), and other complications (5.3%) were reported among liver donors (2016–2020). Among these donors, 0.9% had Clavien Grade 1 complications, 1.5% had Clavien Grade 2%, and 0.4% had Clavien Grade 3 complications.

Outcomes

The short-term and long-term outcomes of liver transplants continued to improve. It was reported in 2019 that 5.9% of deceased donor liver transplant recipients failed at 6 months and 7.9% at 1 year, 14.7% at 3 years following transplants in 2017,

20.7% at 5 years after transplants in 2015, and 40.6% at 10 years after transplants in 2010. Living donor liver transplant recipients had similar, if not better, outcomes, with graft failure occurring in 4.9% at 6 months, 7.4% at 1 year, 12.2% at 3 years, 23.7% at 5 years, and 36.7% at 10 years. The survival rates of patients demonstrated similar patterns, with 4.6% mortality at 6 months, 6.4% at 1 year, 13.1% at 3 years, 18.8% at 5 years, and 38.2% at 10 years.

THE RISE OF TRANSPLANT ONCOLOGY

The rise of transplant oncology has brought about many advances within both transplantation and oncology. The goal of transplant oncology is the use principles of both oncology and transplantation to improve patient mortality rates and quality of life. Hepatobiliary cancers treated by liver transplantation have higher rates of improved outcomes than other treatments. Recent advances and increases in donor pools have allowed transplantation to occur within patients with primary and secondary hepatobiliary malignancies, the most relevant being cholangiocarcinoma, colorectal liver metastases, neuroendocrine liver metastases, and hepatic epithelioid hemangioendothelioma.[13]

Liver transplantation is also being considered for colorectal cancer, the third most common cancer worldwide. With the metastases developed within the liver, for many patients, liver resection is the only chance at survival; however, only a small number of patients with hepatic colorectal cancer are eligible for liver resections. Although liver transplantation may seem viable for patients with nonresectable colorectal liver metastases, initial encounters with these patients show high mortality rates. The 5 year survival rate is lower than 20% without any parallel therapies. The organ shortage also plays a big role in this process; many patients can only utilize living donors for liver transplants, which is gaining momentum.[14]

The Milan criteria heavily influence whether patients receive a liver transplant, and it is proven to be a crucial factor in the reception and survival of a liver transplant recipient regarding cirrhosis and HCC. The Milan criteria state that to receive a liver transplant, a patient must only have either a single tumor with a diameter of ≤ 5 cm (about 1.97 in.) or up to 3 tumors, each with a diameter of ≤ 3 cm (about 1.18 in.), and no major vessel or extrahepatic involvement.[15] The extent of the liver disease and the determination of portal hypertension are also considered. Often, patients presenting with tumor(s) that do not fit the Milan criterion will receive other treatments such as chemotherapy, immunotherapy, or radiotherapy to shrink the tumor(s) so they can fit into the Milan criterion and the patient can be eligible for a transplant. A 2022 study showed that around 52% of people with HCC whose tumors met the Milan criteria after prior treatments were performed to shrink the tumors were alive 10 years postoperatively.[16] Patients whose tumors met the Milan criteria at diagnosis showed a 61% survival rate 10 years postoperatively.

Transplant oncology works to broaden the scope of cancer surgery; transplant and oncology in the hepatobiliary area have evolved together.[17] Mobilization techniques involving multiple abdominal organs used by transplant surgeons for organ acquisition are currently used for large upper abdominal tumor resection.

Recently, there has been much interest in LT for patients with colorectal liver metastatic disease. The SECA-II trial demonstrated the highest overall survival of 100%, 83%, and 83% at 1, 3, and 5 years, respectively, and disease-free survival of 53%, 44%, and 35%, respectively, with a narrow inclusion criterion.[18] Currently, this option is only available at some centers in the United States but is being actively explored by many other centers.

LIVING DONOR LIVER TRANSPLANT

A living donor liver transplantation (LDLT) aims to alleviate organ shortages among deceased donors and, as a consequence, reduce mortality on the liver transplant waiting list. Despite its first description in the Western world, this technique has been more successful in Asian countries with extremely low deceased donor rates. Owing to the higher availability of cadaveric grafts in North America than in Asian countries and unfortunate LDLT outcomes, its growth has been limited in North America (**Fig. 3**). LDLT has been rethought as a valid and useful alternative by the North American community due to the high mortality rate on waiting lists in some regions and the limited access to deceased donor grafts for patients with low MELD scores, the expanding indications for LT. In the United States, the number of adult-to-adult LDLTs has steadily increased since 2013.

MACHINE PERFUSION

Using both hypothermic and normothermic machine perfusions shows potential for increasing the pool of useable livers and providing a solution to the shortage of organ availability compared with the organ demand. Machine perfusion was first introduced in the 1960s and sparked up once again in the 2000s. It has been commonly used since then. However, static hypothermic cold storage remains the main method of liver preservation due to logistics and practicality.

Hypothermic perfusion works by inducing a hypothermic reaction within the organ, which slows cellular metabolism, making the time the organ can survive without oxygen longer. A 2005 study showed that hypothermic perfusion lowered graft injuries; subsequent studies showed similar results with lower serum transaminases, higher allograft function, and lower times spent in the hospital than liver allografts put in cold storage from deceased donors.[19,20] Normothermic perfusion, in contrast, artificially creates a physiologic environment through mechanisms such as maintaining body temperature and providing necessary substrates for processes such as cellular metabolism. The normothermic perfusion systems resemble and contain components used for cardiopulmonary bypasses.[20]

Acknowledged uses of normothermic perfusion can include repeal of hyperfibrinolysis after inflammation or reperfusion, repletion of glycogen, and adenosine triphosphate regeneration, allowing for a variety of interventions that can increase organ quality.[21,22] The research within this type of perfusion focuses heavily on biomarker prediction of allograft quality alongside the risks of injury due to ischemia-reperfusion.[22] Current research shows that normothermic perfusion increases hepatic allograft usage and lowers the risk of ischemia-reperfusion injuries, leading to a lower risk of early allograft dysfunction alongside fewer biliary complications.[22] Although suboptimal, static hypothermic cold storage remains the primary method for liver

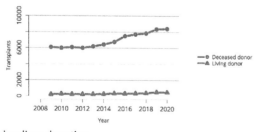

Fig. 3. Trends in living liver donation.

preservation, largely because of its cost effectiveness, simplicity, and logistics. There is a large and apparent need to optimize preservation, particularly for DCD, marginal and extended-criteria donor organs.[23]

CLINICS CARE POINTS

- Patient selection has been a changing target over the years as we've gone to less HCV and more EtOH related liver diseases, older candidates with more comorbidities, and new techniques like robotic transplantation.
- Post transplant rehab care has never been more important to drive long term outcomes (especially EtOH rehab to prevent recidivism) and learning how to assess cardiac risks is a changing landscape with fewer stress tests and more CT calc scoring, etc.
- Resources to address new perfusion technologies have been a major impact on transplant centers from both more flights and transport expenses to device expenses like TransMedics OCS.
- Advantages of new technologies will need to outweigh costs by decreasing LOS, ICU, OR times and blood usage as well as reduce complications.
- Potential for making transplant timing more appealing to surgeons and teams and reduce burden of 24/7 hospital resources and burnout among teams.
- Future will be in improved preservation technologies like XTherma and others as well as perfusion devices, NRP, and more bases for organ perfusion and resuscitation of organs which may shift strategies for OPOs to lease devices from companies, use them to recover organs and bring back to base then allocate after data on organ quality rather than before recovery. This reduces discards and maximizes utilization. Ischemia time limits will become negligible. Ultimately the costs of liver transplants will reduce.
- Finally, will see where xenotransplant will emerge for livers too.

REFERENCES

1. Lué A, Solanas E, Baptista P, et al. How important is donor age in liver transplantation? World J Gastroenterol 2016;22(21):4966–76.
2. Goldberg D, Lynch R. Improvements in organ donation: Riding the coattails of a national tragedy. Clin Transplant 2020;34:e13755.
3. Jones JM, Kracalik I, Levi ME, et al. Assessing Solid Organ Donors and Monitoring Transplant Recipients for Human Immunodeficiency Virus, Hepatitis B Virus, and Hepatitis C Virus Infection — U.S. Public Health Service Guideline, 2020. MMWR Recomm Rep (Morb Mortal Wkly Rep) 2020;69(No. RR-4):1–16.
4. Desai R, Collett D, Watson CJ, et al. Cancer transmission from organ donors-unavoidable but low risk. Transplantation 2012;94(12):1200–7.
5. Khapra AP, Agarwal K, Fiel MI, et al. Impact of donor age on survival and fibrosis progression in patients with hepatitis C undergoing liver transplantation using HCV+ allografts. Liver Transpl 2006;12(10):1496–503.
6. Soma D, PhD1, Park Y, et al. Liver Transplantation in Recipients With Class III Obesity: Posttransplant Outcomes and Weight Gain. Transplantation Direct 2022;8(2):e1242.
7. Gheorghe L, Popescu I, Iacob R, et al. Predictors of death on the waiting list for liver transplantation characterized by a long waiting time. Transpl Int 2005 May; 18(5):572–6.

8. Berenguer M, Prieto M, San Juan F, et al. Contribution of donor age to the recent decrease in patient survival among HCV-infected liver transplant recipients. Hepatology 2002 Jul;36(1):202–10. Erratum in: Hepatology. 2003 Feb;37(2):489.

9. Shaw BW Jr, Gordon RD, Iwatsuki S, et al. Retransplantation of the liver. Semin Liver Dis 1985 Nov;5(4):394–401.

10. Abdelrahim M, Esmail A, Abudayyeh A, et al. Transplant Oncology: An Evolving Field in Cancer Care. Cancers 2021 Sep 29;13(19):4911.

11. Cotter TG, Aronsohn A, Reddy KG, et al. Liver Transplantation of HCV-viremic Donors Into HCV-negative Recipients in the United States: Increasing Frequency With Profound Geographic Variation. Transplantation 2021 Jun 1;105(6):1285–90.

12. Conzen KD, Vachharajani N, Collins KM, et al. Morbid obesity in liver transplant recipients adversely affects longterm graft and patient survival in a single-institution analysis. HPB (Oxford) 2015 Mar;17(3):251–7.

13. Abreu P, Gorgen A, Oldani G, et al. Recent advances in liver transplantation for cancer: The future of transplant oncology. JHEP Rep 2019;1(5):377–91.

14. Moeckli B, Ivanics T, Claasen M, et al. Recent developments and ongoing trials in transplant oncology. Liver Int 2020 Oct;40(10):2326–44.

15. Weerakkody Y, Gajera J, Di Muzio B, et al. Milan criteria in liver transplantation. Reference article, Radiopaedia.org (Accessed on April 24 2023).

16. Tabrizian P, Holzner ML, Mehta N, et al. Ten-Year Outcomes of Liver Transplant and Downstaging for Hepatocellular Carcinoma. JAMA Surg 2022;157(9): 779–88.

17. Sousa Da Silva RX, Weber A, Dutkowski P, et al. Machine perfusion in liver transplantation. Hepatology 2022;76(5):1531–49.

18. Ahmed FA, Kwon YK, Zielsdorf S, et al. Liver Transplantation as a Curative Approach for Patients With Nonresectable Colorectal Liver Metastases. Exp Clin Transplant 2022;20(2):113–21.

19. Guarrera JV, Estevez J, Boykin J, et al. Hypothermic machine perfusion of liver grafts for transplantation: technical development in human discard and miniature swine models. Transplant Proc 2005;37(1):323–5.

20. Reddy SP, Brockmann J, Friend PJ. Normothermic perfusion: a mini-review. Transplantation 2009;87(5):631–2.

21. Dultz G, Graubard BI, Martin P, et al. Liver transplantation for chronic hepatitis C virus infection in the United States 2002–2014: an analysis of the UNOS/OPTN registry. Gruttadauria S. PLoS One 2017;12(10):e0186898.

22. van Beekum CJ, Vilz TO, Glowka TR, et al. Normothermic Machine Perfusion (NMP) of the Liver - Current Status and Future Perspectives. Ann Transplant 2021;26:e931664.

23. Croome KP. Introducing Machine Perfusion into Routine Clinical Practice for Liver Transplantation in the United States: The Moment Has Finally Come. J Clin Med 2023;12(3):909. Published 2023 Jan 23.

Current Use of Immunosuppression in Liver Transplantation

Michie Adjei, MD, Irene K. Kim, MD*

KEYWORDS

- Liver transplant • Immunosuppression • Induction immunosuppression
- Antibody-mediated rejection

KEY POINTS

- The use of induction therapy, immunosuppression used perioperatively during transplant, is highly varied among transplant centers. Induction therapy has been show to reduce the risk of rejection in liver transplant recipients.
- Maintenance therapy regimens in liver transplant patients generally consist of calcineurin inhibitor and steroid therapy, but alternatives, such as mammalian target of rapamycin inhibitors and belatacept, exist.
- Antibody-mediated rejection is a relatively rare occurrence in liver transplantation. Mainstays of treatment depend on rituximab, intravenous immunolgobulin therapy, and plasmapheresis strategies.

INTRODUCTION

The first liver transplant, performed by Dr Thomas Starzl in 1967, used a combination of azathioprine, steroids, and heterolygous antilymphocyte globulin (ALG) for immunosuppression.[1] Mitigating the balance between immunologic rejection of the allograft and vulnerability to opportunistic infection, Starzl and colleagues recognized the importance of tapering immunosuppression (ie, Steroids) and eventual discontinuation of ALG. In 1979, Dr Roy Calne introduced cyclosporine, a calcineurin inhibitor, which enabled a new era in liver transplantation of superior clinical outcomes as an agent with less drug toxicity and fewer infections.[2] With advancement in liver transplantation technique and the introduction of calcineurin inhibitors, 1-year patient survival approached 70% in the initial era.[3]

In the current era of liver transplantation, 1-year adult patient survival now approaches 93.6%, mainly attributed to improvements in immunosuppression and

Comprehensive Transplant Center, Cedars-Sinai Medical Center, 8900 Beverly Boulevard, Los Angeles, CA 90048, USA
* Corresponding author.
E-mail address: Irene.Kim@cshs.org

Surg Clin N Am 104 (2024) 11–25
https://doi.org/10.1016/j.suc.2023.08.004
0039-6109/24/© 2023 Elsevier Inc. All rights reserved.

less toxic medical regimens.[4] (**Fig. 1**). Many debates still exist in optimal approach to immunosuppression for liver transplant recipients, starting with differences in approach with induction therapy to attempts in minimization of maintenance immuno-suppressive therapy to avoid long-term side effects. This review article explores some of the main controversies related to immunosuppression in liver transplantation, pre-sents the data and rationale for immunosuppression approaches, and explores some of the newer advancements in immunosuppressive drug therapy.

INDUCTION THERAPY IN LIVER TRANSPLANTATION

Induction therapy, immunosuppression administered at the time of transplant and routinely used in kidney transplantation, has been shown to decrease rejection, improve graft survival, delay the introduction of calcineurin inhibitors reducing the risk of renal dysfunction, and minimize steroid use in liver transplantation as well.[5-8] Induction therapy remains controversial in liver transplant with only 31.1% of liver transplant recipients in the United States receiving induction therapy, according to the most recent OPTN/SRTR annual reports[9] (**Fig. 2**). Because of the lack of random-ized controlled trials (RCTs) and variability on the utilization of induction therapy, there are no consensus guidelines for induction therapy in liver transplantation by the Amer-ican Association for the Study of Liver Diseases.[10] However, more recent guidelines from the Asian Liver Transplant Network in 2018 recommend induction therapy in all liver transplant patients. Likewise, the European Association for the Study of the Liver recommends induction therapy in liver transplant recipients with pretransplant renal insufficiency.[11,12]

There are 2 main forms of induction therapy used in transplantation: lymphocyte-depleting agents and interleukin-2 receptor antagonists (IL2-RA), started before, at the time of, or immediately following transplantation. In the former category, the 2 most common forms of lymphocytic depletion are thymoglobulin and alemtuzumab. In the latter category, the main agents historically used have been basiliximab and daclizumab. Lymphocyte-depleting agents have been shown to reduce the risk of rejection compared with IL2-RA; however, they increase infection and malignancy risk.[13]

One concern for the use of induction therapy in liver transplantation has been the risk for accelerated disease progression for patients transplanted with active hepatitis C virus (HCV).[14,15] A few studies have demonstrated the contrary.[16,17] A small RCT of 49 patients who underwent liver transplantation for HCV received either rabbit antith-ymocyte globulin (ATG) induction (n = 26) or standard immunosuppression (n = 23).

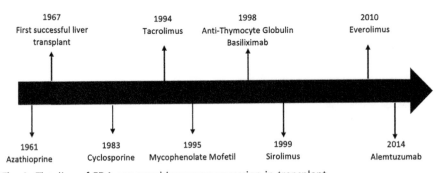

Fig. 1. Timeline of FDA-approved immunosuppression in transplant.

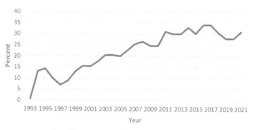

Fig. 2. Induction therapy use by liver transplant centers in the United States (1993–2021); from the SRTR Database. Scientific Registry of Transplant Recipients. OPTN/SRTR 2020 Annual Data Report: Liver. https://srtr.transplant.hrsa.gov/annual_reports/2020/Liver.aspx# LI_tx_ped_imsxn_ind_b64. Accessed 14 August 2023.

They found that induction with ATG had a lower recurrence of HCV when compared with standard therapy (26.9 vs 73.9%, $P = .001$).[18]

Rabbit Antithymocyte Globulin

Rabbit ATG or thymoglobulin, a polyclonal immunoglobulin G (IgG) T-cell depleting antibody, is one of the most common agents used for induction in liver transplant.[19] When compared with IL2-RA, ATG had lower rates of acute cellular rejection (ACR) and improved rates of patient and graft survival.[8,20] In a large retrospective analysis of 595 patients, 322 receiving ATG and 273 receiving IL2-2RA, ACR was higher in patients who received IL2-2RA than in patients who received ATG (27% vs 18%; $P < .03$). At 5 years posttransplant, both patient survival (86% vs 80%) and graft survival (83% vs 78%) were superior with ATG than with IL2-RA ($P < .002$).[20] However, when specifically evaluated in patients who underwent liver transplantation for acute liver failure, those receiving ATG had an increased risk of overall mortality compared with steroid only and IL2-RA regimens, which the investigators hypothesize may be due to the increased risk of infection related to ATG use.[21]

An additional perceived benefit of ATG utilization is the ability to delay the introduction of calcineurin inhibitors (CNI), which has demonstrated improved renal function without an increase in rejection, graft failure, or patient survival.[22–24] Standard regimens using ATG for delayed CNI initiation, starting CNI 3 to 6 days posttransplantation, generally demonstrated significant improvement in renal function throughout the first year posttransplant with lower serum creatinine and higher glomerular filtration rates (GFR) compared with the noninduction groups.[24,25] In a recent multicenter RCT of comparing induction ATG with an extended 10-day delayed CNI initiation (n = 55) to upfront CNI commencement (n = 55), there was a significant difference in delta creatinine between the groups at 9 months ($P = .03$) but not at 12 months ($P = .05$).[22]

The use of ATG has not been associated with an increased recurrence of HCV when using a steroid-free protocol.[26,27] In those undergoing liver transplant for HCV, recipients receiving induction therapy with ATG had comparable recurrence HCV rates to those receiving steroids, as shown by Saidi and colleagues.[28] Similarly, in an RCT comparing ATG induction with standard steroid therapy, lower rates of HCV recurrence were found in the ATG group.[18]

Interleukin-2 Receptor Antagonists

Basiliximab is a monoclonal antibody that binds to the CD25 chain of the IL-2 receptor in activated T cells, inhibiting proliferation of T lymphocytes and reducing acute cellular rejection.[29] Likewise, daclizumab, another IL2-RA and monoclonal antibody that binds CD25, was previously used in kidney transplant induction but drug manufacturing was discontinued in 2009 and removed from market in 2018 secondary to multiple cases of autoimmune encephalitis after use.[30] In the kidney transplant literature, it has been repeatedly shown that induction with IL2-RA led to the reduction of acute rejection and graft loss compared with placebo (ie, no induction). Several RCTs have also studied outcomes in kidney transplantation between IL2-RA and lymphocyte-depleting agents.[31,32] Brennan and colleagues demonstrated no difference in patient or graft survival between ATG versus basiliximab in kidney transplant recipients; however, patients at high risk for acute rejection receiving ATG had reduced incidence and severity of acute rejection.[13]

In the liver transplant literature, several RCTs have demonstrated overall decreased risk of rejection, mortality, and metabolic complications with the utilization of basiliximab.[33–35] Neuhaus and colleagues demonstrated reduced biopsy-confirmed rejection at 6 months posttransplant with basiliximab in a double-blind, randomized placebo-controlled trial in 381 liver transplant patients (35.1% vs 43.5%, $P = .105$). Of note, they saw no differences in infection or other adverse events.[16] Additional benefits in liver recipients also included reduction of de novo diabetes and hypertension with basiliximab in conjunction with steroid-free protocols.[35]

Similar to the benefit seen with ATG induction, multiple studies have demonstrated that delayed calcineurin inhibitor administration after induction with basiliximab results in improved renal function with no increased incidence on rejection or mortality compared with control groups.[29,33,36] A large retrospective cohort study by Cederborg and colleagues compared patients who received either standard treatment consisting of immediate introduction of tacrolimus, target trough levels 10 to 15 ng/mL, corticosteroids (n = 203) or basiliximab induction, reduced-dose tacrolimus starting on day 3, target trough levels 5 to 8 ng/mL, and mycophenolate mofetil 2000 mg/d (n = 343). At 12 months after liver transplant, mean GFR was higher in the induction group (60.9 vs 69.7 mL/min/1.73 m²; $P < .001$). There was a significant difference in graft survival (91% vs 97% at 1 year and 75% vs 84% at 5 years) and rejection (38% vs 21%, $P < .001$ at 1 year, $P = .01$), but no difference in mortality (97% vs 99% at 1 year and 84% vs 87% at 5 years, $P = .16$).[29]

Although the use of basiliximab has been associated with progression of HCV recurrence in HCV-positive recipients, there is no statistically significant difference in HCV recurrence rates when basiliximab was compared with ATG.[37,38]

Alemtuzumab

Alemtuzumab (Campath-1H) is a humanized monoclonal antibody against CD52, an antigen found on both normal and malignant T and B lymphocytes.[39] Because of its profound lymphocytic depleting effects, it has been associated with increased posttransplant infections in renal transplant and rapidly progressive HCV in liver transplant patients.[40,41] There is limited data on the use of alemtuzumab as an induction agent in liver transplant. A retrospective case-control study of 55 HCV-negative liver transplant recipients receiving alemtuzumab induction performed by Levitsky and colleagues showed a decreased number of rejections when compared with the nonalemtuzumab group. Concurrent with alemtuzumab induction, the researchers adopted a steroid-free protocol but used dual immunosuppression with tacrolimus and mycophenolate mofetil (MMF) posttransplant. Not surprisingly, there was a statistical significant difference in viral infections in the alemtuzumab group compared with the nonalemtuzumab group (13 vs 2, $P < .0001$).[39] Smaller studies have demonstrated similar results of decreased rates of rejections, all excluding HCV-positive recipients.[42,43]

MAINTENANCE THERAPY IN LIVER TRANSPLANTATION

Beyond the initial posttransplant period (3–6 months) following liver transplantation, most patients are maintained on a stable, lifelong immunosuppressive regimen. Over the years, immunosuppression in liver transplantation has significantly improved, with lower amounts of graft rejection, graft loss, and increases in patient survival.[12] Most maintenance therapy regimens include a combination of a glucocorticoid, calcineurin inhibitor, and/or a third agent, commonly an antimetabolite such as MMF or azathioprine. In 2021, 71.8% of adult liver transplant recipients received steroid-containing immunosuppressive regimen.[9] Most of the patients were still being discharged on standard triple therapy regimen of tacrolimus + MMF + corticosteroids (68%).[9] The most common dual therapy maintenance immunosuppression combinations for liver transplant were tacrolimus + MMF (17%) and tacrolimus + corticosteroids (6%).[44] The utilization of types of maintenance therapy varies internationally, with center-specific protocol being a strong predictor of immunosuppression selection.[45]

After its introduction in 1981, calcineurin inhibitors, particularly tacrolimus and cyclosporine, became the most common immunosuppressive drugs used for liver transplant recipients.[9] Although, in an RCT of 606 patients randomly assigned to either tacrolimus or cyclosporine, tacrolimus demonstrated superior patient and graft survival outcomes.[46] With subsequent studies demonstrating similar results, tacrolimus became the first-line therapy at most liver transplant centers.[47] One of the most significant side effects of using CNIs is nephrotoxicity.[48] Given that an estimated 20% of liver transplant recipients develop chronic renal failure within 5 years posttransplant, several studies have evaluated minimization of CNI use to decrease CNI-induced renal impairment.[49]

Glucocorticosteroid use has become a cornerstone in liver transplant immunosuppression regimens.[9] But the use of glucocorticoids is associated with several adverse events, including diabetes mellitus, hypertension, and infections, leading to decreased use at some transplant centers. In a systematic review of RCTs examining steroid-free versus steroid-containing immunosuppression, the incidence of diabetes mellitus and hypertension was statistically less seen in steroid-free regimens; however, there were more frequent episodes of acute rejection and steroid-resistant rejection in the steroid-free group. There was no difference in graft survival, mortality, or infection rates between the 2 groups.[50]

Role of Mammalian (Mechanistic) Target of Rapamycin Inhibitors in Maintenance Immunosuppression

mTOR inhibitors (mTORi) have been used to prevent graft rejection since approval for kidney transplant in 1999.[51] The 2 commonly used mTORi are everolimus and sirolimus. Because of wound healing complications, mTORi are not used immediately following transplantation. Furthermore, a higher incidence of hepatic artery thrombosis observed in the early posttransplant period led to a Food and Drug Administration (FDA)–issued black box warning in liver transplant recipients. In liver transplant, mTORi have been used to minimize CNI use in those with renal dysfunction to reduce CNI-related nephrotoxicity.[52,53] Multiple trials have consistently demonstrated improved renal function compared with CNI-based therapy, with follow-up data showing sustained renal advantages up to 5 years posttransplant.[54–59]

One of the suggested benefits of mTORi, due to mTORi activity inhibiting tumor growth and efficacy in treating cancers such as renal cell carcinoma,[60] is the potential of preventing posttransplant malignancy.[61] The large prospective randomized SiLVER trial sought to determine if the utilization of sirolimus minimized hepatocellular carcinoma (HCC) recurrence in those undergoing liver transplant for HCC. The study included 2 groups: mTORi-free immunosuppression (n = 264) and sirolimus-containing immunosuppression regimen (n = 261). When comparing recurrence-free survival between both groups, there was no statistical difference in recurrence-free survival after 5 years (P = .28), although there was an initial significant benefit in recurrence-free survival at 3 years posttransplant.[62] However, an exploratory analysis of the SiLVER trial performed by Schnitzbauer and colleagues suggested that mTORi treatment may be beneficial in those with an elevated alpha fetoprotein greater than 10 ng/mL, finding improved overall survival and recurrence-free survival in that subgroup.[63]

DUAL (CALCINEURIN + ANTIMETABOLITE) THERAPY MAINTENANCE IMMUNOSUPPRESSION

Long-term steroid discontinuation is a common practice and is a recommended practice of the guidelines from the International Liver Transplant Society (ILTS). Many centers maintain postliver transplant patients with CNI monotherapy, also endorsed by the ILTS guidelines. However, rationale for dual, long-term therapy with tacrolimus and an antimetabolite, such as with patients receiving simultaneous liver and kidney transplantation, and other indications exist. Later, 2 additional indications, renal sparing and autoimmune liver diseases, are discussed further for the rationale in using dual maintenance immunosuppression with CNI and MMF.[64]

Patients with Posttransplant Renal Impairment

Chronic renal failure and end-stage renal disease have been recognized to be a major cause of morbidity and mortality after liver transplantation.[48] Reduction and/or withdrawal of CNI in those with renal dysfunction has become common practice.[49] Everolimus plus lowered dose CNI compared with standard dose CNI therapy has been associated with improved renal function at 12 months in multiple studies.[65] In a similar multicenter RCT comparing low-dose sirolimus plus low-dose extended release tacrolimus, compared with standard-dose tacrolimus, there was a higher mean eGFR in the sirolimus group at 6 months posttransplantation (73.1 $\pm$ 15 vs 67.6 $\pm$ 16 mL.min/1.73 m,^{2} P = .02) but no difference at 36 months.[66] A retrospective review of 60 patients who were withdrawn from CNI therapy to either MMF + prednisolone or azathioprine + prednisolone demonstrated improvements in renal function with maintenance 6 years posttransplant.[67]

Patients with Autoimmune Disorders of the Liver

Autoimmune disorders of the liver such as primary biliary cirrhosis (PBC), primary sclerosing cholangitis (PSC), and autoimmune hepatitis (AIH) account for a sizable amount of liver transplants performed in the United States and Europe.[68] Recurrent disease posttransplantation is common, ranging from 12% to 30% in PBC, 12% to 60% in PSC, and 17% to 42% in AIH.[69] Immunosuppression regimens have been developed to prevent both rejection and autoimmune disease recurrence. Interestingly, AIH recurrence has been associated with a history of acute rejection, and tacrolimus monotherapy use has been associated with increased recurrence of PBC after liver transplantation.[70]

Utilization of dual immunosuppression with both tacrolimus and mycophenolate with or without steroid withdrawal may prevent autoimmune liver disease recurrence.[71] In the nontransplant setting, combination tacrolimus and MMF have been used as initial or rescue therapy in the treatment of AIH, especially in patients intolerant or refractory to first-line treatment with steroids and azathioprine.[72] There-fore, it stands to reason that strategic utilization of dual immunosuppression with both tacrolimus and mycophenolate with or without steroid withdrawal may prevent autoimmune liver disease recurrence.[71] Combination therapy with tacrolimus + MMF also allows for the potential withdrawal of steroids in patients with AIH. Junge and colleagues from Charité Hospital in Berlin demonstrated similar graft and patient survival out to 24 months postliver transplant for patients receiving steroids + tacrolimus + MMF versus tacrolimus + MMF alone.[73] Likewise, Satapathy and colleagues presented acceptable long-term outcomes with ATG + maintenance MMR with tacrolimus or mTORi without steroids in liver transplant recipients for auto-immune reasons (PSC, PBC, AIH) from a single-center study.[71] Studies to determine immunologic benefit (ie, time to disease recurrence), if any, with varying immunologic regimens are needed.

BELATACEPT IN LIVER TRANSPLANT

Belatacept is a fusion protein that combines IgG1 with the extracellular domain of CTLA-4 that binds CD80/86 molecules on antigen-presenting cells, blocking a crucial component in T-cell costimulation. This infusion drug inhibits T-cell activation and was initially approved for use in renal transplantation in June 2011.[74] In a phase II trial eval-uating the safety and efficacy of belatacept in liver transplant patients, those receiving belatacept had improved renal function but increased rates of acute rejection, graft loss, and death compared with those treated with a CNI-based regimen.[75] The results of this trial lead to a black box warning issue by the US FDA for belatacept use in liver transplantation. However, there have been a few reports and small studies of belata-cept use in liver transplant recipients with more favorable outcomes.[76,77] In a retro-spective review of 7 adult liver transplant recipients with HCV and renal dysfunction receiving belatacept postliver transplant, the 6-month patient and graft survival was 86%.[74] A study evaluating belatacept use in 8 patients who had a history of liver trans-plantation and then underwent kidney transplantation demonstrated preserved liver graft function in all patients.[78]

WITHDRAWAL OF IMMUNOSUPPRESSION

Given the associated toxicity of immunosuppression regimens, the withdrawal of immunosuppression has been increasingly studied.[79–81] A trial of 102 liver trans-plant patients, at least 3 years posttransplant, was discontinued from immunosup-pression over a 6- to 9-month period. Of the 98 patients evaluated, 41 patients (42%) reached stable biochemical and histologic graft function 1 year after com-plete discontinuation. Although, those more than 10.6 years posttransplant had a 79% success rate compared with the 38% success rate of those 5.7 years posttransplant.[82]

Shaked and colleagues performed a prospective randomized trial of 275 patients to evaluate early immunosuppression minimization and complete withdrawal in those receiving standard immunosuppression drugs (corticosteroids and a calcineurin inhib-itor and/or antimetabolite). Of the 95 patients enrolled in the study, 77 were randomly assigned to withdrawal 1 to 2 years posttransplant. Seventy-one (92%) were able to tolerate once-a-day dosing by study end. For those who had further minimization, 52 (67.5%) were reduced to 50% or less of baseline monotherapy dose without biochemical evidence of graft dysfunction. Ten patients (13%) tolerated complete withdrawal at a mean of 2.8 years after transplantation.[83]

PREGNANCY AND IMMUNOSUPPRESSION IN LIVER TRANSPLANT

Although most immunosuppressive drugs (tacrolimus, corticosteroids, cyclosporine, mTORi, MMF, azathioprine) cross the placenta, only 2 drugs, mycophenolate and mTOR inhibitors, are currently contraindicated in pregnancy.[84] Because of its teratogenic properties, MMF is contraindicated in pregnancy and its use in pregnancy has led to spontaneous abortions, still births, and structural malformations such as cleft lip/palate abnormalities and tetralogy of Fallot.[85,86] It is recommended that women who are or may become pregnant be switched off of MMF and transitioned to azathioprine at least 6 weeks before conceiving. Azathioprine has been demonstrated as a safe immunosuppressive alternative in both transplant and nontransplant populations, due to fetal absence of inosinate pyrophosphorylase, an enzyme required to convert the drug into an active metabolite.[87] Secondary to concerns that the mTORi antiproliferative activity might interfere with fetal maturation, this class of drugs is currently contraindicated in pregnancy.[87]

AGENTS FOR ANTIBODY-MEDIATED REJECTION IN LIVER TRANSPLANTATION

Because of the immune-protective properties of the liver by absorption and neutralization of recipient antibodies, antibody-mediated rejection (AMR) following liver transplantation is uncommon, with a reported incidence of 0.3% to 2%.[88] The histologic definition for acute AMR has been standardized by the Banff criteria, which includes endothelial cell hypertrophy; portal capillary dilation; and monocytic, eosinophilic, and neutrophilic microvasculitis, in the presence of C4d deposition in portal microvasculature, positive serum DSA, following exclusion of other liver diseases.[89] The histologic definition for chronic AMR includes periportal/portal, sinusoidal and/or perivenular fibrosis, mononuclear portal and/or perivenular inflammation, positive serum DSA, greater than 10% CD4 deposition, and exclusion of other liver diseases.[89] Given the rarity of AMR in liver transplant, there is no set algorithm for treatment. Treatment pathways are generally adapted from experience in treating kidney transplant recipients with AMR. Evidence of treatment of AMR in liver transplant is limited to case reports and series, with variable results. Mild AMR is classically managed with an increase in maintenance immunosuppression (eg, calcineurin inhibitors, MMF), with the addition of pulse-dose steroids.[90,91]

Moderate to severe AMR is treated with a combination of rituximab, high-dose intravenous Ig (IVIg), and plasmapheresis.[90,91] IVIg has been proved to be effective treating severe allograft rejection in highly sensitized kidney transplant recipients.[92] Plasmapheresis combined with high-dose IVIg (1–2 g/kg) success in AMR in liver transplantation has been documented with variable success.[91,93] The addition of rituximab, an anti-CD20 monoclonal antibody, to IVIg has demonstrated satisfactory results in select patients.[91,93] A more recent multicenter retrospective study of evaluating the use of rituximab in 13 patients in Japan showed improved liver function tests in 3 adults and 2 pediatric patients with chronic AMR but no therapeutic effect in those with acute AMR.[94]

Treatments that have demonstrated success in other fields of solid organ transplant have demonstrated potential success in liver recipients as well. Eculizumab, a terminal complement inhibitor monoclonal antibody, has been used in AMR in kidney transplant patients and has demonstrated effectiveness in select liver transplant AMR cases.[95] As a proteasome inhibitor, bortezomib has been shown to target plasma cells in late acute AMR. Its use in refractory AMR has been documented in various case reports for liver transplantation, as well as other allografts, however with variable results.[95-97] Prospective randomized studies will be needed to evaluate the therapeutic efficiency of these treatments in AMR in liver transplant recipients.

SUMMARY

There remains considerable variation in the approach to immunosuppression in liver transplant recipients, and larger, multicenter RCTs are needed to determine best practices in the approach to immunosuppression. There remain many opportunities for further optimization of immunosuppressive drugs, which carry risk and long-term toxicities. Current and future research in personalized, patient-directed drug selection with the advent of donor-derived cell-free DNA and gene activation assays are evolving and target real-time analysis of rejection during drug minimization. The holy grail of transplantation, tolerance may depend on the exciting and innovative research surrounding regulatory T-cell therapies.

CLINICS CARE POINTS

- Approximately 30% of liver transplant centers use induction therapy immunosuppression during transplant.
- Thymoglobulin, IL-2 receptor antagonists, and alemtuzumab have all been used in liver transplantation and have all demonstrated a reduced incidence of transplant rejection.
- The mainstay of maintenance immunosuppression continues to be calcineurin inhibitors and steroids.
- Dual immunosuppression with calcineurin inhibitors and mycophenolate has been used to help mitigate effects of recurrent autoimmune diseases of the liver and posttransplantation renal impairment.

DISCLOSURE

Authors have nothing to disclose.

REFERENCES

1. Starzl TE, Groth CG, Brettschneider L, et al. Orthotopic homotransplantation of the human liver. Ann Surg 1968;168(3):392–415.
2. Calne RY, Rolles K, White DJ, et al. Cyclosporin A initially as the only immunosuppressant in 34 recipients of cadaveric organs: 32 kidneys, 2 pancreases, and 2 livers. Lancet 1979;2(8151):1033–6.
3. Calne RY. Immunosuppression for organ grafting. Int J Immunopharmacol 1979; 1(3):163–4.
4. Kwong AJ, Ebel NH, Kim WR, et al. OPTN/SRTR 2020 Annual Data Report: Liver. Am J Transplant 2022;22(Suppl 2):204–309.
5. Moonka DK, Kim D, Kapke A, et al. The influence of induction therapy on graft and patient survival in patients with and without hepatitis C after liver transplantation. Am J Transplant 2010;10(3):590–601.
6. Cai J, Terasaki PI. Induction immunosuppression improves long-term graft and patient outcome in organ transplantation: an analysis of United Network for Organ Sharing registry data. Transplantation 2010;90(12):1511–5.

7. Bittermann T, Hubbard RA, Lewis JD, et al. The use of induction therapy in liver transplantation is highly variable and is associated with posttransplant outcomes. Am J Transplant 2019;19(12):3319–27.
8. Halldorson JB, Bakthavatsalam R, Montenovo M, et al. Differential rates of ischemic cholangiopathy and graft survival associated with induction therapy in DCD liver transplantation. Am J Transplant 2015;15(1):251–8.
9. Kwong AJ, Ebel NH, Kim WR, et al. OPTN/SRTR 2021 Annual Data Report: Liver. Am J Transplant 2023;23(2S1):S178–263.
10. Lucey MR, Im GY, Mellinger JL, et al. Introducing the 2019 American Association for the Study of Liver Diseases Guidance on Alcohol-Associated Liver Disease. Liver Transpl 2020;26(1):14–6.
11. Tan PS, Muthiah MD, Koh T, et al. Asian Liver Transplant Network Clinical Guidelines on Immunosuppression in Liver Transplantation. Transplantation 2019; 103(3):470–80.
12. easloffice@easloffice.eu EAftSotLEa. EASL Clinical Practice Guidelines: Liver transplantation. J Hepatol 2016;64(2):433–85.
13. Brennan DC, Daller JA, Lake KD, et al. Rabbit antithymocyte globulin versus basiliximab in renal transplantation. N Engl J Med 2006;355(19):1967–77.
14. Uemura T, Schaefer E, Hollenbeak CS, et al. Outcome of induction immunosuppression for liver transplantation comparing anti-thymocyte globulin, daclizumab, and corticosteroid. Transpl Int 2011;24(7):640–50.
15. Ghanekar A, Kashfi A, Cattral M, et al. Routine induction therapy in living donor liver transplantation prevents rejection but may promote recurrence of hepatitis C. Transplant Proc 2012;44(5):1351–6.
16. Neuhaus P, Clavien PA, Kittur D, et al. Improved treatment response with basiliximab immunoprophylaxis after liver transplantation: results from a double-blind randomized placebo-controlled trial. Liver Transpl 2002;8(2):132–42.
17. Horton PJ, Tchervenkov J, Barkun JS, et al. Antithymocyte globulin induction therapy in hepatitis C-positive liver transplant recipients. J Gastrointest Surg 2005; 9(7):896–902.
18. Garcia-Saenz-de-Sicilia M, Olivera-Martinez MA, Grant WJ, et al. Impact of antithymocyte globulin during immunosuppression induction in patients with hepatitis C after liver transplantation. Dig Dis Sci 2014;59(11):2804–12.
19. Turner AP, Knechtle SJ. Induction immunosuppression in liver transplantation: a review. Transpl Int 2013;26(7):673–83.
20. Montenovo MI, Jalikis FG, Li M, et al. Superior Patient and Graft Survival in Adult Liver Transplant with Rabbit Antithymocyte Globulin Induction: Experience with 595 Patients. Exp Clin Transplant 2017;15(4):425–31.
21. Anugwom CM, Parekh JR, Hwang C, et al. Comparison of Clinical Outcomes of Induction Regimens in Patients Undergoing Liver Transplantation for Acute Liver Failure. Liver Transpl 2021;27(1):27–33.
22. Nair A, Coromina Hernandez L, Shah S, et al. Induction Therapy With Antithymocyte Globulin and Delayed Calcineurin Inhibitor Initiation for Renal Protection in Liver Transplantation: A Multicenter Randomized Controlled Phase II-B Trial. Transplantation 2022;106(5):997–1003.
23. Yoo MC, Vanatta JM, Modanlou KA, et al. Steroid-free Liver Transplantation Using Rabbit Antithymocyte Globulin Induction in 500 Consecutive Patients. Transplantation 2015;99(6):1231–5.
24. Soliman T, Hetz H, Burghuber C, et al. Short-term induction therapy with antithymocyte globulin and delayed use of calcineurin inhibitors in orthotopic liver transplantation. Liver Transpl 2007;13(7):1039–44.

25. Bajjoka I, Hsaiky L, Brown K, et al. Preserving renal function in liver transplant recipients with rabbit anti-thymocyte globulin and delayed initiation of calcineurin inhibitors. Liver Transpl 2008;14(1):66–72.

26. Nair S, Loss GE, Cohen AJ, et al. Induction with rabbit antithymocyte globulin versus induction with corticosteroids in liver transplantation: impact on recurrent hepatitis C virus infection. Transplantation 2006;81(4):620–2.

27. De Ruvo N, Cucchetti A, Lauro A, et al. Preliminary results of a "prope" tolerogenic regimen with thymoglobulin pretreatment and hepatitis C virus recurrence in liver transplantation. Transplantation 2005;80(1):8–12.

28. Saidi RF, Hertl M, Chung RT, et al. Induction with Rabbit Antithymocyte Globulin following Orthotopic Liver Transplantation for Hepatitis C. Int J Organ Transplant Med 2011;2(4):160–5.

29. Cederborg A, Norén Å, Barten T, et al. Renal function after liver transplantation: Real-world experience with basiliximab induction and delayed reduced-dose tacrolimus. Dig Liver Dis 2022;54(8):1076–83.

30. Daclizumab withdrawn from the market worldwide. Drug Ther Bull 2018;56(4):38.

31. Sollinger H, Kaplan B, Pescovitz MD, et al. Basiliximab versus antithymocyte globulin for prevention of acute renal allograft rejection. Transplantation 2001; 72(12):1915–9.

32. Tullius SG, Pratschke J, Strobelt V, et al. ATG versus basiliximab induction therapy in renal allograft recipients receiving a dual immunosuppressive regimen: one-year results. Transplant Proc 2003;35(6):2100–1.

33. Hashim M, Alsebaey A, Ragab A, et al. Efficacy and safety of basiliximab as initial immunosuppression in liver transplantation: A single center study. Ann Hepatol 2020;19(5):541–5.

34. Kathirvel M, Mallick S, Sethi P, et al. Randomized trial of steroid free immunosuppression with basiliximab induction in adult live donor liver transplantation (LDLT). HPB (Oxford) 2021;23(5):666–74.

35. Zhang GQ, Zhang CS, Sun N, et al. Basiliximab application on liver recipients: a meta-analysis of randomized controlled trials. Hepatobiliary Pancreat Dis Int 2017;16(2):139–46.

36. Lange NW, Salerno DM, Sammons CM, et al. Delayed calcineurin inhibitor introduction and renal outcomes in liver transplant recipients receiving basiliximab induction. Clin Transplant 2018;32(12):e13415.

37. Hanouneh IA, Zein NN, Lopez R, et al. IL-2 Receptor Antagonist (Basiliximab) Is Associated with Rapid Fibrosis Progression in Patients with Recurrent Hepatitis C after Liver Transplantation Using Serial Biopsy Specimens. Int J Organ Transplant Med 2010;1(1):7–14.

38. Kamar N, Borde JS, Sandres-Saune K, et al. Induction therapy with either anti-CD25 monoclonal antibodies or rabbit antithymocyte globulins in liver transplantation for hepatitis C. Clin Transplant 2005;19(1):83–9.

39. Levitsky J, Thudi K, Ison MG, et al. Alemtuzumab induction in non-hepatitis C positive liver transplant recipients. Liver Transpl 2011;17(1):32–7.

40. Descourouez JL, Jorgenson MR, Parajuli S, et al. Alemtuzumab induction for retransplantation after primary transplant with alemtuzumab induction. Clin Nephrol 2020;93(2):77–84.

41. Marcos A, Eghtesad B, Fung JJ, et al. Use of alemtuzumab and tacrolimus monotherapy for cadaveric liver transplantation: with particular reference to hepatitis C virus. Transplantation 2004;78(7):966–71.

42. Tzakis AG, Tryphonopoulos P, Kato T, et al. Preliminary experience with alemtuzumab (Campath-1H) and low-dose tacrolimus immunosuppression in adult liver transplantation. Transplantation 2004;77(8):1209–14.
43. Tryphonopoulos P, Madariaga JR, Kato T, et al. The impact of Campath 1H induction in adult liver allotransplantation. Transplant Proc 2005;37(2):1203–4.
44. Nelson J, Alvey N, Bowman L, et al. Consensus recommendations for use of maintenance immunosuppression in solid organ transplantation: Endorsed by the American College of Clinical Pharmacy, American Society of Transplantation, and the International Society for Heart and Lung Transplantation. Pharmacotherapy 2022;42(8):599–633.
45. Nazzal M, Lentine KL, Naik AS, et al. Center-driven and Clinically Driven Variation in US Liver Transplant Maintenance Immunosuppression Therapy: A National Practice Patterns Analysis. Transplant Direct 2018;4(7):e364.
46. O'Grady JG, Hardy P, Burroughs AK, et al. Randomized controlled trial of tacrolimus versus microemulsified cyclosporin (TMC) in liver transplantation: poststudy surveillance to 3 years. Am J Transplant 2007;7(1):137–41.
47. McAlister VC, Haddad E, Renouf E, et al. Cyclosporin versus tacrolimus as primary immunosuppressant after liver transplantation: a meta-analysis. Am J Transplant 2006;6(7):1578–85.
48. Farkas SA, Schnitzbauer AA, Kirchner G, et al. Calcineurin inhibitor minimization protocols in liver transplantation. Transpl Int 2009;22(1):49–60.
49. Kong Y, Wang D, Shang Y, et al. Calcineurin-inhibitor minimization in liver transplant patients with calcineurin-inhibitor-related renal dysfunction: a meta-analysis. PLoS One 2011;6(9):e24387.
50. Fairfield C, Penninga L, Powell J, et al. Glucocorticosteroid-free versus glucocorticosteroid-containing immunosuppression for liver transplanted patients. Cochrane Database Syst Rev 2018;4(4):CD007606.
51. Miller JL. Sirolimus approved with renal transplant indication. Am J Health Syst Pharm 1999;56(21):2177–8.
52. Campsen J, Zimmerman MA, Mandell S, et al. A Decade of Experience Using mTor Inhibitors in Liver Transplantation. J Transplant 2011;2011:913094.
53. Uhlmann D, Weber T, Ludwig S, et al. Long-term outcome of conversion to sirolimus monotherapy after liver transplant. Exp Clin Transplant 2012;10(1):30–8.
54. De Simone P, Nevens F, De Carlis L, et al. Everolimus with reduced tacrolimus improves renal function in de novo liver transplant recipients: a randomized controlled trial. Am J Transplant 2012;12(11):3008–20.
55. Saliba F, Duvoux C, Gugenheim J, et al. Efficacy and Safety of Everolimus and Mycophenolic Acid With Early Tacrolimus Withdrawal After Liver Transplantation: A Multicenter Randomized Trial. Am J Transplant 2017;17(7):1843–52.
56. Saliba F, Duvoux C, Dharancy S, et al. Five-year outcomes in liver transplant patients receiving everolimus with or without a calcineurin inhibitor: Results from the CERTITUDE study. Liver Int 2022;42(11):2513–23.
57. Fischer L, Klempnauer J, Beckebaum S, et al. A randomized, controlled study to assess the conversion from calcineurin-inhibitors to everolimus after liver transplantation–PROTECT. Am J Transplant 2012;12(7):1855–65.
58. Teperman L, Moonka D, Sebastian A, et al. Calcineurin inhibitor-free mycophenolate mofetil/sirolimus maintenance in liver transplantation: the randomized spare-the-nephron trial. Liver Transpl 2013;19(7):675–89.
59. Nashan B, Schemmer P, Braun F, et al. Early Everolimus-Facilitated Reduced Tacrolimus in Liver Transplantation: Results From the Randomized HEPHAISTOS Trial. Liver Transpl 2022;28(6):998–1010.

60. Motzer RJ, Escudier B, Oudard S, et al. Efficacy of everolimus in advanced renal cell carcinoma: a double-blind, randomised, placebo-controlled phase III trial. Lancet 2008;372(9637):449–56.
61. Klintmalm GB, Saab S, Hong JC, et al. The role of mammalian target of rapamycin inhibitors in the management of post-transplant malignancy. Clin Transplant 2014; 28(6):635–48.
62. Geissler EK, Schnitzbauer AA, Zülke C, et al. Sirolimus Use in Liver Transplant Recipients With Hepatocellular Carcinoma: A Randomized, Multicenter, Open-Label Phase 3 Trial. Transplantation 2016;100(1):116–25.
63. Schnitzbauer AA, Filmann N, Adam R, et al. mTOR Inhibition Is Most Beneficial After Liver Transplantation for Hepatocellular Carcinoma in Patients With Active Tumors. Ann Surg 2020;272(5):855–62.
64. Charlton M, Levitsky J, Aqel B, et al. International Liver Transplantation Society Consensus Statement on Immunosuppression in Liver Transplant Recipients. Transplantation 2018;102(5):727–43.
65. Lin M, Mittal S, Sahebjam F, et al. Everolimus with early withdrawal or reduced-dose calcineurin inhibitors improves renal function in liver transplant recipients: A systematic review and meta-analysis. Clin Transplant 2017;31(2).
66. Mulder MB, van Hoek B, van den Berg AP, et al. Three-year results of renal function in liver transplant recipients on low-dose sirolimus and tacrolimus: a multicenter, randomized, controlled trial. Liver Transpl 2023;29(2):184–95.
67. Mackay AJ, Angus PW, Gow PJ. Long-term outcomes of calcineurin inhibitor withdrawal for post-liver transplant renal dysfunction. Transplant Proc 2011;43(10): 3802–6.
68. Liberal R, Zen Y, Mieli-Vergani G, et al. Liver transplantation and autoimmune liver diseases. Liver Transpl 2013;19(10):1065–77.
69. Montano-Loza AJ, Bhanji RA, Wasilenko S, et al. Systematic review: recurrent autoimmune liver diseases after liver transplantation. Aliment Pharmacol Ther 2017;45(4):485–500.
70. Jacob DA, Neumann UP, Bahra M, et al. Long-term follow-up after recurrence of primary biliary cirrhosis after liver transplantation in 100 patients. Clin Transplant 2006;20(2):211–20.
71. Satapathy SK, Jones OD, Vanatta JM, et al. Outcomes of Liver Transplant Recipients With Autoimmune Liver Disease Using Long-Term Dual Immunosuppression Regimen Without Corticosteroid. Transplant Direct 2017;3(7):e178.
72. Efe C, Hagström H, Ytting H, et al. Efficacy and Safety of Mycophenolate Mofetil and Tacrolimus as Second-line Therapy for Patients With Autoimmune Hepatitis. Clin Gastroenterol Hepatol 2017;15(12):1950–6.e1.
73. Junge G, Neuhaus R, Schewior L, et al. Withdrawal of steroids: a randomized prospective study of prednisone and tacrolimus versus mycophenolate mofetil and tacrolimus in liver transplant recipients with autoimmune hepatitis. Transplant Proc 2005;37(4):1695–6.
74. LaMattina JC, Jason MP, Hanish SI, et al. Safety of belatacept bridging immunosuppression in hepatitis C-positive liver transplant recipients with renal dysfunction. Transplantation 2014;97(2):133–7.
75. Klintmalm GB, Feng S, Lake JR, et al. Belatacept-based immunosuppression in de novo liver transplant recipients: 1-year experience from a phase II randomized study. Am J Transplant 2014;14(8):1817–27.
76. Klintmalm GB, Trotter JF, Demetris A. Belatacept Treatment of Recurrent Late-onset T Cell-mediated Rejection/Antibody-mediated Rejection With De Novo

Donor-specific Antibodies in a Liver Transplant Patient. Transplant Direct 2022; 8(7):e1076.

77. Klintmalm GB, Gunby RT. Successful Pregnancy in a Liver Transplant Recipient on Belatacept. Liver Transpl 2020;26(9):1193–4.

78. Cristea O, Karadkhele G, Kitchens WH, et al. Belatacept Conversion in Kidney After Liver Transplantation. Transplant Direct 2021;7(11):e780.

79. Pons JA, Ramírez P, Revilla-Nuin B, et al. Immunosuppression withdrawal improves long-term metabolic parameters, cardiovascular risk factors and renal function in liver transplant patients. Clin Transplant 2009;23(3):329–36.

80. Londoño MC, Rimola A, O'Grady J, et al. Immunosuppression minimization vs. complete drug withdrawal in liver transplantation. J Hepatol 2013;59(4):872–9.

81. Feng S, Ekong UD, Lobritto SJ, et al. Complete immunosuppression withdrawal and subsequent allograft function among pediatric recipients of parental living donor liver transplants. JAMA 2012;307(3):283–93.

82. Benítez C, Londoño MC, Miquel R, et al. Prospective multicenter clinical trial of immunosuppressive drug withdrawal in stable adult liver transplant recipients. Hepatology 2013;58(5):1824–35.

83. Shaked A, DesMarais MR, Kopetskie H, et al. Outcomes of immunosuppression minimization and withdrawal early after liver transplantation. Am J Transplant 2019;19(5):1397–409.

84. Rahim MN, Long L, Penna L, et al. Pregnancy in Liver Transplantation. Liver Transpl 2020;26(4):564–81.

85. Kamarajah SK, Arntdz K, Bundred J, et al. Outcomes of Pregnancy in Recipients of Liver Transplants. Clin Gastroenterol Hepatol 2019;17(7):1398–404.e1.

86. Sifontis NM, Coscia LA, Constantinescu S, et al. Pregnancy outcomes in solid organ transplant recipients with exposure to mycophenolate mofetil or sirolimus. Transplantation 2006;82(12):1698–702.

87. Coscia LA, Armenti DP, King RW, et al. Update on the Teratogenicity of Maternal Mycophenolate Mofetil. J Pediatr Genet 2015;4(2):42–55.

88. Kim PT, Demetris AJ, O'Leary JG. Prevention and treatment of liver allograft antibody-mediated rejection and the role of the 'two-hit hypothesis'. Curr Opin Organ Transplant 2016;21(2):209–18.

89. Demetris AJ, Bellamy C, Hübscher SG, et al. Comprehensive Update of the Banff Working Group on Liver Allograft Pathology: Introduction of Antibody-Mediated Rejection. Am J Transplant 2016;16(10):2816–35.

90. Lee M. Antibody-Mediated Rejection After Liver Transplant. Gastroenterol Clin North Am 2017;46(2):297–309.

91. Baradaran H, Dashti-Khavidaki S, Taher M, et al. Antibody-Mediated Rejection in Adult Liver Transplant Recipients: A Case Series and Literature Review. J Clin Pharmacol 2022;62(2):254–71.

92. Jordan SC, Peng A, Vo AA. Therapeutic strategies in management of the highly HLA-sensitized and ABO-incompatible transplant recipients. Contrib Nephrol 2009;162:13–26.

93. Lee BT, Fiel MI, Schiano TD. Antibody-mediated rejection of the liver allograft: An update and a clinico-pathological perspective. J Hepatol 2021;75(5):1203–16.

94. Sakamoto S, Akamatsu N, Hasegawa K, et al. The efficacy of rituximab treatment for antibody-mediated rejection in liver transplantation: A retrospective Japanese nationwide study. Hepatol Res 2021;51(9):990–9.

95. Wozniak LJ, Naini BV, Hickey MJ, et al. Acute antibody-mediated rejection in ABO-compatible pediatric liver transplant recipients: case series and review of the literature. Pediatr Transplant 2017;21(1).

96. Tajima T, Hata K, Okajima H, et al. Bortezomib Against Refractory Antibody-Mediated Rejection After ABO-Incompatible Living-Donor Liver Transplantation: Dramatic Effect in Acute-Phase? Transplant Direct 2019;5(10):e491.

97. Komagome M, Maki A, Nagata R, et al. Refractory Acute Antibody Mediated Rejection in Liver Transplant After Desensitization of Preformed Donor Specific Antibody-Validity of Bortezomib and Everolimus: A Case Report. Transplant Proc 2022;54(1):147–52.

Donation After Circulatory Death Liver Transplantation

Early Challenges, Clinical Improvement, and Future Directions

Brianna Ruch, MD, Kayla Kumm, MD, Sandra Arias, MD, Nitin N. Katariya, MD, Amit K. Mathur, MD, MS*

KEYWORDS

- Liver transplantation • Donation after circulatory death • Donor and recipient pairing
- Clinical outcomes • Machine perfusion

KEY POINTS

- Donation after circulatory death (DCD) liver transplantation is a rapidly evolving field.
- Despite initially inferior outcomes, careful selection of donor and recipient pairs and rapid donor recovery allow for successful transplantation.
- Clinical perfusion modalities are set to potentially transform the field, by redefining the current guidelines for DCD selection and utilization, and improving clinical outcomes.

INTRODUCTION

Donation after circulatory death (DCD) liver transplantation (LT) is one of the fastest evolving fields in transplantation today. DCD refers to the donation of organs after the irreversible cessation of circulation. This is applicable for potential donors not meeting strict brain death criteria, but for whom further medical intervention is determined to be futile. DCD donors are classified by the modified Maastricht criteria, which are based on the clinical status and location of the intended donor[1,2] (**Table 1**). In the United States, Maastricht Category III donors, those who are controlled donors, constitute nearly all of the DCD donor activity. Maastricht Category III DCD donation occurs when a potential donor undergoes planned withdrawal of life support therapy (WLST) and confirmation of irreversible circulatory cessation, declaration of death, followed by super rapid organ recovery after a stand-down period to ensure the absence of auto-resuscitation.[1]

Department of Surgery, Division of Transplant Surgery, Mayo Clinic, Phoenix, AZ, USA
* Corresponding author. Mayo Clinic, 5777 East Mayo Boulevard, Phoenix, AZ 85054.
E-mail address: Mathur.Amit@mayo.edu
Twitter: @BriannaCRuch (B.R.); @Kayla_Kumm (K.K.); @nnk_tx_hpb (N.N.K.); @MathurAmitK (A.K.M.)

Surg Clin N Am 104 (2024) 27–44
https://doi.org/10.1016/j.suc.2023.08.001
0039-6109/24/© 2023 Elsevier Inc. All rights reserved.

Table 1	
The modified Maastricht classification	
Modified Maastricht Classification	
Category I: Found dead	Uncontrolled
IA: In hospital	
IB: Out of hospital	
Category II: Death after unsuccessful resuscitation	Uncontrolled
IIA: In hospital	
IIB: Out of hospital	
Category III: Awaiting cardiac death	Controlled
Category IV: Cardiac arrest while brain dead	Uncontrolled

Although the first liver transplants performed by Starzl in 1967 utilized DCD organs,[3] the legal adoption of the declaration of death based on neurologic criteria led to almost exclusive use of donation after brain death (DBD) organs for liver transplantation.[4] In an attempt to alleviate the critical organ shortage, DCD donors were reintroduced in the United States in the 1990s after considerable efforts by donation and transplant professionals to ensure ethical, legal, and clinical standards of death were met in the timeline after withdrawal of care and before initiation of donation surgery. Despite initial enthusiasm, early DCD grafts were found to have inferior outcomes compared with DBD LT. Patient mortality, primary nonfunction (PNF), graft failure, repeat transplant and delayed biliary complications such as ischemic cholangiopathy (IC) occurred at an alarmingly high rate that was met with trepidation despite the ongoing organ shortage.[5–13]

Reports of these poor outcomes and the concomitant obligation of transplant center public reporting led to hesitation by transplant programs to use DCD livers in many US centers. Progress in the field was made incrementally via low-volume single-center experiences, and in a few larger programs. Over the last decade, DCD LT has been shown to have dramatically better outcomes that those initial reports, owing to the identification of best practices in high-volume programs, honing of procurement techniques and donor selection criteria, optimization of donor and recipient matching, and familiarization with postoperative recipient management. Even more recently, adjuncts in clinical perfusion such as normothermic regional perfusion and machine perfusion have begun to be implemented, thus precipitating further expedited change and improved outcomes.

EARLY EXPERIENCE: CLINICAL OUTCOMES

The initial outcomes of DCD grafts for liver transplantation from the 1990s were largely inferior with regards to patient and graft survival, primary nonfunction, need for repeat transplant, hepatic artery thrombosis, and ischemic biliary complications when compared with DBD.[5,7,8,10,12,14]

One of the earliest reviews of the UNOS (United Network for Organ Sharing) data from 1993 to 2001 found significant inferiority in the 1- and 3-year graft survival rates when comparing DCD (n = 144) with DBD (n = 26,856) (70.2% and 63.3% for DCD vs 80.4% and 72.1% for DBD $P=.003$ and $P=.012$).[6] Several reports demonstrated similarly poor patient and graft survival with DCD LT until the early 2000s (**Table 2**). An interval review of SRTR (Scientific Registry of Transplant Recipients) data spanning from 2001 to 2009 by Mathur and colleagues showed that even after almost a decade of performing DCD liver transplant in the United States, only 64.9% of DCD recipients

Table 2				
Early outcomes of donation after circulatory death liver transplant between 1993 and 2007				
	Timeframe	Patient Survival (1 y)	Graft Survival (1 y)	Repeat Transplant
Abt UNOS review DCD = 144	1993–2001	DCD 79.7% DBD 85.0% P=.082	DCD 70.2% DBD 80.4% P=.003	DCD 13.9% DBD 8.3% P = .04
Foley Single center DCD = 36	1993–2002	DCD 80% DBD 91% P=.002	DCD 67% DBD 86% P=.001	
De Vera Single center DCD = 141	1993–2007	DCD 79% DBD 85% P=.08	DCD 69% DBD 82% P<.0001	DCD 18% DBD 7% P<.001
Jay SRTR review DCD = 1113	1996–2007	DCD 82% DBD 86% P<.001		DCD 14.7% DBD 6.8% P<.001

were alive with a functioning graft; 13.6% required repeat transplant, and 21.6% were dead by 3 years after transplant.[11]

Concerns regarding poor DCD LT survival has been based on early reports of poor outcomes, attributed largely to a higher associated rate of PNF, biliary complications, and hepatic artery thrombosis.[7,8,12,15] In a single-center review of 141 DCD cases, De Vera and colleagues found that PNF and biliary complications accounted for 67% of the early DCD graft failures.[12] Biliary complications were common in this period. Reports quoted 1-year biliary complications occurring as frequently as 33% in DCD LT compared with only in 10% in DBD LT.[7] More specifically, DCD grafts had a 35.8% higher risk of ischemic cholangiopathy, which had significant morbidity including frequent invasive endoscopic and radiological interventions, hospital time, and the possibility of surgically challenging liver repeat transplantation.[8] Hepatic artery stenosis was also documented as occurring 3 times as frequently in DCD grafts compared with DBD (16.6% vs 5.4% P=.001).[7]

By the late 2000s, between the implementation of center of excellence requirements for programs, and the overwhelming consensus of DCD graft inferiority, DCD LT stalled in the United States save few LT centers.[16–24] This precipitated a nationwide focus on outcomes improvement in order to use this valuable resource given the continued critical organ shortage.[20,25–27]

MODERN APPROACH

Following initial DCD outcomes, there has been a systematic approach to improvement through donor and recipient matching, procurement optimization, and better management of DCD-attributable complications. Several clinical risk factors are summarized and are accompanied by respective current standards of practice based on clinical consensus.

Donor Selection

Several donor risk factors have been associated with an increased risk of patient and graft loss. First, increasing donor age has early on been linked with decreased graft survival. Older grafts may be more vulnerable to ischemia reperfusion injury (IRI) due to having less regenerative capability.[28] Several studies found a donor age greater than 50 to be associated with increased risk of graft loss.[11,29,30] Over time, some studies suggest that donors over the age of 60 years old may be used with acceptable graft outcomes should other risk factors be modified, as has been done abroad.[26,31,32] However, even with risk factor modification, these older grafts were still subject to increased rates of biliary complications and anastomotic strictures.[26,31–33] A 2021 ILTS (International Liver Transplantation Society) consensus statement and other studies recommend the use of all DCD organs less than or equal to 60 years old. Selective use of donors older than 60 may be considered if other risk factors are mitigated.[24,28,31,33–35]

Donor weight or body mass index (BMI) has also been linked with worse outcomes. The specific mechanism within this association is unknown, but has been theorized to be linked to hepatic macrosteatosis and metabolic disease-associated steatohepatitis, surgical challenges related to body size during procurement, and hepatomegaly and difficulties of organ cooling. Causality has not been proven. An early SRTR review found donor weight greater than 100 kg served as a predictor of patient mortality (hazard ratio [HR] 1.39, $P=.035$).[11] Croome and colleagues have identified potential mechanisms in their institutional study; DCD donors with macrosteatosis greater than 30% also had higher rates of post-reperfusion syndrome, primary nonfunction, post-reperfusion cardiac arrest, early allograft dysfunction (EAD), and acute kidney injury (AKI).[16,36]

Finally, cold ischemic times (CITs) are possibly one of the greatest modifiable donor factors linked with graft outcomes. CIT is disproportionately detrimental to DCD compared with DBD, with each hour of CIT being associated with a 6% increase in graft failure (HR 1.06, $P<.001$).[11] Even moderate CIT of 6 to 10 hours was associated with 64% higher graft failure risk compared to allografts with CIT less than 6 hours.[11] In addition to graft failure, longer CIT has been linked to a longer hospital stay, higher PNF rate, EAD, and cholestasis.[37] By minimizing donor CIT to less than 6 hours, 3-year liver survival rates can be increased by 4%, leading to an equivalent graft survival compared with DBD.[13,29] As such, logistics to minimize DCD CIT are critical when planning a potential case. Factors to consider include procurement process efficiencies and best practices, timing and location of donor withdrawal of life support, donor surgical recovery efficiency, expeditious donor hepatectomy and liver assessment, understanding door-to-door travel time, the preemptive admission of the recipient and operating room availability, and commitment to initiating recipient surgery before DCD organ arrival.

The ILTS released a consensus on donor risk factors in 2021 (**Table 3**).[28,38,39] In large-volume centers with frequent experience with DCD organs, these criteria are often viewed in terms of summative risks, not strictly prohibitive. Exceptions can be made if other risk factors are minimized. Of note, strict donor requirements have likely contributed to the high nonutilization rate of DCD livers.

Table 3
Donation after circulatory death donor risk factors, 2021 International Liver Transplantation Society consensus

DCD Donor Risk Factors: ILTS 2021 Consensus	
Donor age	< or equal 60 y/o *
Donor BMI	< or equal 30 kg/m^2 *
Steatosis	Avoid grafts with macrosteatosis > 30%
Cold Ischemia	Keep CIT < 8 h * Do not use if CIT > 12 h

* May selectively go over the general recommendations with consideration of other potential risks such as: fDWIT, donor hospital stay, liver tests, hepatectomy time

Procurement

Maastricht Category 3 donors are donors who undergo controlled withdrawal of life support therapy, confirmation of circulatory cessation, and super rapid cannulation and cold preservation flush. The hepatectomy is then expeditiously performed. A schematic of the anticipated procurement flow is illustrated in **Fig. 1**. There are several factors at time of procurement that can be modified to improve outcomes. As such it is the authors' single center's preference, if logistics allow, to send their own procurement surgeon to each DCD to mitigate these risks.

First, and before any surgical conduct begins, it is of utmost importance in DCD procurements to ensure that the public trust is maintained in the donation process. Frequently, DCD organ recoveries occur at donor hospitals that have rarely or never participated in this approach to donation, and may be unfamiliar with the goals and surgical conduct in super rapid recovery. To this end, It is key before each recovery to review the donor's wishes, consent, clinical documentation, and conditions of organ acceptance, and discuss the details of surgical conduct with the organ procurement organization (OPO) and operating room (OR) staff. Description of the surgical conduct should include the need for rapid aortic cannulation, equipment and personnel readiness, and team communication of critical donor information with the recipient center. Although each hospital and OPO may adopt different policies, some of which may impact expected donor warm ischemia time (DWIT), at no time should the donor recovery team participate in or influence the care of the patient whose life support is being withdrawn. There is a bright line of demarcation between care delivered to the intended donor before and during withdrawal of life-sustaining therapy (WLST) and any actions taken after he or she is declared dead.

As the recovery is initiated, the first factor affecting graft outcomes is DWIT.[11,28,39] There is no consensus definition of what constitutes DWIT that has been universally adopted by transplant programs in the United States, despite efforts to gain consensus by the American Society of Transplant Surgeons, ILTS, and the Association of Organ Procurement Organizations.[39–41] This is primarily related to a lack of agreement as to when warm ischemia begins in the donor during the WLST process. DWIT can be broken down into several subcategories but largely encompasses the time from WLST to the initiation of cold perfusion (total DWIT [tDWIT]). Not all of the tDWIT is truly ischemic, as perfusion can be normal after WLST depending on the underlying donor condition and other factors. tDWIT can further include a period of functional DWIT (fDWIT), which also lacks a consensus, universally adopted definition across all centers. fDWIT typically is defined by when the donor hemodynamics or oxygenation drop below a certain threshold following withdrawal. Recent efforts to convene a consensus around DWIT defines fDWIT as the period from when the donor

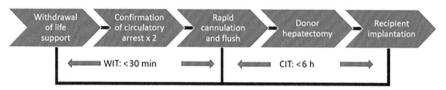

Fig. 1. Ischemia time trajectories in the DCD donation and preservation process with cold storage. This figure shows events in DCD donation, recovery, and preservation. Notably, in the United States, there is a mandatory no touch stand down period after declaration of circulatory death to observe for auto-resuscitation in the donor. After this, organ recovery procedures are initiated.

peripheral oxygen saturation (Spo2) drops below 80% or mean arterial pressure (MAP) drops below 60 mm Hg.[39,40] Each transplant center has different acceptance guidelines based on either the tDWIT, the fDWIT, or a combination of the two. The authors' large-volume center prefers to base acceptance decisions on tDWIT for several reasons, including challenges in assessing what physiologic conditions constitute true ischemia to the donor biliary tree.

Longer DWITs have been linked with increased rates of graft failure and ischemic cholangiopathy.[8,10–12,40,42,43] One SRTR registry study identified a DWIT greater than 35 minutes correlated with increased graft failure rates (HR 1.84, P=.002) compared with dWIT less than 15 minutes.[11] In addition, every minute of added WIT between asystole and cross clamp increased IC risk by 16.1%.[44,45] The exact time leading to prohibitive risk is difficult to define, as many studies have shown stepwise increases in risk with longer WIT.[12,42,44] Furthermore, some centers and studies define their cutoffs by either the fWIT, the tWIT, or both.[44,45] A recent ILTS consensus statement defined donors with fWIT greater than 30 minutes as being considered increased risk DCD livers.[39] When combined with other risk modifications, allografts with dWIT less than 30 minutes can achieve similar survival outcomes as DBD.[10,42]

Methods to minimize donor WIT include a procurement team familiar with super rapid recovery, pre-recovery consideration of anatomically difficult donors (eg, obesity, prior surgeries, presence of sternal wires, or need for abdominal or thoracic cannulation), review of donor imaging, and WLST in the OR when permissible based on OPO and donor hospital policies. In particular, withdrawal in the OR has been independently linked with 1-year patient survival similar to DBD.[46] Other DCD donor ILTS consensus guidelines include completing the portal flush after the aortic, a short hepatectomy time less than 60 minutes, no fibrinolytic administration, heparin before WLST, and histidine-tryptophan-ketoglutarate (HTK) avoidance in grafts anticipating greater than 8 hours CIT.[38,39] The authors emphasize rapid aortic cannulation after incision, within 2 to 3 minutes, which allows for timely organ cooling relative to the declaration of death and mandatory stand-down periods.

Candidate Selection

Early DCD liver utilization patterns suggest use of these grafts in the most critically ill LT candidates (higher model for end-stage liver disease [MELD] score) was more likely to have a survival benefit, whereas lower MELD patients could afford to remain on the list pending a better offer.[47–52] Because of the ongoing donor shortage and allocation policy design, there has been a clear shift in the patterns of use of DCD organs with regard to identifying the appropriate candidate. DCD organs used in lower MELD (<20) patients function better,[30] and these recipients have a lower risk-adjusted hazard of death compared with candidates remaining on the waitlist (HR 0.55; 95% CI 1.40 - 1.94).[53] In addition, DCD grafts provide a survival benefit to HCC patients without exception points.[54–57] In response, the selection approach for the appropriate DCD LT candidate has drastically changed over the last decade.

The current main tenets of DCD recipient selection center on

The ability of the recipient to tolerate IRI to the allograft and its clinical sequelae including post-reperfusion syndrome during the intraoperative course (PRS), early allograft dysfunction, secondary organ dysfunction, such as AKI, mechanical ventilation, or vasopressor requirements; decompensated cirrhotic patients with vasodilated vascular tone who are critically ill or have secondary comorbidities such as cardiac disease may not have the capacity to withstand DCD-associated IRI and its clinical sequelae

The recipient does not have factors that would extend the possible CIT; these factors may include clinical and logistical factors, such as complex abdominal surgery history, portal vein thrombosis, repeat transplantation, challenges with vascular access, or long travel time to the hospital

In practical terms, these lower-risk LT candidates tend to be younger (<60 years old), not in the intensive care unit (ICU) or on life support, not on dialysis, and have had no prior transplants or complicated surgeries. A review of the UNOS data by Mateo and colleagues found that low-risk DCD donor organs placed into such low-risk LT candidates were able to achieve 1 year graft survival (81%) not significantly different from DBD grafts (80%).[42] A more recent review of the SRTR by Mathur and colleagues found recipient predictors of graft failure included a MELD score greater than 35 at transplant. This study similarly found repeat transplant was independently associated with a 45% higher risk of graft failure. Recipient age greater than 55 years was associated with 26% higher adjusted graft failure rate.[11]

Other surgical considerations when selecting a DCD LT candidate include the planned biliary reconstruction. Given the risk of ischemic cholangiopathy associated with DCD LT, and the possible need for multiple endoscopic interventions,[58,59] future endoscopic retrograde cholangiopancreatography (ERCP) access should be planned for at the time of LT. Patients who have a choledochocholedochostomy have normal anatomic configurations that are amenable to typical ERCP approaches. Patients who require Roux-en-Y biliary reconstruction should be avoided, as the reconstruction been associated with higher risk of DCD graft loss.[35] In cases where duct-to-duct continuity is not feasible because of biliary disease or other factors, the authors prefer to perform biliary reconstruction via a choledochoduodenostomy to the first portion of the duodenum over a Roux-en-Y configuration to preserve reliable ERCP access to the duct.[60–63] Patients with prior Roux anatomy such as gastric bypass patients may still be DCD LT candidates, but duct access should be planned for in advance. Advanced endoscopy may be necessary to assist in accessing the biliary tree, which may be achieved by endoscopic access of the gastric remnant percutaneously, operatively, or via EDGE (EUS-directed transgastric ERCP) procedures.[64]

Management of the Donation After Circulatory Death Liver Transplant Recipient and Management of Complications

Although the total number of DCD livers transplanted has increased over time, only select centers routinely perform DCD transplants. An analysis of the OPTN (Organ Procurement and Transplantation Network) data found that almost half of all DCD transplants in the United States are performed at 11 of the approximately 100 US LT centers, and that only 3 centers performed more than 100 DCD transplants over a 5 year period.[18] This is likely related to the broader discomfort with the management of DCD LT intraoperative and postoperative complications and the ability to rescue patients from these complications.[13,65,66] Given the lack of broad utilization of DCD livers across the United States, the clinical management of the DCD recipient is driven by local practices or derived and extrapolated from high-volume centers. Several practice pearls have been identified to optimize DCD LT outcomes and facilitate rescue when complications occur.

Intraoperative safety in DCD LT is critically important. A strong LT anesthesia team comfortable managing postreperfusion syndrome (PRS) is imperative for the successful intraoperative management of DCD recipients.[67,68] PRS carries significant risk of abrupt and significant bradycardia, hypotension, and coagulopathy. Further comfort with advanced techniques including Swan-Ganz catheters and transesophageal echocardiography, familiarity with use of thromboelastography, high-volume blood product resuscitation, and expertise in managing patients in vasodilatory shock are necessary.[67] Dedicated LT anesthesia teams are able to achieve these goals in clinical management in conjunction with surgical teams. Additional surgical maneuvers may help lessen effects of PRS. Reduction of portal venous and organ perfusate potassium load is routinely used in the authors' practice, as well as maneuvers to lessen hypothermic effects on the myocardium at reperfusion. The authors routinely perform a room temperature saline flush through the portal vein followed by a generous blood flush to allow the organ to warm immediately before reperfusion.

These grafts are also associated with higher rates of intraoperative and postoperative bleeding.[69] Management often requires more blood product transfusion, temporary intraoperative packing, and a greater likelihood of planned and unplanned returns to the operating room compared with analogous DBD graft cases.[70] Goal-directed resuscitation based on thromboelastography is 1 approach the authors' group has used in DCD LT.[71]

Although not exclusive to DCD organs, biliary complications such as IC are considered the Achilles heel of DCD LT.[72,73] Ischemic cholangiopathy represents a clinical and radiographic continuum of nonanastomotic biliary stricture phenotypes with a spectrum of severity.[72,73] For formal diagnosis, IC must be present within 12 months of LT and occur without concomitant hepatic artery thrombosis.[20] A key study by Croome and colleagues from Mayo Clinic described 4 main radiographic phenotypes of IC at presentation – minor form, confluence dominant, multifocal progressive, and diffuse necrosis. The associated risk of stent dependence and retransplantation depends on variable and type (**Table 4**).

Initial DCD outcomes quoted IC rates as high at 30%[7,8] and identified it as one of the greater risk factors leading to graft failure and repeat LT. With donor and recipient matching optimization and selectivity with donor characteristics, IC risk has decreased, with some single centers reporting IC rates from 2% to 5%, similar to the rates seen in DBD recipients.[28,35,74]

RECENT EXPERIENCE: CLINICAL OUTCOMES AND DONATION AFTER CIRCULATORY DEATH UTILIZATION

Since the latter part of the 2000s, national DCD acceptance practices have evolved to mitigate risks observed and reported in the previous decade. High-volume DCD LT centers have targeted DCD liver utilization in lower-risk recipients with medical conditions that justify the risks.[35] These recipients are typically patients with relatively lower laboratory MELD scores, and consistently has been CIT less than 6 hours and WIT less than 30 minutes.[30,75]In response, there has been a significant improvement in DCD liver allograft clinical outcomes, with several large single centers describing DCD graft survival outcomes equivalent to DBD.[29,76,77]

In a large review of the OPTN database, Haque and colleagues compared DCD outcomes before and after 2009. Recipients of DCD liver allografts saw improvement in hospital length of stay and rate of repeat transplant (a difference of only 1.2% between DCD and DBD by 2019), and a precipitous drop in ischemic cholangiopathy resulting in graft failure from 9.1% in 2002 to 0.92% in 2019. By 2019, the difference in DCD versus DBD biliary complications causing graft failure was only 0.77%.[78] It is generally now accepted that appropriately matched patients who receive a DCD transplant have a lower risk-adjusted hazard of death than those who remain on the waitlist (HR 0.55; 95% CI 1.40-1.94).[53,79] With aggressive management of complications, outcomes have improved but could precipitate excess health care utilization. From a

Table 4
Types of ischemic cholangiopathy, risk of stent dependence, and retransplantation

	Diffuse Necrosis	Multifocal Progressive	Confluence Dominant	Minor
Radiologic Patterns				
Description	Severe abnormalities throughout	Mild-to-moderate stenosis with progression over time	Strictures limited to confluence	Mild irregularities without progression
Stent dependent at 1 y	100%	86.7%	62.5%	11.1%
Listed for repeat transplant	84.2%	64.7%	16.7%	0%

patient-centered outcomes perspective, DCD and DBD LT recipients have been shown to spend similar numbers of days alive and out of the hospital within the first year after LT.[77]

With these promising outcomes, the interest in DCD transplantation has been reinvigorated. Between 2009 and 2019, DCD liver transplantation numbers grew 147% compared with only a 32.3% increase for DBD.[75,78] Despite this growth, the total number of DCD LTs performed remains significantly less than that of DBD (**Fig. 2**A).[80,81] DCD LT activity constitutes less than 15% of all US LT activity in 2022, and most US centers perform fewer than 5 DCD LT procedures per year. Most DCD transplants are continuing to occur at only a handful of centers across the United States.[18] Frequently, DCD livers are recovered and not used, occurring in 25% to 30% DCD livers per year (**Fig. 2**B).[81] The lack of DCD utilization is likely attributable to several factors. Donor risk perception is magnified in DCD LT, leading to avoidance of these grafts.[13] DCD livers are also not used related to center protocols to mitigate risk, including issues related to donor age, steatosis, procurement and technical issues, excess DWIT, and global perceptions of liver quality, as discussed. Some large centers have published promising outcomes using DCD organs outside these risk guidelines; however, this carries a stigma relative to current national practice patterns.[26,31,35,82]

LIVER PERFUSION AND FUTURE DIRECTIONS

The most exciting area of DCD LT innovation has been the introduction of perfusion therapies to reduce organ injury and restore organ function. Clinical liver perfusion therapy aims to minimize the inherent ischemic injury DCD organs sustained by perfusing the organs either before (in situ) or following procurement (ex situ). Multiple perfusion innovations have been identified in practice and in clinical trials internationally. In situ perfusion of DCD liver allografts is performed through normothermic regional perfusion (NRP). Ex situ perfusion has had the greatest concentration of technological innovation in clinical transplantation over the last 2 decades. Ex situ perfusion includes hypothermic and normothermic approaches. Hypothermic perfusion includes hypothermic machine perfusion and hypothermic oxygenated perfusion (HOPE). HOPE devices are currently used in Europe and are in US clinical trial investigation at this time. At present, 2 liver normothermic machine perfusion (NMP) devices carry US Food and Drug Administration (FDA) approval.

Normothermic regional perfusion has been a known technique to recover abdominal organs (A-NRP) since the early 2000s,[83–86] but gained significant favor in 2020 after

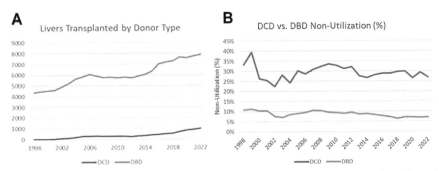

Fig. 2. Trends in US liver transplantation, 1998 to 2022. Fig. 2A shows the total number of deceased donor liver transplants by donor type per year for DBD and DCD livers. Fig. 2B shows the nonutilization rate of DBD and DCD liver allografts per year.

reports emerged of successful utilization of DCD hearts using a thoracoabdominal NRP (TA-NRP) technique.[87–90] NRP is a means of normothermic perfusion and is achieved through immediate and rapid donor cannulation and in situ organ perfusion following WLST and confirmed cessation of circulation with exclusion of perfusion from non-recovered organs.[91] Early outcomes of NRP livers have found an increase in DCD liver utilization rate from 39.0% to 70.6% ($P<.001$), while maintaining comparable graft survival.[92] DCD LT outcomes using either A-NRP or TA-NRP are significantly better than standard rapid recovery DCD LT, based on US and European data.[93–95] Although NRP has promising outcomes and has been increasing in popularity because of beneficial effects on all perfused organs and its relatively lower cost, several groups have raised ethical and legal concerns around NRP practices and whether this contravenes the cessation of circulation in the definition of death.[96–98] The ongoing discourse on these issues continues to coexist with the growing NRP practice in the United States.

NMP involves the ex situ perfusion of the liver graft following donor hepatectomy as an end-ischemic modality. NMP modalities involve oxygenated perfusion of the portal venous and arterial systems and the use of pH, lactate, and bile production as biomarkers for allograft viability. Both the TransMedics OCS system and the OrganOx metra have undergone extensive clinical testing and rigorous trials to achieve FDA approval.[99–101] The OCS Liver PROTECT randomized clinical trial found NMP was able to significantly reduce the risk of EAD, increase DCD liver utilization, and reduce the incidence of ischemic biliary complications.[99] Nasralla and colleagues demonstrated that the OrganOx metra, compared with static cold storage (SCS), was also associated with decreased EAD in DCD livers and increased rate of organ utilization. OrganOx, however, did not show decreased rates of biliary complications compared with SCS.[101] At present, real-world utilization of NMP modalities is hampered by the costs associated with use of the technology.

Few comparisons between NRP and NMP modalities have been conducted. One international observational study by Mohkam and colleagues was not able to provide any evidence showing superiority of 1 method over the other. Both DCD perfusion methods were, however, able to achieve similar outcomes to expected DBD benchmarks.[95] As these technologies are used more and are associated with their respective commercial interests, head-to-head clinical trials are unlikely to occur unless they are investigator initiated, and several groups have reported their use in complementary fashion, with NRP followed by NMP for DCD LT.[102]

How HOPE will be applied to US DCD LT is unknown at this time, as clinical trials needed for FDA approval are completing accrual. There is undoubtedly a clinical benefit with HOPE after a period of SCS back-to-base, as has been demonstrated in European studies,[34,103,104] but its translation to the US context is heretofore not widely known. HOPE is associated with a 16% absolute risk reduction in tumor-censored 5-year graft loss compared with SCS, despite longer fWIT times (HOPE-DCD 94% vs DCD-SCS 78%).[103] Other advantages of HOPE have also been touted including ease of surgical application, lower cost, and shorter perfusion duration. There have been no head-to-head trial designs of HOPE versus NMP modalities published in the current literature, but this is a promising area of investigation.

The authors' single large-volume center has used NMP over the last 18 months for DCD liver allografts, and their experience has been presented at national and international transplant meetings and is pending publication. The authors have observed improvement in PRS, EAD, IC, and hospital use. This has enabled the authors' center to expand and continuously reassess DCD liver allograft acceptance (currently up to donor age 70 and tWIT 40 minutes) and candidate eligibility for DCD LT (DCD LT can be used for any candidate). Using DCD livers for retransplantation, higher biologic MELD recipients and patients with acute decompensation no longer are taboo. The authors expect with the increased adoption of liver perfusion, the growing LT waiting list, and the availability of multiple clinical modalities aimed at organ restoration after donor death, the entire definition of appropriate donor and recipient matching will be redefined in DCD LT.

SUMMARY

DCD allografts for LT remain a widely underutilized means to increase access to LT. With suitable donor and LT candidate selection criteria, appropriate donor and recipient matching, good surgical technique, and appropriate perioperative management, these grafts can achieve patient and graft survival equivalent to that observed in DBD LT. Current limitations in further growth of DCD LT are driven by risk aversion, and the current US DCD LT experience has largely been sequestered in large centers. With time, and the advent of regional and machine perfusion promises to completely redefine the definition of a viable DCD liver allograft and hopefully will encourage more widespread usage of and comfort with these organs.

CLINICS CARE POINTS

- DCD liver allografts provide a viable means to help alleviate the critical organ shortage.
- Despite initially inferior outcomes, careful selection of donor and recipient pairs, rapid donor recovery, and appropriate perioperative management allow for successful transplantation.
- Machine and in situ normothermic perfusion are set to redefine the current guidelines for DCD selection and utilization.

DISCLOSURE

The authors have no conflicts of interest to disclose.

REFERENCES

1. Thuong M, et al. New classification of donation after circulatory death donors definitions and terminology. Transpl Int 2016;29(7):749–59.
2. Kootstra G, Daemen JH, Oomen AP. Categories of non-heart-beating donors. Transplant Proc 1995;27(5):2893–4.
3. Starzl TE, et al. Orthotopic homotransplantation of the human liver. Ann Surg 1968;168(3):392–415.
4. A definition of irreversible coma. Report of the Ad Hoc Committee of the Harvard Medical School to Examine the Definition of Brain Death. JAMA 1968;205(6): 337–40.
5. Abt P, et al. Liver transplantation from controlled non-heart-beating donors: an increased incidence of biliary complications. Transplantation 2003;75(10): 1659–63.
6. Abt PL, et al. Survival following liver transplantation from non-heart-beating donors. Ann Surg 2004;239(1):87–92.
7. Foley DP, et al. Donation after cardiac death: the University of Wisconsin experience with liver transplantation. Ann Surg 2005;242(5):724–31.

8. Skaro AI, et al. The impact of ischemic cholangiopathy in liver transplantation using donors after cardiac death: the untold story. Surgery 2009;146(4): 543–52 [discussion: 552-3].

9. Jay CL, et al. The increased costs of donation after cardiac death liver transplantation: caveat emptor. Ann Surg 2010;251(4):743–8.

10. Jay CL, et al. Ischemic cholangiopathy after controlled donation after cardiac death liver transplantation: a meta-analysis. Ann Surg 2011;253(2):259–64.

11. Mathur AK, et al. Donation after cardiac death liver transplantation: predictors of outcome. Am J Transplant 2010;10(11):2512–9.

12. de Vera ME, et al. Liver transplantation using donation after cardiac death donors: long-term follow-up from a single center. Am J Transplant 2009;9(4): 773–81.

13. Sher L, et al. Attitudes and barriers to the use of donation after cardiac death livers: comparison of a United States transplant center survey to the United Network for Organ Sharing data. Liver Transplant 2017;23(11):1372–83.

14. Skaro AI, et al. Trends in donation after cardiac death and donation after brain death–reading between the lines. Am J Transplant 2010;10(11):2390–1.

15. Wells M, et al. Comparing outcomes of donation after cardiac death versus donation after brain death in liver transplant recipients with hepatitis C: a systematic review and meta-analysis. Chin J Gastroenterol Hepatol 2014;28(2): 103–8.

16. Croome KP, Muiesan P, Taner CB. Donation after circulatory death (DCD) liver transplantation: a practical guide. Cham, Switzerland: Springer; 2020.

17. Croome KP, Taner CB. Expanding role of donation after circulatory death donors in liver transplantation. Clin Liver Dis 2021;25(1):73–88.

18. Hobeika MJ, et al. United States donation after circulatory death liver transplantation is driven by a few high-utilization transplant centers. Am J Transplant 2020;20(1):320–1.

19. Goldberg DS, et al. Liver transplant center variability in accepting organ offers and its impact on patient survival. J Hepatol 2016;64(4):843–51.

20. Goldberg DS, et al. Interpreting Outcomes in DCDD Liver Transplantation: first report of the multicenter IDOL Consortium. Transplantation 2017;101(5): 1067–73.

21. Sonnenberg EM, Goldberg DS. Donation after circulatory death liver procurement: time to consider more options? Liver Transplant 2019;25(4):533–4.

22. Sonnenberg EM, et al. Wide variation in the percentage of donation after circulatory death donors across donor service areas: a potential target for improvement. Transplantation 2020;104(8):1668–74.

23. Kumar SR, Chyou D, Goldberg D. Effect of acuity circles allocation policy on local use of donation after circulatory death donor livers. Liver Transplant 2022;28(6):1103–7.

24. Giorgakis E, et al. Centre volume impact on graft survival and waiting list time in donation after circulatory death liver transplantation in the USA. Br J Surg 2021; 108(12):e404–6.

25. Schenk AD, et al. Textbook outcome as a quality metric in liver transplantation. Transplant Direct 2022;8(5):e1322.

26. Ivanics T, et al. Outcomes after liver transplantation using deceased after circulatory death donors: a comparison of outcomes in the UK and the US. Liver Int 2023;43(5):1107–19.

27. Giorgakis E, et al. Acuity circles allocation policy impact on waitlist mortality and donation after circulatory death liver transplantation: a nationwide retrospective analysis. Health Sci Rep 2023;6(2):e1066.

28. Schlegel A, et al. Recommendations for donor and recipient selection and risk prediction: working group report from the ILTS Consensus Conference in DCD Liver Transplantation. Transplantation 2021;105(9):1892–903.

29. Scalea JR, Redfield RR, Foley DP. Liver transplant outcomes using ideal donation after circulatory death livers are superior to using older donation after brain death donor livers. Liver Transplant 2016;22(9):1197–204.

30. Croome KP, et al. Improving national results in liver transplantation using grafts from donation after cardiac death donors. Transplantation 2016;100(12):2640–7.

31. Giorgakis E, et al. Disparities in the use of older donation after circulatory death liver allografts in the United States versus the United Kingdom. Transplantation 2022;106(8):e358–67.

32. Croome KP, et al. Outcomes of donation after circulatory death liver grafts from donors 50 years or older: a multicenter analysis. Transplantation 2018;102(7): 1108–14.

33. Giorgakis E, et al. Comparable graft survival is achievable with the usage of donation after circulatory death liver grafts from donors at or above 70 years of age: a long-term UK national analysis. Am J Transplant 2021;21(6):2200–10.

34. Schlegel A, et al. A multicentre outcome analysis to define global benchmarks for donation after circulatory death liver transplantation. J Hepatol 2022;76(2): 371–82.

35. Croome KP, Taner CB. The changing landscapes in DCD liver transplantation. Curr Transplant Rep 2020;7(3):194–204.

36. Croome KP, et al. Perioperative and long-term outcomes of utilizing donation after circulatory death liver grafts with macrosteatosis: a multicenter analysis. Am J Transplant 2020;20(9):2449–56.

37. Paterno F, et al. Clinical implications of donor warm and cold ischemia time in donor after circulatory death liver transplantation. Liver Transplant 2019;25(9): 1342–52.

38. Hessheimer AJ, Kalisvaart M. Creation of the ILTS consensus statements on DCD and liver perfusion: defining the future of liver transplantation by returning to the past. Transplantation 2021;105(4):695–6.

39. Kalisvaart M, et al. Donor warm ischemia time in DCD liver transplantation-working group report from the ILTS DCD, liver preservation, and machine perfusion consensus conference. Transplantation 2021;105(6):1156–64.

40. Croome KP, et al. American Society of Transplant Surgeons recommendations on best practices in donation after circulatory death organ procurement. Am J Transplant 2023;23(2):171–9.

41. Hobeika MJ, et al. A step toward standardization: results of two national surveys of best practices in donation after circulatory death liver recovery and recommendations from The American Society of Transplant Surgeons and Association of Organ Procurement Organizations. Clin Transplant 2020;34(10):e14035.

42. Mateo R, et al. Risk factors for graft survival after liver transplantation from donation after cardiac death donors: an analysis of OPTN/UNOS data. Am J Transplant 2006;6(4):791–6.

43. Skaro AI, et al. Donation after cardiac death liver transplantation: time for policy to catch up with practice. Liver Transplant 2012;18(1):5–8.

44. Taner CB, et al. Asystole to cross-clamp period predicts development of biliary complications in liver transplantation using donation after cardiac death donors. Transpl Int 2012;25(8):838–46.

45. Taner CB, et al. Events in procurement as risk factors for ischemic cholangiopathy in liver transplantation using donation after cardiac death donors. Liver Transplant 2012;18(1):100–11.

46. Cao Y, et al. Donation after circulatory death for liver transplantation: a meta-analysis on the location of life support withdrawal affecting outcomes. Transplantation 2016;100(7):1513–24.

47. Merion RM, et al. The survival benefit of liver transplantation. Am J Transplant 2005;5(2):307–13.

48. Schaubel DE, et al. The survival benefit of deceased donor liver transplantation as a function of candidate disease severity and donor quality. Am J Transplant 2008;8(2):419–25.

49. Schaubel DE, et al. Survival benefit-based deceased-donor liver allocation. Am J Transplant 2009;9(4 Pt 2):970–81.

50. Merion RM, et al. Evidence-based development of liver allocation: a review. Transpl Int 2011;24(10):965–72.

51. Perry DK, et al. Should donation after cardiac death liver grafts be used for re-transplantation? Ann Hepatol 2011;10(4):482–5.

52. Taner CB, et al. Liver transplantation in the critically ill: donation after cardiac death compared to donation after brain death grafts. Ann Hepatol 2012;11(5):679–85.

53. Taylor R, et al. Survival advantage for patients accepting the offer of a circulatory death liver transplant. J Hepatol 2019;70(5):855–65.

54. Croome KP, et al. The use of donation after cardiac death allografts does not increase recurrence of hepatocellular carcinoma. Am J Transplant 2015;15(10):2704–11.

55. Jay CL, et al. Comparative effectiveness of donation after cardiac death versus donation after brain death liver transplantation: recognizing who can benefit. Liver Transplant 2012;18(6):630–40.

56. Silverstein J, et al. Donation after circulatory death is associated with similar posttransplant survival in all but the highest-risk hepatocellular carcinoma patients. Liver Transplant 2020;26(9):1100–11.

57. Lee DD, Cotler SJ. Finding the right balance for the use of donation after circulatory death livers for patients with hepatocellular carcinoma. Liver Transplant 2020;26(9):1081–2.

58. Kohli DR, et al. Outcomes of endoscopic retrograde cholangiography and percutaneous transhepatic biliary drainage in liver transplant recipients with a Roux-en-Y biliary-enteric anastomosis. Ann Hepatobiliary Pancreat Surg 2023;27(1):49–55.

59. Croome KP, et al. Endoscopic management of biliary complications following liver transplantation after donation from cardiac death donors. Can J Gastroenterol 2012;26(9):607–10.

60. Bennet W, et al. Choledochoduodenostomy is a safe alternative to Roux-en-Y choledochojejunostomy for biliary reconstruction in liver transplantation. World J Surg 2009;33(5):1022–5.

61. Wigmore SJ. Choledochoduodenostomy as an alternative to choledochojejunostomy in liver transplantation. World J Surg 2009;33(5):1026–7.

62. Wu Q, et al. Choledochoduodenostomy as an alternative to choledochojejunostomy for biliary reconstruction in liver transplantation. World J Surg 2010;34(7):1727 [author reply 1728-9].
63. Schmitz V, Neuhaus P. Choledochoduodenostomy is a safe alternative to Roux-en-Y choledochojejunostomy for biliary reconstruction in liver transplantation. World J Surg 2011;35(3):696-7.
64. Vanek P, et al. Single-session endoscopic ultrasound-directed transgastric ERCP ("EDGE") in a bariatric patient with pancreatic mass and biliary obstruction. Obes Surg 2020;30(11):4681-3.
65. Ghaferi AA, Birkmeyer JD, Dimick JB. Hospital volume and failure to rescue with high-risk surgery. Med Care 2011;49(12):1076-81.
66. Ghaferi AA, Birkmeyer JD, Dimick JB. Variation in hospital mortality associated with inpatient surgery. N Engl J Med 2009;361(14):1368-75.
67. Chadha RM, et al. Intraoperative events in liver transplantation using donation after circulatory death donors. Liver Transplant 2019;25(12):1833-40.
68. Croome KP, et al. The impact of postreperfusion syndrome during liver transplantation using livers with significant macrosteatosis. Am J Transplant 2019;19(9):2550-9.
69. Liang TB, et al. Early postoperative hemorrhage requiring urgent surgical reintervention after orthotopic liver transplantation. Transplant Proc 2007;39(5):1549-53.
70. Dunn R, Voleti S, Rowley S, et al. Risk factors associated with urgent surgical reintervention due to postoperative hemorrhage after orthotopic liver transplantation. Journal of Liver Transplantation 2022;8.
71. Hawkins RB, et al. Review: the perioperative use of thromboelastography for liver transplant patients. Transplant Proc 2018;50(10):3552-8.
72. Croome KP, et al. Classification of distinct patterns of ischemic cholangiopathy following DCD liver transplantation: distinct clinical courses and long-term outcomes from a multicenter cohort. Transplantation 2022;106(6):1206-14.
73. Giesbrandt KJ, et al. Radiologic characterization of ischemic cholangiopathy in donation-after-cardiac-death liver transplants and correlation with clinical outcomes. AJR Am J Roentgenol 2015;205(5):976-84.
74. Kollmann D, et al. Expanding the donor pool: donation after circulatory death and living liver donation do not compromise the results of liver transplantation. Liver Transplant 2018;24(6):779-89.
75. Haque O, et al. Evolving utilization of donation after circulatory death livers in liver transplantation: The day of DCD has come. Clin Transplant 2021;35(3):e14211.
76. Bohorquez H, et al. Safety and outcomes in 100 consecutive donation after circulatory death liver transplants using a protocol that includes thrombolytic therapy. Am J Transplant 2017;17(8):2155-64.
77. Frasco PE, et al. Days alive and out of hospital after liver transplant: comparing a patient-centered outcome between recipients of grafts from donation after circulatory and brain deaths. Am J Transplant 2023;23(1):55-63.
78. Haque OJ, et al. Long-term outcomes of early experience in donation after circulatory death liver transplantation: outcomes at 10 years. Ann Transplant 2021;26:e930243.
79. McLean KA, et al. Decision modeling in donation after circulatory death liver transplantation. Liver Transplant 2017;23(5):594-603.
80. Kwong AJ, et al. OPTN/SRTR 2021 annual data report: liver. Am J Transplant 2023;23(2 Suppl 1):S178-263.

81. Network O.P.a.T. National Data. 2022; Available at: https://optn.transplant.hrsa. gov/data/view-data-reports/national-data/#. Accessed March 1, 2023.
82. Nunez-Nateras R, et al. Simultaneous liver-kidney transplantation from donation after cardiac death donors: an updated perspective. Am J Transplant 2020; 20(12):3582–9.
83. Magliocca JF, et al. Extracorporeal support for organ donation after cardiac death effectively expands the donor pool. J Trauma 2005;58(6):1095–101 [discussion: 1101-2].
84. Englesbe MJ, et al. Salvage of an unstable brain dead donor with prompt extracorporeal support. Transplantation 2005;79(3):378.
85. Gravel MT, et al. Kidney transplantation from organ donors following cardiopulmonary death using extracorporeal membrane oxygenation support. Ann Transplant 2004;9(1):57–8.
86. Rudich SM, et al. Extracorporeal support of the non-heart-beating organ donor. Transplantation 2002;73(1):158–9.
87. Nistal JF, et al. Heart transplantation from controlled donation after circulatory death using thoracoabdominal normothermic regional perfusion and cold storage. J Card Surg 2021;36(9):3421–4.
88. Minambres E, et al. Spanish experience with heart transplants from controlled donation after the circulatory determination of death using thoraco-abdominal normothermic regional perfusion and cold storage. Am J Transplant 2021; 21(4):1597–602.
89. Jawitz OK, et al. Increasing the United States heart transplant donor pool with donation after circulatory death. J Thorac Cardiovasc Surg 2020;159(5):e307–9.
90. Perez Redondo M, et al. Transplantation of a heart donated after circulatory death via thoraco-abdominal normothermic regional perfusion and results from the first Spanish case. J Cardiothorac Surg 2020;15(1):333.
91. Frontera JA, et al. Thoracoabdominal normothermic regional perfusion in donation after circulatory death does not restore brain blood flow. J Heart Lung Transplant 2023. https://doi.org/10.1016/j.healun.2023.05.010.
92. Bekki Y, et al. Normothermic regional perfusion can improve both utilization and outcomes in DCD liver, kidney, and pancreas transplantation. Transplant Direct 2023;9(3):e1450.
93. Croome KP, et al. Development of a portable abdominal normothermic regional perfusion (A-NRP) program in the United States. Liver Transplant 2023. https:// doi.org/10.1097/LVT.0000000000000178.
94. Schurink IJ, et al. Salvage of declined extended-criteria DCD livers using in situ normothermic regional perfusion. Ann Surg 2022;276(4):e223–30.
95. Mohkam K, et al. In situ normothermic regional perfusion versus ex situ normothermic machine perfusion in liver transplantation from donation after circulatory death. Liver Transplant 2022;28(11):1716–25.
96. Bernat JL, et al. Understanding the brain-based determination of death when organ recovery is performed with DCDD in situ normothermic regional perfusion. Transplantation 2023;107(8):1650–4.
97. Glazier AK, Capron AM. Normothermic regional perfusion and US legal standards for determining death are not aligned. Am J Transplant 2022;22(5): 1289–90.
98. Peled H, Bernat JL. Why arch vessel ligation is unethical for thoracoabdominal normothermic regional perfusion. J Thorac Cardiovasc Surg 2022;164(2):e93.

99. Markmann JF, et al. Impact of portable normothermic blood-based machine perfusion on outcomes of liver transplant: the OCS Liver PROTECT randomized clinical trial. JAMA Surg 2022;157(3):189–98.

100. Nasralla D, et al. A randomized trial of normothermic preservation in liver transplantation. Nature 2018;557(7703):50–6.

101. Chapman WC, et al. Normothermic machine perfusion of donor livers for transplantation in the United States - a randomized controlled trial. Ann Surg 2023. https://doi.org/10.1097/SLA.0000000000005934.

102. Ghinolfi D, et al. The role of sequential normothermic regional perfusion and end-ischemic normothermic machine perfusion in liver transplantation from very extended uncontrolled donation after cardiocirculatory death. Artif Organs 2023;47(2):432–40.

103. Schlegel A, et al. Outcomes of DCD liver transplantation using organs treated by hypothermic oxygenated perfusion before implantation. J Hepatol 2019; 70(1):50–7.

104. Schlegel A, Muller X, Dutkowski P. Hypothermic machine preservation of the liver: state of the art. Curr Transplant Rep 2018;5(1):93–102.

Role of Machine Perfusion in Liver Transplantation

Alban Longchamp, MD, PhD[a,b,1], Tsukasa Nakamura, MD, PhD[a,1],
Korkut Uygun, PhD[a,b], James F. Markmann, MD, PhD[a,b],*

KEYWORDS

- Liver transplantation • Surgical techniques • Post-transplant • Machine perfusion
- Liver

KEY POINTS

- One of the strategies to increase the number of available livers for transplantation is to improve organ utilization through the use of marginal organs, including elderly, overweight, or organs donated after circulatory death.
- The utilization of these "marginal" organs was associated with an increased risk of early allograft dysfunction, primary nonfunction, ischemic-type biliary complications, or even re-transplantation.
- One of the most promising strategies is the utilization of ex vivo machine perfusion.
- Although tremendous progress has been made over the past years in the fields of procurement, preservation, surgical techniques, and post-transplant immunosuppression, the mortality on the waiting list remains high due to an ever-increasing shortage of suitable donor organs.

INTRODUCTION

Liver transplantation stands as the sole curative treatment for individuals suffering from end-stage liver disease. Although tremendous progress has been made over the past years in the fields of procurement, preservation, surgical techniques, and post-transplant immunosuppression, the mortality on the waiting list remains high due to an ever-increasing shortage of suitable donor organs.[1] This current shortage of organs led to an increase in the utilization of extended criteria donors (ECDs) for transplantation, which has the potential to address the unmet needs in liver transplantation. Unfortunately, ECD livers have a higher likelihood of developing early allograft

a Division of Transplant Surgery, Massachusetts General Hospital, Harvard Medical School, Boston, MA, USA; b Department of Surgery, Center for Engineering in Medicine, Massachusetts General Hospital, Harvard Medical School, Boston, MA, USA
1 Contributed equally.
* Corresponding author. Massachusetts General Hospital, Mass General Brigham, 55 Fruit Street, WHT 517, Boston, MA 02114.
E-mail address: jmarkmann@mgh.harvard.edu

Surg Clin N Am 104 (2024) 45–65
https://doi.org/10.1016/j.suc.2023.07.001
0039-6109/24/© 2023 Elsevier Inc. All rights reserved.

surgical.theclinics.com

dysfunction (EAD), primary nonfunction (PNF), or serious late-onset complications such as ischemic cholangiopathy (IC).[2] In the recent years, ex vivo liver machine perfusion before transplantation has emerged as an attractive approach. Using machine perfusion, the rate of complications observed with donation after circulatory death (DCD) livers was found to be comparable to that of livers obtained following brainstem death (donation after brain death [DBD]).[3,4] In addition to graft preservation, machine perfusion offers an opportunity to assess the organ viability, increase organ sharing, and treat or repair livers historically considered unsuitable for transplantation. Moreover, studies have also reported positive impact of machine perfusion on graft rejection[5] and the recurrence of hepatocellular carcinoma.[6] The latter highlights potential broader therapeutic effects machine perfusion. Although machine perfusion has not yet surpassed the advantages of the simple and inexpensive static cold storage (SCS) (in particular for standard or DBD organs), the rapid increase in the utilization of ECD livers for transplantation has led to a significant interest in the use and development of machine perfusion technologies. These advancements are expected to revolutionize the field in the near future. In this review, the authors discuss the role of machine perfusion in liver transplantation with a particular focus on its clinical application.

MACHINE PERFUSION
General Principles of Machine Perfusion

In the current practice of organ transplantation, the process of procurement and storage of organs ultimately leads to ischemia–reperfusion (IR) injury. The extent of this injury varies depending on the duration of both cold and warm ischemia times. Compared with standard criteria donor livers, ECD livers, which include DCD livers, livers with severe steatosis, elderly livers, or livers infected with hepatitis C are at a greater risk of IR injury, clinically manifest as EAD or PNF.[7] The mechanisms suggested to underlie the benefits of machine perfusion include the suppression of IR injury, providing continous nutritional supplementation to the graft, and improvement in the clearance of deleterious metabolites during perfusion.[8,9] Machine perfusion of liver transplants can be categorized into three types based on the target temperature.[10] (1) Hypothermic machine perfusion (HMP), which typically involves temperatures of 4°C to 12°C HMP can be used to perfuse the portal vein only or both portal and arterial systems. In addition, HMP can be performed with or without the use of oxygen. HMP with oxygen is known as hypothermic oxygenated machine perfusion (HOPE). (2) Normothermic machine perfusion (NMP), which mimics the human body temperature (34–37°C) and requires the use of an oxygen carrier (blood or artificial hemoglobin). (3) Subnormothermic machine perfusion (SNMP), an intermediate approach between HMP and NMP. SNMP is performed at temperatures between 20°C and 22°C. The purpose of SNMP is to reduce the oxygen demand to a level that does not require the use of an oxygen carrier while still maintaining metabolic activity and the ability to assess liver function. In addition to the temperature-based categorization, machine perfusion of liver transplants can further be classified into ex situ machine perfusion and in situ machine perfusion. Ex situ machine perfusion refers to the perfusion procedure that takes place after the liver has been recovered from the donor's body. In this approach, the liver is transported to a specialized perfusion system where it is perfused with the desired solution and maintained under controlled conditions. Ex situ machine perfusion allows for extended preservation and assessment of the liver outside of the donor's body before transplantation. On the other hand, in situ machine perfusion, also known as normothermic regional perfusion

(NRP), involves perfusing the liver with a preservation solution, whereas it is still inside the donor's body, before organ recovery. This technique allows for the assessment and treatment of the liver in its native environment, providing a more realistic representation of the organ's function and response to perfusion. In situ machine perfusion, or NRP, might also offers the advantage of maintaining near physiological conditions during the perfusion process. Finally, machine perfusion can be initiated at the donor hospital using a portable device, allowing for limited ischemic time, immediate preservation, and assessment of the liver graft.[3] Alternatively, the liver graft can be transferred on ice and machine perfusion started at the recipient site. This is known as end-ischemic perfusion. Finally, combinations of different therapies/types of machine perfusion techniques have gained popularity in recent years. These combinations involve using different perfusion modalities, such as incorporating hypothermic, normothermic, or subnormothermic perfusion at various stages of the transplantation process.[11,12] An overview of clinical devices available is presented in **Table 1**.

Hypothermic Machine Perfusion

Until very recently, the transplantation field heavily relied on SCS as the primary method for preserving livers intended for transplantation. However, despite its ability to slow down metabolism, SCS does not completely suspend cellular metabolism, resulting in the continued consumption of cellular energy stores during storage. Moreover, SCS is characterized by the absence of flow, whereas pulsatile preservation was shown to upregulate nitric oxide (NO) production by the vascular endothelium and faciliate the clearance of debris and toxic metabolites.[13] HMP works by providing a continuous flow to the portal circulation with or without hepatic artery perfusion. The role of oxygen will be discussed later (see below). The perfusates commonly used during liver HMP are based on the original or modified University of Wisconsin (UW) solution or UW machine perfusion solution. Perfusion studies have also been conducted using IGL-1 (Institut Georges Lopez), Celsior solution, or HTK (Histidine-Tryptophan-Ketoglutarate) solutions, but there is no direct comparison available. Lower potassium concentrations decrease vascular resistance during hypothermia, whereas the presence of starch increases viscosity. Therefore, solutions with low potassium and without starch seem advantageous.[14,15] In a pig model, single portal perfusion, the perfusate reaches all hepatocytes within less than 1 minute after initiating low-pressure cold perfusion. Considering the low oxygen demand at 4°C, supplying oxygen through single portal perfusion seems to be adequate, at least for hepatocytes, endothelial cells, Kupffer cells, and intrahepatic interlobular biliary branches.[16] Consistently, studies on discarded human livers undergoing HMP showed no significant difference in perfusion quality between singular perfusion of the portal vein or the hepatic artery alone compared with dual perfusion.[17] Another aspect of HMP is optimal perfusion pressure, aimed at maximizing perfusion while minimizing endothelial injury. Liver sinusoids are highly sensitive to endothelial shear stress. Previous studies in rat livers have indicated that reducing the portal perfusion pressure to 4 mm Hg allows for complete perfusion without endothelial injury, whereas perfusion at 8 mm Hg leads to endothelial damage.[17,18] In human livers, a low portal perfusion pressure around 3 mm Hg ensures complete perfusion without any signs of sinusoidal impairment.[18] Finally, it should be noted that hypothermia does not completely halt aerobic metabolism, and even at 4°C, the oxygen demand of the liver may exceed the available supply. Although dissolved oxygen may be adequate at standard DBD livers, DCD livers exposed to warm ischemia before organ procurement, have higher oxygen demands.[19,20] The optimal level of oxygenation also remains unclear, and high O_2 during HMP might increase oxidative stress.[21] Of

Table 1
Perfusion devices

Manufacture	OrganOx	Xvivo	TransMedics	Organ Recovery System	Bridge to Life
Name	Metra	Liver Assist	OCS liver	Lifeport Liver	Vitasmart
Type	NMP	HOPE & NMP	NMP	HMP	HMP & HOPE
Perfusion Temperature	37°C	12–38°C	34°C	4°C	4°C
Arterial Flow/ Pressure	Pressure controled (artery)	Pressure controlled. Artery and portal flows independent	Flow controlled. Total distributed to arterial and portal cannula	Continuous Flow	Continuous Flow
Portal Flow/ Pressure	Not adjustable	Pressure controlled. Artery and portal flows independent	Flow controlled. Total distributed to arterial and portal cannula	Continuous Flow	Continuous Flow
Transportable	Yes	No. Battery operated for 20-min	Yes	Yes	Yes

interest, the rate of oxygen consumption during HMP rapidly decreases within the first hour and is eventually arrested after 90 minutes of perfusion,[15] despite sufficient levels of substrate (adenosine diphosphate [ADP], oxygen). Currently, there is no randomized trial evaluating HMP without oxygen.

In a retrospective study, HMP with UW reduced the length of hospitalization and peak aspartate aminotransferase (AST) serum levels compared with SCS.[19] Subsequently, the same group showed that HMP was associated with fewer biliary complications, compared with SCS in ECD livers initially declined by the originating United Network for Organ Sharing region. HMP did not affect patient survival in this study[22] (**Table 2**).

Hypothermic Oxygenated Machine Perfusion

HMP with oxygen supplementation can be delivered via the portal vein only (HOPE) or both the hepatic artery and portal vein (dual HOPE [DHOPE]). These techniques aim to safely preserve the liver and enhance mitochondrial recovery and function. In ECD livers, oxygenation was suggested to restore endothelial cell viability,[23] demonstrated by increased nitric oxide (NO) levels and lower thrombomodulin. In addition, it was shown in rats that HOPE not only protects against IR injury but also dampens the immune response.[24] Finally, oxygen-rich perfusion allows for intracellular ATP regeneration and reduces lactate production via glycolysis.[25] In the first comparison of SCS versus HOPE, 25 DCD livers underwent end-ischemic HOPE solely via the portal vein, compared to 50 DCD liver transplantations after SCS.[26] HOPE was associated with a reduction in graft injury (peak alanine transaminase [ALT]), IC, biliary complications and improved 1-year graft survival (90% vs 69%, $P = 0.035$). Of importance, HOPE-perfused DCD livers achieved similar results as control DBD livers in all investigated endpoints. Subsequently, Rijn and colleagues,[27] compared 20 control patient with matched 10 DCD liver grafts, were treated with end-ischemic DHOPE. DHOPE was associated with increased ATP content and a twofold reduction in peak serum alanine transaminase (ALT) and bilirubin levels. IC and graft survival were similar in both groups.[27] Of interest, the 5-year outcomes of HOPE-treated DCD liver transplants were similar to those of DBD primary transplants and superior to those of untreated DCD liver transplants, despite much higher risk.[28] This led to two much larger RCT comparing HOPE to SCS that enrolled 160[29] and 177[30] livers, respectively. In the study led by R Porte,[29] HOPE reduced the rate of IC (6% vs 18%) and EAD occurred (26% vs 40%) in DCD livers. Similarly, the Zurich team reported a significant reduction in graft loss in DBD liver treated with HOPE compared with SCS.[30] Overall, HOPE is an effective strategy that has the potential to enable the safe utilization of extended DCD liver grafts, thereby expanding the pool of available livers for transplantation (**Table 2**).

Subnormothermic machine perfusion

SNMP has been developed, as a convenient, intermediate approach between blood-based NMP (see below) and HMP. SNMP offers the advantage to lower metabolic demands at sub-physiological temperatures while still providing adequate metabolism for viability testing and improving graft function. In addition, the utilization of acellular perfusate during SNMP minimize the presence of leukocytes, platelets, and cytokines that could potentially lead to adverse outcomes upon reperfusion/transplantation. Previously, our team demonstrated that 3 hours acellular SNMP improved DCD graft survival post-transplantation in rats compared to SCS.[31] In a porcine model, a 3-hour SNMP using an albumin-based perfusate (Steen solution) supplemented with leukocyte-depleted washed erythrocytes reduced serum ALP and bilirubin levels

Table 2
Clinical studies

RCT		Donor Type	Intervention Arm (#)	Control Arm (#)	Primary End Points	Secondary End Points	Main Outcomes	References
NMP								
No	2016	DBD and DCD	NMP (20)	SCS (40)	30-d graft survival	Biochemical measures of liver function, patient and graft survival, and graft function at 6-mo	Meadian peak AST after transplant was lower in the NMP group	PMID: 26752191
Yes	2017	DBD and DCD	NMP (120)	SCS (100)	Peak AST witihn 7-d	Organ discard rate, post-reperfusion syndrome, PNF, EAD, length of hospital/ICU stay, renal replacement therapy, IC by MRCP at 6 mo after transplant, graft/patient survival at 1-y	A 50% lower level of graft injury and 50% reduction in organ discard rate and 54% longer preservation time, but the comparable patient and graft survival	PMID: 29670285
Yes	2018	Elder than 70 DBD	NMP (10)	SCS (10)	Graft and patient survival at 6-mo posttransplantation	Liver and bile duct biopsies; IRI by means of peak transaminases within 7-d after surgery; and incidence of biliary complications at 6-mo	Older liver grafts after NMP is associated with histologic evidence of reduced IRI	PMID: 30362649
No	2019	DBD and DCD	NMP back to base (26)	NMP local (17)	The safety and efficacy of NMP for liver preservation applied in a back-to-base strategy	Opatient/graft survival at 90-d and 6-mo, LFTs, incidence of EAD, IC at 6 mo	The back-to-base approach was safe, did not compromise the overall benefit of NMP	PMID: 30938039

No/Yes	Year	Donor	Group 1	Group 2	Primary outcome	Secondary outcomes	Results	PMID
No	2019	DBD and DCD	Post static cold storage and NMP (31)	Continuous NMP (104)	30-d graft survival	LFTs, incidence of EAD, post-reperfusion syndrome, adverse events, length of hospital/ICU stay, biliary complication, 12-mo graft survival	Applying NMP after SCS is feasible and safe with a 30-d graft survival rate of 94%	PMID: 31206217
No	2020	DBD and DCD	NMP(31)		Feasibility of NMP in discarded organ recovery and achievement of successful transplantation	LFTs, incidence of PNF, EAD, length of hospital/ICU stay, incidence of vascular complications, biliary complications by MRCP at 6-mo, 90-d graft survival	Viability testing with NMP is feasible and enabled successful transplantation of 71% of discarded livers, with 100% 90-d patient and graft survival	PMID: 32546694
Yes	2022	DBD and DCD	NMP (151)	SCS (142)	The incidence of EAD, PNF, graft related significant events	The ability of NMP to monitor donor liver function, incidenc of IC/bile leak, reperfusion syndrome, and histology of the graft	Reduction in the incidence of EAD (18% vs 31%) and IC (1.3% and 2.6% vs 8.5% and 9.9% at 6 and 12-mo after transplant) in the NMP group	PMID: 34985503
No	2022	DBD and DCD	NMP DCD (123)	NMP DBD (80)	To identify perfusion variables relate to EAD/PNF		Perfusate ALT and lactate at 2-h, the amount of supplementary bicarbonate required to keep the perfusate pH > 7.2 in the first 4-h, and peak bile pH were associated with early graft function	PMID: 36044364

(continued on next page)

Table 2
(continued)

RCT		Donor Type	Intervention Arm (#)	Control Arm (#)	Primary End Points	Secondary End Points	Main Outcomes	References
No	2022	DCD	NMP(34)	NRP (157)	Liver utilization rate, 30-d and 12 and 24-mo patient and graft survival, incidence of biliary complications and EAD, and peak transaminase levels		Both NMP and NRP achieved similar results for recipients after brain death livers	PMID: 35662403
No	2022	DCD	NMP(67)/NRP (69)	SCS (97)	The incidence of EAD, PNF, model for early allograft function, biliary complications, postoperative AKI, chronic kidney injury at 6-mo, length of hospital/ICU stay, hepatic artery thrombosis, surgical complication rates within 30 d, patient/graft survival at 6-mo, 1 and 3-y		NRP and NMP were associated with better early liver function compared to SCS, whereas NRP was associated with superior preservation of the biliary system	PMID: 35258511
Yes	2023	DBD	NMP(32)	SCS (33)	The incidence of early allograft dysfunction	Complications related to graft IRI	Ischemia free liver transplant decreased the incidence of EAD, reperfusion syndrome, IC	PMID: 37086919

No	Year	Donor type	Intervention	Comparator	Outcomes	Secondary outcomes	Results	PMID
No	2023	DBD and DCD	NMP(79)	SCS (386)	Graft survival	Mortality rate, the incidence of EAD, vascular/biliary complications, length of hospital/ICU stay	NMP could extend the total preservation time of livers without increasing complications	PMID: 37086951
No	2023	DBD and DCD	NMP (165)	SCS (4270)	Length of hospital/ICU stay, rates of PNF and graft failure, graft survival		NMP mitigated donor risk factors, which were relative contraindications for transplant in elderly liver recipients	PMID: 36906889
NRP								
No	2012	DBD and uncontrolled DCD	Potential DCD(400), transplant (34)	DBD (538)	Feasibility of NRP for uncontrolled DCD		NRP expands donor criteria albeit <10% applicability	PMID: 22070538
No	2014	Controlled DCD	NRP (37)		Feasibility of NRP for controlled DCD		13 out of 37 (61.9%) livers were utilized	PMID: 24825520
No	2019	Controlled DCD	NRP (70)	Non-NRP(187)	EAD and cholangiopathy		A reduction in EAD, 30-d graft loss, the incidence of IC, an anastomotic strictures in the NRP group. A multivariable analysis showed that NRP had a protective effect on IC	PMID: 30589499
No	2019	Controlled DCD	NRP (95)	Non-NRP (117)	PNF, EAD and IC		Incidence of overall biliary complications, IC, and graft loss were lower in the NRP group with 0.14, 0.11, and 0.39 odds ratio, respectively	PMID: 30582980

(continued on next page)

Table 2
(continued)

RCT	Donor Type	Intervention Arm (#)	Control Arm (#)	Primary End Points	Secondary End Points	Main Outcomes	References
No 2020	DBD and controlled DCD	NRP (50)	DBD (100)	Death noncensored/censored graft survival, patient survival, PNF, EAD, AKI, biliary complications, IC		Similar results in the incidence of EAD, AKI, arterial and biliary complications and 2-y graft and patient survival were obtained between controlled DCD and DBD liver transplants	PMID: 32639402
No 2021	DBD and controlled DCD	NRP (144)	DBD (447)	RBC transfusion, 1-y graft/patient survival		No differences in the number of RBC units transfused, graft and patient survival between controlled DCD and DBD liver transplants	PMID: 34848373
No 2021	DBD and controlled DCD	NRP (100)	DBD (200)	Overall and death-censored graft survival	Biliary complications, incidence of postreperfusion syndrome, ALT peak, EAD and AKI	No differences in ALT peaks, the incidence of EAD and the 1 and 3-y graft survival between controlled DCD and DBD liver transplants	PMID: 34455694
No 2022	Controlled DCD	NRP (545)	Non-NRP (258)	Biliary complications, IC, graft/patient survival		Incidence of overall biliary complications, IC, and patient death were lower in the NRP group with 0.30, 0.112, and 0.54 odds ratio, respectively	PMID: 34856070

HMP

	Year	Donor	Intervention	Control	Primary outcome	Secondary outcome	Results	PMID
No	2010	DBD	HMP (20)	SCS (20)	The incidence of PNF, EAD and patient and graft survival at 1 mo and 1 y	Biliary and vascular complications and LFTs and renal function	Lower incidence of EAD with low LFTs and short hospitalization were observed in the HMP group	PMID: 19958323
Yes	2015	DCD	HOPE (25)	SCS (50)	The incidence and severity of biliary complications within 1 y after transplantation	Liver ischemia reperfusion injury and function as well as graft survival	HOPE provided low ALT peak and incidence of IC, and higher 1-y graft survival	PMID: 26583664
No	2015	ECD	HMP (31)	SCS (30)	The incidences of PNF, EAD and vascular complications, graft and patient survival at 1-y	The incidence of biliary complications, AKI, hospital length of stay, LFTs and complications including reoperations	Lower incidence of IC and shorter hospitalization were observed in the HMP group.	PMID: 25521639
No	2017	DCD	DHOPE (10)	SCS (20)	Graft survival at 6-mo	Graft and patient survival rates at 1-y, the safety of machine perfusion, microbiological testing of perfusate and post transplant complications	Twofold lower in ALT and Bil 1-wk after transplant and none of the DHOPE livers required retransplantation due to IC	PMID: 28394402
No	2018	DCD	DHOPE (10)	SCS (9)	To dermine K/Na shifts during machine perfusion to reperfusion		Potassium level in recipients who received DHOPE preserved livers decreased after reperfusion Requirement of noradrenaline was less in the DHOPE group	PMID: 30411502

(continued on next page)

Table 2
(continued)

RCT		Donor Type	Intervention Arm (#)	Control Arm (#)	Primary End Points	Secondary End Points	Main Outcomes	References
No	2019	DBD and DCD	HOPE (50)	SCS DCD (50) and SCS DBD (50)	Post transplant complications, and non-tumor related patient death or graft loss	Intraoperative parameters, lactate clearance at the end of transplant, complications, length of hospital/ICU stay	5 y graft survival in the HOPE group was equivalent with that of the DBD cohort and superior to the SCS DCD group	PMID: 30342115
No	2020	ECD DBD	HOPE (10)	SCS (30)	The incidence of EAD	1, 3, and 12-mo graft and patient survival and length of hopitalization	Peak AST within 7-d and INR on post operative day 7 were significantly lower in the HOPE group	PMID: 32269237
Yes	2021	DCD	DHOPE (78)	SCS (78)	The incidence of nonanastomotic biliary strictures within 6-mo after transplantation	Intraoperative postreperfusion syndrome, PNF, EAD, thrombosis of the hepatic artery or portal vein, anastomotic biliary stricture or leakage, and renal replacement therapy within 6-mo after transplant	Reduction in the incidence of IC (OR 0.35), postreperfusion syndrome (OR 0.43), and EAD (OR 0.61) in the DHOPE group.	PMID: 33626248
No	2021	ECD DBD	HOPE (25)	SCS (69)	The incidence of EAD	Determined by intraoperative/ biological/ postoperative parameters and economic impact frrom the hospital's perspective	HOPE improved AST/ ALT/lactate/Cr after transplant and reduced ICU and hospital stay	PMID: 33237618

Abbreviations: AKI, acute kidney injury; ALT, alanine transaminase; AST, aspartate transaminase; DBD, donation after brain death; DCD, donation after circulatory death; DHOPE, dual hypothermic oxygenated perfusion; EAD, early allograft dysfunction; HMP, hypothermic machine perfusion; HOPE, hypothermic oxygenated perfusion; IC, ischemic cholangiopathy; ICU, intensive care unit; IRI, ischemia reperfusion injury; LFTs, liver function tests; NMP, normothermic machine perfusion; NRP, normothermic regional perfusion; PNF, primary non function; RBC, red blood cells; RCT, randomized control trial; SCS, static cold storage.

compared with SCS. Graft survival was similar.[32] In discarded human grafts, SNMP improved energy status, TCA cycle intermediate, and lactate clearance.[33] Of interest, this study further demonstrated that steatotic human livers with 3 hours SNMP resulted in higher ATP stores compared with NMP. However, SNMP was associated with lower antioxidative capacity (assessed by glutathione, and N-acetylcysteine level).[34] In summary, SNMP effectively supports human liver ex vivo with minimal injury, and stable, if not improved, metabolic activity. Moreover, SNMP can be performed using an acellular perfusate, thus avoiding the need for complex machinery required for perfusion at normothermic temperature. To date, no clinical trial has examined the benefits of liver SNMP.

Normothermic machine perfusion

NMP creates an ex situ environment that closely mimics physiological conditions by using a perfusate containing red blood cells as an oxygen carrier and essential substrates. Additional components of the perfusate include insulin and steroids (dexamethasone) to support glucose metabolism and reduce inflammation, respectively. This approach allows for the maintenance of metabolic homeostasis in the liver graft during preservation and assessment. One of the significant advantages of NMP is the ability to evaluate the function of the liver graft before transplantation. Several parameters are assessed to determine the viability and functionality of the liver during NMP. These assessments include (1) Homogeneous perfusion on visual inspection: The perfusion of the liver graft should appear even and consistent throughout the parenchyma. (2) Adequate portal and arterial flow, as well as resistance to assess the vascular integrity and functionality of the liver graft. (3) Lactate clearance: Lactate levels in the perfusate are measured to evaluate the metabolic activity of the liver graft. A slow or fluctuating decrease in lactate levels during NMP may indicate insufficient or compromised perfusion. Such deviations from the expected downward trend should be thoroughly investigated to identify the underlying issue and appropriate measures to optimize perfusion and metabolic activity should be taken. (4) Bile production: The presence of bile production is an indicator of hepatocyte function. Monitoring bile production during NMP provides insights into the functionality of the biliary system and liver secretory function. In general, a steady decrease in lactate levels below 2.5 mmol/L and the presence of new bile production soon after initiating NMP are considered favorable markers of viability.[35,36] Based on the evaluation of these parameters, transplant teams can make informed decisions regarding the suitability of the liver graft for transplantation.[35]

The optimal initiation location for NMP, whether local or back-to-base, is unknown. Although back-to-base NMP is associated with longer cold ischemia time (CIT) compared with local NMP, both strategies were associated with similar lactate clearance. Importantly, there was no difference in the incidence of EAD, PNF, or graft and patient survival[37] between the two approaches. These results are also supported by a study that showed the feasibility of a 6-hour SCS followed by 8.5 hours NMP.[38] Of importance, the initiation of NMP at the donor sites carries a risk of additional warm ischemia if some areas of the liver where to be non/mal-perfused. It is crucial to closely monitor the liver graft during NMP, identify promptly any non-perfused areas, and take appropriate measures to ensure homogenous to minimize potential graft damage.

The Liver Assist machine is designed to support both HMP and NMP. It is not transportable, meaning it is typically used within the hospital or transplantation center. The Metra machine and Organ Care System (OCS) are only designed for NMP and are transportable machine, allowing for the initiation of perfusion at the donor site. Currently, three randomized clinical trial (RCT) evaluated NMP in the context of liver transplantation (**Table 2**). In the UK NMP study, using the Metra (OrganOx, London, UK) was associated with a 50% lower level of graft injury, a 50% reduction in organ discard rate despite 54% longer preservation time compared with SCS. Patient and graft survival were similar.[39] In a recent study using the OCS, our team found that NMP significantly decreased the incidence of EAD compared with SCS (18% vs 31%). In addition, the development of IC, assessed by magnetic resonance cholangiopancreatography (MRCP) at 6 and 12 months post-transplant was reduced. Importantly, the OCS Liver resulted in significantly higher use of DCD livers.[3] In the most recent RCT, recipients of livers from donors after brain death (DBD) were randomly assigned to receive either an ischemia-free liver transplant using combined in situ and ex vivo NMP with the Liver Assist machine or a "conventional" transplant. Here, NMP ischemia-free liver transplant group had lower rates of EAD and post-reperfusion syndrome compared with the conventional transplant group.[40] These findings are consistent with other RCTs discussed previously. In addition to its clinical effectiveness, the introduction of NMP also seems to be a cost-effective approach in the current health care system.[41]

There are several important surgical considerations to review during NMP. To avoid kinking of the portal vein, it is preferable to recover a long segment. Sufficient dissection below the confluence of the superior mesenteric vein and splenic vein can help achieve this goal The hepatic arteries are perfused through the celiac trunk. Similarly, obtaining a long vessel will prevent any tension and prevent potential dissection. Of note, when the right hepatic artery is replaced, or when an hepatic artery arise separately, it should be reconstructed with the common hepatic artery to create one conduit for machine perfusion. There are several methods to achieve this. Ideally, it is the best to have a reconstructed artery so that it is ready for implantation without additional procedures. We believe it is ideal to perform the anastomosis between the splenic artery (SPA) and the replaced right hepatic artery with or without the superior mesenteric artery (SMA) cuff or the gastroduodenal artery and the replaced right hepatic artery. In addition, the aortic segment, with the celiac artery and the SMA, can be anastomosed and perfused from the SPA. Finally, the bile duct cannula should be secured and position to avoid kinking. A pediatric feeding tube can be used for cannulation in small bile ducts.

Normothermic regional perfusion

NRP refers to donor in situ normothermic perfusion. Similar to NMP, NRP aims to provide oxygenated flow and nutrients to mitigate warm ischemic damage, before organ procurement, using extra corporeal membrane oxygenation and pump. This approach can also potentially increase the number of DCD organs. NRP also enables the evaluation of each organ before procurements.[42] During DCD procurement, the donor warm ischemic time (DWIT) is an important consideration. Total DWIT encompasses the period from withdrawal of life support to cold preservation flush, whereas asystolic DWIT refers to the period from circulatory arrest to the flush. To determine clinically significant warm ischemia, functional DWIT is often used during DCD procurements. The duration of functional DWIT varies depending on the country or organ procurement organization. Typically, it starts when certain thresholds are met, such as a drop in SpO2 (peripheral oxygen saturation <80%–70%) or systolic/mean arterial pressure below specific values (eg, <60–50 mm Hg) and continues until the initiation of cold systemic perfusion.[43] Under these circumstances, NRP aims to minimize functional DWIT. In a cohort of Maastricht type 2 (DCD, suffering sudden and unexpected cardiac arrest), NRP allowed a recovery of 34 additional livers in 8 years (9%). In those, 1-year recipient and graft survivals were 82% and 70%, respectively (median follow-up 24 months). Although less than 10% livers were transplantable, these reports indicate that NRP is effective in expanding the donor population.[44] The potential of NRP for uncontrolled DCD was also described in a report from Spain where only one out of 10 (10%) uncontrolled DCD liver transplants developed IC.[45] According to a retrospective cohort study involving 803 controlled DCD liver transplants in Spain, NRP was superior to SCS followed by super-rapid recovery. The study demonstrated significant reductions in overall biliary complications, IC, and patient death in the NRP group compared with SCS.[46] Moreover, several studies have supported that the outcomes of liver transplantation after NRP are comparable to those of traditional DBD livers.[46–49] It has been debated whether NRP is superior to NMP. In a study from the Netherlands,[50] NRP was used to salvage 20 variable livers out of 43 donors initially deemed unsuitable for transplantation. The results showed a 95% 1-year graft and patient survival rate, along with a comparable 11% incidence of IC, indicating the effectiveness of NRP in rescuing discarded livers. An international observational study from Europe, using propensity score matching, found similar graft and patient survival, rate of EAD, and IC when comparing NRP to NMP. In this study, NRP livers had higher peak AST levels.[51] However, a single-center retrospective study suggested that NRP reduces the incidence of IC compared with NMP.[52] Overall, NRP seems to be a reasonable approach to improve outcomes in DCD liver transplant, provided that ethical issues surrounding NRP are properly addressed.[53]

Combination Therapy

The ideal duration of perfusion, timing, and perfusate composition in NMP and NRP is still under intense research. There is no consensus on a standardized protocol, and it may vary depending on the specific clinical scenario. Combining therapies and using different approaches may be necessary to achieve optimal outcomes. R. Porte's team showed that a 1 hour of HOPE, followed by stepwise increase in temperature, and subsequent NMP led to a 20% increase in transplantable livers with favorable outcomes.[54,55] The mechanism proposed was an improvement in ATP store during HOPE and adequate viability assessment during NMP. Finally, a study using a 1:2 propensity score matching method, the effectiveness of NRP and HOPE interventions in DCD liver showed that these interventions increased the number of livers suitable for implantation by 59.5%. Importantly, the combination of NRP and HOPE resulted in outcomes equivalent to DBD liver transplant in terms of 1-year patient and graft survival and incidence of IC. It is noteworthy that in this study, DCD procurements was characterized by a 20 minutes asystole prior to the recovery. Despite the prolonged warm ischemic time, NRP and HOPE resulted in improving the outcomes of DCD liver transplant.[56]

Molecular Markers of Viability

The improvement of organ quality through liver perfusion is directly linked to the development of a reliable methodology to assess organ viability before implantation. In fact, a critical barrier in expanding the number of available livers for transplantation is that there are no reliable tests for viability.[57,58] The viability decision is often based on texture of organ and quality of perfusion at retrieval[59] and in some cases histology.[60] Routine blood gas or biochemical analysis has been incorporated into organ preservation for a long time, with measurements taken from either the cold storage solution or machine perfusates.[60] However, most of these markers lack specificity, as they are adapted from clinical practices for patients with liver diseases, such as pH, lactate, or liver transaminases. However, in a study of human discarded liver, viability defined as lactate clearance to levels ≤ 2.5 mmol/L within 4 hour of perfusion enabled successful transplantation of 71% of discarded livers (n = 22), with 100% 90-day patient and graft survival.[35] Composite/multiparameter index has also been developed, which incorporates not only lactate clearance but also factors pH maintenance, bile production, vascular flow patterns, and liver macroscopic appearance.[61] Such comprehensive index might provide a more holistic assessment of liver viability during NMP ensuring a thorough evaluation of organ function and suitability for transplantation. Throughout perfusion modalities, various samples can be obtained, including perfusates, bile, and tissues. These samples offer opportunities for a wide range of tests, such as quantification of microRNA, mitochondrial DNA, Damage-associated molecular patterns and cytokines, as well as metabolomic, proteomic, genomic analyses, and ATP quantification.[60–62] However, the clinical implementation of these modalities is constrained by the extended time required to obtain results or the necessity for tissue biopsies. Evidence from our laboratory showed in rats and humans that preservation of energy status was of utmost importance during the peri-transplant period. In this context, the ratios of ATP/ADP/adenosine monophosphate (AMP) prior to and following reperfusion correlated with graft function.[33,63,64] In a rat study, we measured various metabolites during NMP, which was used to develop an ischemia index. This index was able to discriminate livers that experienced previous ischemia with a sensibility and specificity of over 0.98.[65] A consistent metabolomic analysis of perfusate has identified a specific protein called flavinmononucleotid (FMNH2). Under normal physiological conditions, flavin mononucleotide (FMN) is tightly bound to mitochondrial complex I.[66] However, during ischemia and subsequent reoxygenation, FMN is released into the perfusate, which was associated with degree of mitochondrial injury as well as post-transplant in rodent and human.[67] During HOPE, if the concentration of perfusate FMN at 30 minutes are below 8800 arbitrary units, the liver is generally accepted for transplant. Interestingly, this threshold was applied for both DBD and ECD livers of all types. Altogether, these are promising approaches to improve graft assessment during machine perfusion and increase organ utilization.

THE FUTURE OF MACHINE PERFUSION: CONCLUSION

Machine perfusion is a revolutionary technology that has the potential to significantly enhance the safety and efficacy of liver transplantation. During the past decade, there has been a significant research interest in optimizing organ preservation using machine perfusion, especially for DCD and ECD organs. Both hypothermic and NMP techniques offer the ability to restore and preserve energy stores while minimizing the adverse effects of IR injury after transplantation. Standardizing machine perfusion protocols remains a major challenge and should continue to be an area of intense research. Recent clinical trials[3,29,39] have highlighted the potential benefits of machine perfusion in reducing the risk of IC and EAD. Future work will also help determine the long-term efficacy of machine perfusion and develop viability markers to aid in matching each organ to the appropriate recipient.

CLINICS CARE POINTS

- Machine perfusion has the potential to enhance the safety, efficacy, and number of liver available for transplantation.
- HOPE reduces nonanastomotic biliary strictures following DCD liver transplantation.

- NMP reduces posttransplant early liver allograft dysfunction and ischemic biliary complications.

FUNDING

AL: The Swiss National Science Foundation (SNSF PZ00P3-185927).

DISCLOSURE

Authors have no conflict of interest to declare.

REFERENCES

1. Black CK, Termanini KM, Aguirre O, et al. Solid organ transplantation in the 21. Ann Transl Med 2018;6(20):409.
2. Schlegel A, Kalisvaart M, Scalera I, et al. The UK DCD risk score: a new proposal to define futility in donation-after-circulatory-death liver transplantation. J Hepatol 2018;68(3):456–64.
3. Markmann JF, Abouljoud MS, Ghobrial RM, et al. Impact of portable normothermic blood-based machine perfusion on outcomes of liver transplant: the OCS Liver PROTECT randomized clinical trial. JAMA Surg 2022;157(3):189–98.
4. Okumura K, Dhand A, Misawa R, et al. Outcomes of liver transplantation using machine perfusion in donation after cardiac death vs brain death in the US. J Am Coll Surg 2023;236(1):73–80.
5. Maspero M, Ali K, Cazzaniga B, et al. Acute rejection after liver transplantation with machine perfusion versus static cold storage: a systematic review and meta-analysis. Hepatology 2023. https://doi.org/10.1097/HEP.0000000000000363.
6. Mueller M, Kalisvaart M, O'Rourke J, et al. Hypothermic oxygenated liver perfusion (HOPE) prevents tumor recurrence in liver transplantation from donation after circulatory death. Ann Surg 2020;272(5):759–65.
7. Gilbo N, Catalano G, Salizzoni M, et al. Liver graft preconditioning, preservation and reconditioning. Dig Liver Dis 2016;48(11):1265–74.
8. Jassem W, Xystrakis E, Ghnewa YG, et al. Normothermic machine perfusion (NMP) inhibits proinflammatory responses in the liver and promotes regeneration. Hepatology 2019;70(2):682–95.
9. Panconesi R, Flores Carvalho M, Dondossola D, et al. Impact of machine perfusion on the immune response after liver transplantation - a primary treatment or just a delivery tool. Front Immunol 2022;13:855263.
10. Serifis N, Matheson R, Cloonan D, et al. Machine perfusion of the liver: a review of clinical trials. Front Surg 2021;8:625394.
11. Liu Q, Del Prete L, Ali K, et al. Sequential hypothermic and normothermic perfusion preservation and transplantation of expanded criteria donor livers. Surgery 2023;173(3):846–54.
12. van Leeuwen OB, Bodewes SB, Lantinga VA, et al. Sequential hypothermic and normothermic machine perfusion enables safe transplantation of high-risk donor livers. Am J Transplant 2022;22(6):1658–70.
13. Gallinat A, Fox M, Lüer B, et al. Role of pulsatility in hypothermic reconditioning of porcine kidney grafts by machine perfusion after cold storage. Transplantation 2013;96(6):538–42.
14. Schlegel A, Dutkowski P. Role of hypothermic machine perfusion in liver transplantation. Transpl Int 2015;28(6):677–89.

15. Schlegel A, Kron P, Dutkowski P. Hypothermic oxygenated liver perfusion: basic mechanisms and clinical application. Curr Transplant Rep 2015;2(1):52–62.
16. de Vries Y, Brüggenwirth IMA, Karangwa SA, et al. Dual versus single oxygenated hypothermic machine perfusion of porcine livers: impact on hepatobiliary and endothelial cell injury. Transplant Direct 2021;7(9):e741.
17. Jomaa A, Gurusamy K, Siriwardana PN, et al. Does hypothermic machine perfusion of human donor livers affect risks of sinusoidal endothelial injury and microbial infection? A feasibility study assessing flow parameters, sterility, and sinusoidal endothelial ultrastructure. Transplant Proc 2013;45(5):1677–83.
18. Schlegel A, de Rougemont O, Graf R, et al. Protective mechanisms of end-ischemic cold machine perfusion in DCD liver grafts. J Hepatol 2013;58(2):278–86.
19. Guarrera JV, Henry SD, Samstein B, et al. Hypothermic machine preservation in human liver transplantation: the first clinical series. Am J Transplant 2010;10(2):372–81.
20. Dutkowski P, Furrer K, Tian Y, et al. Novel short-term hypothermic oxygenated perfusion (HOPE) system prevents injury in rat liver graft from non-heart beating donor. Ann Surg 2006;244(6):968–76 [discussion: 976-7].
21. Rauen U, Petrat F, Li T, et al. Hypothermia injury/cold-induced apoptosis–evidence of an increase in chelatable iron causing oxidative injury in spite of low O2-/H2O2 formation. FASEB J 2000;14(13):1953–64.
22. Guarrera JV, Henry SD, Samstein B, et al. Hypothermic machine preservation facilitates successful transplantation of "orphan" extended criteria donor livers. Am J Transplant 2015;15(1):161–9.
23. Burlage LC, Karimian N, Westerkamp AC, et al. Oxygenated hypothermic machine perfusion after static cold storage improves endothelial function of extended criteria donor livers. HPB (Oxford) 2017;19(6):538–46.
24. Schlegel A, Kron P, Graf R, et al. Hypothermic Oxygenated Perfusion (HOPE) downregulates the immune response in a rat model of liver transplantation. Ann Surg 2014;260(5):931–7 [discussion: 937-8].
25. Marecki H, Bozorgzadeh A, Porte RJ, et al. Liver ex situ machine perfusion preservation: a review of the methodology and results of large animal studies and clinical trials. Liver Transplant 2017;23(5):679–95.
26. Dutkowski P, Polak WG, Muiesan P, et al. First comparison of hypothermic oxygenated perfusion versus static cold storage of human donation after cardiac death liver transplants: an international-matched case analysis. Ann Surg 2015;262(5):764–70 [discussion: 770-1].
27. van Rijn R, Karimian N, Matton APM, et al. Dual hypothermic oxygenated machine perfusion in liver transplants donated after circulatory death. Br J Surg 2017;104(7):907–17.
28. Schlegel A, Muller X, Kalisvaart M, et al. Outcomes of DCD liver transplantation using organs treated by hypothermic oxygenated perfusion before implantation. J Hepatol 2019;70(1):50–7.
29. van Rijn R, Schurink IJ, de Vries Y, et al. Hypothermic machine perfusion in liver transplantation - a randomized trial. N Engl J Med 2021;384(15):1391–401.
30. Schlegel A, Mueller M, Muller X, et al. A multicenter randomized-controlled trial of hypothermic oxygenated perfusion (HOPE) for human liver grafts before transplantation. J Hepatol 2023;78(4):783–93.
31. Berendsen TA, Bruinsma BG, Lee J, et al. A simplified subnormothermic machine perfusion system restores ischemically damaged liver grafts in a rat model of orthotopic liver transplantation. Transplant Res 2012;1(1):6.

32. Knaak JM, Spetzler VN, Goldaracena N, et al. Subnormothermic ex vivo liver perfusion reduces endothelial cell and bile duct injury after donation after cardiac death pig liver transplantation. Liver Transplant 2014;20(11):1296–305.

33. Bruinsma BG, Sridharan GV, Weeder PD, et al. Metabolic profiling during ex vivo machine perfusion of the human liver. Sci Rep 2016;6:22415.

34. Karimian N, Raigani S, Huang V, et al. Subnormothermic machine perfusion of steatotic livers results in increased energy charge at the cost of anti-oxidant capacity compared to normothermic perfusion. Metabolites 2019;9(11). https://doi. org/10.3390/metabo9110246.

35. Mergental H, Laing RW, Kirkham AJ, et al. Transplantation of discarded livers following viability testing with normothermic machine perfusion. Nat Commun 2020;11(1):2939.

36. Olumba FC, Zhou F, Park Y, et al. Normothermic machine perfusion for declined livers: a strategy to rescue marginal livers for transplantation. J Am Coll Surg 2023;236(4):614–25.

37. Bral M, Dajani K, Leon Izquierdo D, et al. A back-to-base experience of human normothermic ex situ liver perfusion: does the chill kill? Liver Transplant 2019; 25(6):848–58.

38. Ceresa CDL, Nasralla D, Watson CJE, et al. Transient cold storage prior to normothermic liver perfusion may facilitate adoption of a novel technology. Liver Transplant 2019;25(10):1503–13.

39. Nasralla D, Coussios CC, Mergental H, et al. A randomized trial of normothermic preservation in liver transplantation. Nature 2018;557(7703):50–6.

40. Guo Z, Zhao Q, Jia Z, et al. A randomized-controlled trial of ischemia-free liver transplantation for end-stage liver disease. J Hepatol 2023. https://doi.org/10. 1016/j.jhep.2023.04.010.

41. Webb AN, Lester ELW, Shapiro AMJ, et al. Cost-utility analysis of normothermic machine perfusion compared to static cold storage in liver transplantation in the Canadian setting. Am J Transplant 2022;22(2):541–51.

42. Oniscu GC, Randle LV, Muiesan P, et al. In situ normothermic regional perfusion for controlled donation after circulatory death–the United Kingdom experience. Am J Transplant 2014;14(12):2846–54.

43. Kalisvaart M, Croome KP, Hernandez-Alejandro R, et al. Donor warm ischemia time in DCD liver transplantation-working group report from the ILTS DCD, liver preservation, and machine perfusion consensus conference. Transplantation 2021;105(6):1156–64.

44. Fondevila C, Hessheimer AJ, Flores E, et al. Applicability and results of Maastricht type 2 donation after cardiac death liver transplantation. Am J Transplant 2012;12(1):162–70.

45. Herrero Torres MA, Domniguez Bastante M, Molina Raya A, et al. Eight years of extracorporeal membrane oxygenation in liver transplantation: our experience. Transplant Proc 2020;52(2):572–4.

46. Hessheimer AJ, de la Rosa G, Gastaca M, et al. Abdominal normothermic regional perfusion in controlled donation after circulatory determination of death liver transplantation: outcomes and risk factors for graft loss. Am J Transplant 2022;22(4):1169–81.

47. Ruiz P, Valdivieso A, Palomares I, et al. Similar results in liver transplantation from controlled donation after circulatory death donors with normothermic regional perfusion and donation after brain death donors: a case-matched single-center study. Liver Transplant 2021;27(12):1747–57.

48. Savier E, Lim C, Rayar M, et al. Favorable outcomes of liver transplantation from controlled circulatory death donors using normothermic regional perfusion compared to brain death donors. Transplantation 2020;104(9):1943–51.

49. Viguera L, Blasi A, Reverter E, et al. Liver transplant with controlled donors after circulatory death with normothermic regional perfusion and brain dead donors: a multicenter cohort study of transfusion, one-year graft survival and mortality. Int J Surg 2021;96:106169.

50. Schurink IJ, de Goeij FHC, Habets LJM, et al. Salvage of declined extended-criteria DCD livers using in situ normothermic regional perfusion. Ann Surg 2022;276(4):e223–30.

51. Mohkam K, Nasralla D, Mergental H, et al. In situ normothermic regional perfusion versus ex situ normothermic machine perfusion in liver transplantation from donation after circulatory death. Liver Transplant 2022;28(11):1716–25.

52. Gaurav R, Butler AJ, Kosmoliaptsis V, et al. Liver transplantation outcomes from controlled circulatory death donors: SCS vs in situ NRP vs ex situ NMP. Ann Surg 2022;275(6):1156–64.

53. Schiff T, Koziatek C, Pomerantz E, et al. Extracorporeal cardiopulmonary resuscitation dissemination and integration with organ preservation in the USA: ethical and logistical considerations. Crit Care 2023;27(1):144.

54. van Leeuwen OB, de Vries Y, Fujiyoshi M, et al. Transplantation of high-risk donor livers after ex situ resuscitation and assessment using combined hypo- and normothermic machine perfusion: a prospective clinical trial. Ann Surg 2019; 270(5):906–14.

55. de Vries Y, Matton APM, Nijsten MWN, et al. Pretransplant sequential hypo- and normothermic machine perfusion of suboptimal livers donated after circulatory death using a hemoglobin-based oxygen carrier perfusion solution. Am J Transplant 2019;19(4):1202–11.

56. Patrono D, Zanierato M, Vergano M, et al. Normothermic regional perfusion and hypothermic oxygenated machine perfusion for livers donated after controlled circulatory death with prolonged warm ischemia time: a matched comparison with livers from brain-dead donors. Transpl Int 2022;35:10390.

57. Vilca Melendez H, Rela M, Murphy G, et al. Assessment of graft function before liver transplantation: quest for the lost ark? Transplantation 2000;70(4):560–5.

58. Longchamp A, Klauser A, Songeon J, et al. Ex vivo analysis of kidney graft viability using 31P magnetic resonance imaging spectroscopy. Transplantation 2020. https://doi.org/10.1097/TP.0000000000003323.

59. Casavilla A, Ramirez C, Shapiro R, et al. Experience with liver and kidney allografts from non-heart-beating donors. Transplantation 1995;59(2):197–203.

60. Panconesi R, Flores Carvalho M, Mueller M, et al. Viability assessment in liver transplantation-what is the impact of dynamic organ preservation? Biomedicines 2021;9(2). https://doi.org/10.3390/biomedicines9020161.

61. Stephenson BTF, Afford SC, Mergental H, et al. Lactate measurements in an integrated perfusion machine for human livers. Nat Biotechnol 2020;38(11):1259.

62. Berendsen TA, Izamis ML, Xu H, et al. Hepatocyte viability and adenosine triphosphate content decrease linearly over time during conventional cold storage of rat liver grafts. Transplant Proc 2011;43(5):1484–8.

63. Bruinsma BG, Avruch JH, Sridharan GV, et al. Peritransplant energy changes and their correlation to outcome after human liver transplantation. Transplantation 2017;101(7):1637–44.

64. Martins PN, Berendsen TA, Yeh H, et al. Oxygenated UW solution decreases ATP decay and improves survival after transplantation of DCD liver grafts. Transplantation 2019;103(2):363–70.
65. Perk S, Izamis ML, Tolboom H, et al. A metabolic index of ischemic injury for perfusion-recovery of cadaveric rat livers. PLoS One 2011;6(12):e28518.
66. Kahl A, Stepanova A, Konrad C, et al. Critical role of flavin and glutathione in complex i-mediated bioenergetic failure in brain ischemia/reperfusion injury. Stroke 2018;49(5):1223–31.
67. Schlegel A, Muller X, Mueller M, et al. Hypothermic oxygenated perfusion protects from mitochondrial injury before liver transplantation. EBioMedicine 2020; 60:103014.

Donor Viral Hepatitis and Liver Transplantation

Sara-Catherine Whitney Zingg, MD[a], Kristina Lemon, MD[a,b],*

KEYWORDS

- Liver • Transplantation • Hepatitis B • Hepatitis C

KEY POINTS

- Utilization of allografts from hepatitis B and hepatitis C donors has provided additional support for the supply and demand mismatch.
- Liver transplantation using allografts with acute or chronic hepatitis C virus (HCV) followed by novel direct acting antivirals has proven to be safe in both HCV positive and negative recipients.
- Liver transplantation with hepatitis B positive allografts requires life-long antiviral treatment but may be safely used in hepatitis B virus positive or negative recipients.

INTRODUCTION

Liver transplantation remains the mainstay of treatment of patients with end-stage liver disease (ESLD) worldwide. Although 9528 liver transplants were performed in 2022 across the United States, another 10,445 candidates remained on the waiting list at the end of the year.[1] Despite increases in the number of deceased donors and liver transplantations performed each year, the demand for liver transplant continues to exceed the organ supply.[1,2] Over the last 10 years, the use of "marginal" livers, including those from donors who are hepatitis C virus (HCV) or hepatitis B virus (HBV) positive, has been used to help combat the supply and demand mismatch. This article will provide a review of the use of HCV(+) and HBV(+) donors in liver transplantation.

THE HISTORY: HEPATITIS C VIRUS

The terminology "HCV(+) donors" has been used to encompass donors at any stage of the HCV infection. However, the risk of transmission of the virus varies significantly

a Department of Surgery, University of Cincinnati College of Medicine, 231 Albert Sabin Way, ML 0558, Cincinnati, OH 45267, USA; b Division of Transplantation, University of Cincinnati School of Mediicne, 231 Albert Sabin Way, ML 0558, Cincinnati, OH 45267, USA
* Corresponding author. 231 Albert Sabin Way, ML 0558, Cincinnati, OH 45267-0558.
E-mail address: lemonkh@ucmail.uc.edu
Twitter: @transplant_u (S.-C.W.Z.); @kristinalemon22 (K.L.)

Surg Clin N Am 104 (2024) 67–77
https://doi.org/10.1016/j.suc.2023.07.002
0039-6109/24/© 2023 Elsevier Inc. All rights reserved.

surgical.theclinics.com

based on the stage of the infection. Therefore, it is important that we are specific with the terminology we use when discussing these types of donors. Those donors who are referred to as "seropositive" are those that are positive for the anti-HCV antibody. This can further be subdivided into donors that are actively "viremic" or "NAT(+)" indicating detection of HCV ribonucleic acid (RNA) or those that are "NAT(−)" to help distinguish acute and chronic phases of infection (**Table 1**).[3–5] This distinction becomes important during consideration of use for transplantation in uninfected recipients as the risk of disease transmission can be significantly different.[3,5]

The use of HCV seropositive donors was traditionally reserved for HCV seropositive or infected recipients as the reinfection rate was almost universal. Wright and colleagues noted a 95% reinfection rate in their study of 89 patients as demonstrated by post-transplant viremia.[6] However, despite this almost guaranteed reinfection rate, Vargas and colleagues followed by Marroquin demonstrated that transplantation with HCV seropositive livers into HCV(+) recipients did not confer a worse overall survival.[7,8]

Ballarin and colleagues looked at 63 patients with HCV-related cirrhosis who underwent transplantation with HCV seropositive allografts. They again demonstrated comparable graft and patient survival rates; however, they noted more rapid recurrence of HCV as well as higher rates of acute cellular rejection and biliary complications.[9] They noted that those who received HCV NAT(+) allografts trended toward more advanced stages of fibrosis and subsequent earlier development of hepatitis recurrence.[9] Although graft and patient survivals were comparable, there were concerns regarding the indiscriminate use of HCV(+) allografts.

THE FIRST STEP: UTILIZATION OF HEPATITIS C VIRUS (+) DONORS IN HEPATITIS C VIRUS(+) RECIPIENTS

The initial introduction of direct-acting antivirals (DAAs) in 2011 allowed for increased use of HCV seropositive livers in all recipients. Bowring and associates were the first to demonstrate the efficacy of transplanting HCV seropositive allografts into HCV(+) recipients in the era of DAAs.[10] They used the Scientific Registry of Transplant Recipients (SRTR) to identify over 25,000 HCV(+) deceased donor liver transplant (DDLT) recipients between 2005 and 2015. At the beginning of the study period, approximately 6% of patients were receiving HCV(+) livers, but with the advent of DAAs this number increased to almost 17%. Although they demonstrated increased utilization of HCV(+) donors, these grafts were still being discarded at a rate 1.7 times higher than HCV(−) livers. Importantly, they demonstrated no difference in all-cause graft loss for recipients of HCV(+) allografts versus those recipients of HCV(−) allografts at either 6-month or 1-year follow up.[10] Cotter and colleagues then expanded on this by looking at longer term outcomes in HCV(+) recipients in the DAA era.[11] Using

Table 1
Terminology used for hepatitis C positive donors

HCV Antibody "Seropositivity"	HCV RNA "Viremic"/"NAT Positivity"	Interpretation
+	−	No active infection/ resolved infection
−	+	Acute infection
+	+	Chronic infection

Abbreviations: HCV, hepatitis C virus; NAT, nucleic acid amplification testing; RNA, ribonucleic acid.

the SRTR, they identified 2378 HCV(+) recipients that received HCV(+) allografts between 2008 and 2018. They noted an improved 3-year graft survival in the post-DAA era compared with the pre-DAA era (85% vs 78%).[11] Bowring and Cotter paved the way for increased utilization of HCV(+) organs by demonstrating the efficacy and long-term viability of HCV(+) DDLT with the advent of DAAs.[10,11]

Subsequently, there were several studies that published the efficacy of transplanting not only HCV seropositive organs but NAT(+) or "viremic" organs into both seropositive and viremic recipients.[7-9,12,13] Ultimately in 2017, the American Society of Transplantation convened to review the current state of utilization of HCV(+) allografts.[3] They concluded that organs from HCV viremic individuals represented an underused resource, and HCV allograft use was acceptable if the donor biopsy demonstrated less than stage 2 fibrosis. The University of Colorado convened an expert panel in 2019 and reiterated the efficacy of HCV(+) allografts in the post-DAA era.[14] They also supported the use of HCV(+) allografts in HCV(−) recipients, but outlined essential criteria for use including guaranteed access to DAA therapy as well as rigorous recipient education.[14]

THE CULTURE SHIFT: UTILIZATION OF HEPATITIS C VIRUS(+) ALLOGRAFTS IN HEPATITIS C VIRUS(−) RECIPIENTS

With the advent of DAAs offering a relatively easy and reliable cure for HCV, interest continued to grow for using HCV(+) donors in HCV(−) recipients. The utilization of HCV(+) allografts followed by DAA therapy became an approach at select centers to avoid discarding these "marginal" livers. Danford and associates noted that from 2016 to 2019 there was a 35-fold increase in utilization of HCV(+) livers transplanted into HCV(−) recipients.[15] However, there was growing concern regarding the efficacy and safety of this practice.

Ting and colleagues out of Johns Hopkins evaluated 26 HCV(−) recipients who received HCV(+) allografts between 2017 and 2019.[16] Of these 26 patients, 20 received allografts from HCV NAT(+) "viremic" donors. All patients were initiated on DAA therapy within 12 weeks of transplantation. Twelve recipients completed their DAA courses and reached sufficient follow-up to evaluate sustained virologic response after 12 weeks of treatment (SVR12). These 12 patients all reached SVR12 and had normal graft function. They concluded that HCV(+) allografts could be used in HCV(−) individuals with good short-term outcomes.[16]

A larger, single-center study performed by Luckett, from the University of Cincinnati, described 55 HCV(−) recipients of HCV Ab(+)/NAT(−) livers.[17] Per their institutional protocol, all patients underwent HCV nucleic acid amplification testing (NAT) at 3 months follow-up unless indicated earlier by rising liver enzymes. At 3 months, 9.4% of patients were HCV NAT(+). All viremic patients received DAA therapy and achieved SVR12. They also demonstrated no difference in 3-month or 1-year outcomes which included liver enzymes, graft loss, and mortality.[17] Larger database studies have also been encouraging regarding outcomes in HCV(−) individuals. In 2019, Cholankeril performed a retrospective review using the Organ Procurement and Transplantation Network/United Network for Organ Sharing (UNOS) database to identify HCV seropositive DDLT recipients and demonstrated comparable patient and graft survival at 1-year follow-up.[18]

THE FUTURE OF HEPATITIS C VIRUS LIVER TRANSPLANTATION

Although the transmission rates among all HCV seropositive allografts may be relatively low ranging from 9% to 16%,[17,19] HCV NAT(+) allografts almost universally transmit HCV infection to their recipients.[5,16] The safety of HCV Ab(+)/NAT(−) allografts in the era of DAAs has allowed for the usage of HCV Ab(+)/NAT(+) or "viremic" allografts to become the reality. Cotter and colleagues used the SRTR database and identified 87 seronegative recipients of HCV NAT(+) allografts. They demonstrated no difference in patient or graft survival at 1- or 2-year when compared with recipients of seronegative allografts.[20]

Although the post-DAA era has allowed for increased use of HCV seropositive allografts for transplantation into recipients regardless of their HCV status, long-term data are still needed. The number of new HCV infections has increased threefold between 2010 and 2016 secondary to the opioid epidemic and the number of deaths among patients with chronic HCV without cirrhosis is projected to increase.[21] One could conclude that the number of donors with HCV is also likely to increase and further data derived from HCV(+) organ utilization are needed. The combination of the organ shortage, increasing numbers of HCV NAT(+) donors, and the advent of DAAs has resulted in a rapid increase in HCV viremic organ transplants into HCV(−) recipients. Although studies have proven early safety and efficacy, it is necessary to continue to provide full informed consent, adequate preoperative education, and ensuring adequate access to DAA therapy after transplantation.

CURRENT HEPATITIS C VIRUS TREATMENT STRATEGIES

The initial treatment of HCV relied on interferon-based therapy; however, these therapies had low SVR12 and were very poorly tolerated.[22] DAA therapy was first introduced in 2011, and these first-generation protease inhibitors, such as telaprevir and boceprevir, were used initially in conjunction with interferon and ribavirin therapy. These first combination therapies were not ideal for patients with decompensated cirrhosis due to the high risk of further decompensation or death.[23] There were also significant initial concerns with the use of DAAs due to concern over drug interactions most importantly with calcineurin inhibitors resulting in potentially significant toxicity.[5] Finally, new combination antivirals were made that eliminated the need for interferon therapy and proved to have high efficacy and safety protocols. There have been several studies since that attest to the efficacy and safety of these therapies.[5,24,25]

Glecaprevir/pibrentasvir and sofosbuvir/velpatasvir have both been developed as once daily oral combination therapy for patients with chronic HCV infection. Several phase 2 and 3 clinical trials demonstrate their tolerability, high SVR12 rates, and efficacy among all HCV genotypes.[26–31] With the increased availability and high efficacy of these agents in patients with chronic HCV, the discussion moved toward whether to treat pre- or post-transplantation. Patient with low baseline Model for End-Stage Liver Disease (<16), a low baseline Child-Pugh score, and absence of complications from portal hypertension should be considered for treatment pre-transplant, whereas those patients with advanced liver disease are unlikely to benefit from pre-transplant treatment.[32,33] Subsequently, several studies also evaluated these DAA regimens in seronegative recipients of seropositive or viremic allografts and have again demonstrated favorable outcomes.[34–36]

The American Association for the Study of Liver Diseases (AASLD) current recommendations included treatment with either glecaprevir/pibrentasvir or sofosbuvir/velpatasvir for 12 weeks in the post-transplant patient.[25] There are no consensus guidelines on the timing of treatment. Most of the clinical trials conducted in patients with chronic HCV are treated 6 to 12 months post-transplant and there have been little data to support earlier initiation of DAA therapy in this patient population. However, seronegative patients who receive seropositive or NAT(+) allografts should receive

DAA therapy early. Several studies have demonstrated detectable HCV RNA levels as early as 3 days post-transplant.[37,38] Terrault and colleagues evaluated 13 seronegative recipients of NAT(+) liver allografts treated with sofosbuvir/velpatasvir, which was initiated at a median of 7 days post-transplant. All liver transplants in this study demonstrated SVR12.[37] Aqel and colleagues evaluated a larger recipient cohort of viremic liver allografts who received DAA therapy at a median of 27 days post-transplant and again all patients demonstrated SVR12.[38] Although more robust data are needed on timing of DAA initiation in this population, the AASLD recommends early treatment initiation within the first week after transplantation provided the patient is clinically stable.[25]

HEPATITIS B VIRUS

Although the national shortage of donor livers has led to the increased use of HCV seropositive allografts, HBV positive donors are another potential opportunity to expand the donor pool. When discussing transplantation of HBV allografts, it is again important to define infection based on serology. Patients with resolved infections are defined as hepatitis B core antibody (HBcAb) positive but hepatitis B surface antigen (HBsAg) negative. Those donors with evidence of acute or chronic infection are defined as HBcAb positivity and HBsAg positivity. HBV NAT detects trace amounts of circulating HBV DNA and represents viremia. Like those patients with HCV, HBV(+) allografts have traditionally been reserved for HBV(+) recipients. The most widely used and studied groups are those allografts from donors of resolved HBV infections (**Table 2**). Allografts with acute or chronic infection were rarely used due to prohibitively high transmission risks.[39,40]

Before the advent of antiviral therapy, transplantation of individuals with chronic HBV cirrhosis demonstrated almost universal HBV recurrence and rapid graft loss.[40–42] Ultimately, the risk of transmission was stratified based on the recipients HBV serologic status as well as the organ transplanted, with liver being higher risk than other solid organ transplantation. Transplantation into a recipient without evidence of prior infection or vaccine-mediated immunity [HBcAb(−)/HBsAb(−)] poses the highest risk of transmission.[4,40] Cholongitas and colleagues completed a systematic review of recipients of HBcAb(+) donors and demonstrated the importance of vaccination status or evidence of immunity on transmission. They noted an almost 50% rate of transmission in HBV naïve recipients compared with 15% and 9% in patients with evidence of past infection and vaccination, respectively.[43] To decrease transmission rates, current recommendations include administration of hepatitis B

Table 2
Terminology used for hepatitis B positive recipients and donors

HBsAg	HBcAb (Anti-HBc IgG)	NAT	HBsAb	Interpretation
−	−	−	−	"HBV naïve," susceptible
−	−	−	+	Vaccinated individual
−	+	−	−	Resolved infection
+	+/−	+	−	Acute infection
+	+	+/−	−	Chronic infection

Abbreviations: HBsAg, hepatitis B surface antigen; HBcAb, hepatitis B core antibody; NAT, nucleic acid amplification test; HBsAb, hepatitis B surface antibody.

vaccine to all eligible organ transplant candidates before transplantation to allow for vaccine response.[4,40]

HEPATITIS B CORE ANTIBODY LIVER TRANSPLANTATION:

Before the advent of nucleos(t)ide analog therapies, transplantation of HBcAb(+) donors into HBcAb(−) or HBsAg(−) recipients carried an extremely high rate of transmission with reported rates ranging from 58% to 77%.[43,44] In the 2000s, effective nucleos(t)ide analog therapies were introduced and were being used as post-transplant prophylaxis to decrease the rate of transmission.[40] This allowed for utilization of HBcAb(+) livers with relatively low rates of de novo hepatitis B (DNH) as defined by HBsAg(+) in a previously HBsAg(−) patient. Skagen and colleagues performed a systematic review and noted that in HBV naïve patients transplanted with HBcAb(+) livers, post-transplant prophylaxis resulted in a decrease in DNH rate from 58% to 11%. In vaccinated recipients, the DNH went from 18% to 0% with prophylaxis, again stressing the importance of pre-transplant vaccination.[44]

Wong and associates published a single-center study evaluating 416 recipients of HBcAb(+) liver grafts and demonstrated equivalent long-term outcomes after transplantation followed by antiviral monotherapy prophylaxis. They demonstrated similar 1-, 5-, and 10-year graft and patient survival rates when compared with HBcAb(−) grafts. Furthermore, they demonstrated only a 2.8% DNH rate in recipients of HBcAb(+) grafts when either lamivudine or entecavir post-transplant prophylaxis was used.[39] Ultimately, in 2015, a consensus guideline for organ transplantation from HBV(+) donors was published and concluded that organs from HBsAg(−)/HBcAb(+) donors should be considered for all adult transplant candidates with appropriate risk benefits discussion and informed consent.[45]

HEPATITIS B SURFACE ANTIGEN LIVER TRANSPLANTATION

Historically HBsAg(+) donors were infrequently used in the United States. However, they do hold importance in other regions of the world but have preferentially been transplanted into chronically infected individuals. Ju and colleagues evaluated 23 patients with ESLD secondary to HBV infection who underwent liver transplantation with HBsAg(+) allografts. They demonstrated no difference in short-term survival among recipients and concluded that the use of HBsAg(+) allograft was safe for patients with ESLD secondary to HBV.[46] A study out of China by Wei and associates looked at 282 patients who received a liver transplant from an HBsAg(+) donor. They noted higher HBV recurrence of 17.9% compared with 4.4% in the control group; however, they showed no difference in 1-, 3-, and 5-year patient or graft survival.[47]

Saidi and colleagues used the UNOS database to review 92 recipients of HBsAg(+) allografts. Of note, most recipients (74%) required liver transplantation for HBV-related disease. They noted that allograft and patient survival were comparable between HBsAg(+) allografts and HbsAg(−) allografts.[48] Li and colleagues conducted a similar study using UNOS database and identified 78 recipients of HBsAg(+) allografts and similarly demonstrated comparable graft and patient survival rates. However, in contrast to the previous study, only 19% of these patients required liver transplantation for HBV-related liver failure.[49]

More recently, Yu and colleagues published a retrospective study using the China Liver Transplant Registry to evaluate 503 patients who received HBsAg(+) liver transplants. They noted that compared with matched patients receiving HBsAg(−) allografts, there was comparable allograft and patient survival at 1, 3, and 5 years. They concluded that in the era of antiviral prophylaxis, transplantation with HBsAg(+)

allografts was not associated with inferior outcomes irrespective of the recipients HBsAg status.[50]

HEPATITIS B VIRUS NUCLEIC ACID AMPLIFICATION TESTING POSITIVE ALLOGRAFTS

The transplantation of HBV NAT(+) allografts into HBV naïve or susceptible patients has been met with significant hesitation due to concerns for acute and chronic HBV infection and its sequela, including acute fulminant hepatic failure. Delman and colleagues demonstrated the early safety of using NAT(+) liver allografts into seronegative recipients. They performed 33 NAT(+) liver transplants followed by daily antiviral therapy, they noted no difference in 30-day, 90-day, or 1-year patient or graft survival. They had three patients (9.1%) who developed de novo HBcAb(+) response, indicating a resolved infection, and two patients (6.1%) who developed de novo HBsAg(+)/HBcAb(+) response, indicating chronic infection. They concluded that HBV NAT(+) allografts could be used without a significant risk of HBV viremia or early de novo HBV hepatitis.[51] Although data are just beginning to emerge regarding transplantation of HBV NAT(+) allografts, new nucleos(t)ide analogs allow for the successful suppression of HBV post-transplantation.

CURRENT HEPATITIS B VIRUS TREATMENT STRATEGIES

Hepatitis B immune globulin (HBIG) was introduced in the 1900s and subsequently has been critical in the prevention of HBV recurrence after liver transplant. With the introduction of nucleos(t)ide analogs, combination therapy resulted in very successful prevention of reinfection with HBV after transplantation. Historically, lamivudine was the primary antiviral agent used for the treatment of chronic hepatitis B both before or after transplantation; however, recent advances have produced more potent nucleos(t)ide analogs with better resistance profiles such as entecavir and tenofovir.

There is a wide variation among transplant centers regarding their use and the combination of HBIG with antivirals during the early post-transplant period for chronically infected HBV patients. In patients deemed low risk for recurrence antiviral regimens are often used alone or in combination with short course of HBIG. The AASLD 2018 Hepatitis B Guidance suggested criteria for long-term HBIG versus perioperative only which include both patient factors and virologic factors including HBV DNA levels in the recipient at the time of transplantation.[52] For seronegative HBV recipients of HBcAb(+) or HBV NAT(+) allografts, antiviral therapy should be initiated immediately post-transplantation.[52] There have not been any significant studies that look at the optimal frequency to monitor the development of de novo HBV after transplantation. The consensus guidelines of recipient management recommend initial monitoring every 1 to 3 months for the first year followed by every 3 to 6 months.[45]

SUMMARY

Over the last 20 years, many studies have demonstrated the safety and efficacy of using both HCV(+) and HBV(+) allografts. While using these previously discarded organs is one step toward combating the organ shortage, it may also allow for decreased wait times and decreased waitlist mortality. Croome and colleagues noted a 136% increase in mortality waitlist for individuals who declined these "marginal" livers compared with those who accepted one.[53] There is still need for continued long-term research and we should ensure continued dedication to patient care as we expand our use of these organs by providing thorough informed consent and education as well as ensuring adequate access to HCV and HBV treatment.

CLINICS CARE POINTS

- The post-DAA era has allowed for increased use of seropositive allografts regardless of the recipient HCV status with comparable graft survival and short term outcomes.
- The usage of HBV allografts has been met with more resistance, however several studies have demonstrated the early safety of using HBV allografts in seronegative recipients.
- Despite the early efficacy demonstrated in utilizing HCV and HBV allografts long-term research is still needed.

DISCLOSURE

The authors have no disclosures financial or otherwise.

REFERENCES

1. Services USDoHaH. Organ Procurement and Transplantation Network 2023 (updated 30 March 2023). Available at: https://optn.transplant.hrsa.gov/data/. Accessed 30 March 2023.
2. Kwong AJ, Ebel NH, Kim WR, et al. OPTN/SRTR 20121 Annual Data Report: Liver. Am J Transplant 2023;23(Issue 2):S178–263.
3. Levitsky J, Formica RN, Bloom RD, et al. The American Society of Transplantation Consensus Conference on the use of hepatitis C viremic donors in solid organ transplantation. Am J Transplant 2017;17:2790–802.
4. Delman AM, Ammann AM, Shah SA. The Current Status of Virus-Positive Liver Transplantation. Curr Opin Organ Transplant 2021;26:160–87.
5. Crismale JF, Ahmad J. Expanding the donor pool: hepatitis C, hepatitis B and human immunodeficiency virus-positive donors in liver transplantation. World J Gastroenterol 2019;25:6799–812.
6. Wright TL, Donegan E, Hsu HH, et al. Recurrent and Acquired Hepatits C Viral Infection in Liver Transplant Recipients. Gastroenterology 1992;103:317–22.
7. Vargas HE, Laskus T, Wang LF, et al. Outcome of liver transplantation in hepatitis C virus-infected patients who received hepatitis C virus-infected grafts. Gastroenterology 1999;117:149–53.
8. Marroquin CE, Marino G, Kuo PC, et al. Transplantation of hepatitis C-positive livers in hepatitis C-positive patients is equivalent to transplanting hepatitis Cnegative livers. Liver Transpl 2001;7:762–8.
9. Ballarin R, Cucchetti A, Spaggiari M, et al. Long-term follow-up and outcome of liver transplantation from antihepatitis C virus-positive donors: a European multicentric case-control study. Transplantation 2011;91:1265–72.
10. Bowring MG, Kucirka LM, Massie AB, et al. Changes in utilization and discard of hepatitis C-infected donor livers in the recent era. Am J Transplant 2017;17:519–27.
11. Cotter TG, Paul S, Sandikci B, et al. Improved graft survival after liver transplantation for recipients with hepatitis C virus in the direct-acting antiviral era. Liver Transpl 2019;25:598–609.
12. Kapila N, Khalloufi KA, Flocco G, et al. Transplantation of HCV viremic livers into HCV viremic recipients followed by direct-acting antiviral therapy. J Clin Transl Hepatol 2019;7:122–6.
13. Saab S, Ghobrial RM, Ibrahim AB, et al. Hepatitis C positive grafts may be used in orthotopic liver transplantation: a matched analysis. Am J Transplant 2003;3:1167–72.

14. Burton JR Jr, Terrault NA, Goldberg DS, et al. Liver and kidney recipient selection of hepatitis C virus viremic donors: meeting Consensus Report from the 2019 controversies in transplantation. Transplantation 2020;104:476–81.
15. Danford CJ, Redman JS, Alonso D. Hepatitis C-positive Liver Transplantation: Outcomes and Current Practice. Curr Opin Organ Transplant 2021;26:115–20.
16. Ting PS, Hamilton JP, Gurakar A, et al. Hepatitis C-positive donor liver transplantation for hepatitis C seronegative recipients. Transpl Infect Dis 2019;21:e13194.
17. Luckett K, Kaiser TE, Bari K, et al. Use of hepatitis C virus antibody-positive donor livers in hepatitis C nonviremic liver transplant recipients. J Am Coll Surg 2019; 228:560–7.
18. Cholankeril G, Li AA, Dennis BB, et al. Increasing trends in transplantation of HCV-positive livers into uninfected recipients. Clin Gastroenterol Hepatol 2019; 17:1634–6.
19. Bari K, Luckett K, Kaiser T, et al. Hepatitis C Transmission from Seropositive, Nonviremic Donors to Non-Hepatitis C Liver Transplant Recipients. Hepatology 2018; 67(5):1673–82.
20. Cotter TG, Paul S, Sandikci B, et al. Increasing utilization and excellent initial outcomes following liver transplant of hepatitis C virus (HCV)-viremic donors into HCV-negative recipients: outcomes following liver transplant of HCVviremic donors. Hepatology 2019;69:2381–95.
21. Centers for Disease Control and Prevention. Surveillance for viral hepatitis—United States, 2016. Available at: https://www.cdc.gov/hepatitis/statistics/2016 surveillance/pdfs/2016Hep SurveillanceRpt.pdf. Accessed 30 March 2023.
22. Reau N, Kwo PY, Rhee S, et al. Glecaprevir/Pibrentasvir Treatment in Liver or Kidney Transplant Patients with Hepatitis C Virus Infection. Hepatology 2018;64(4): 1298–307.
23. Fink SA, Jacobson IM. Managing patients with hepatitis-B-related or hepatitis-C-related decompensated cirrhosis. Nat Rev Gastroenterol Hepatol 2011;8:285–95.
24. Naggie S, Muir J. Oral Combination Therapies for Hepatitis C Virus Infection: Successes, Challenges, and Unmet Needs. Annu Rev Med 2017;68:345–58.
25. American Association for the Study of Liver Disease and Infectious Disease Society of America. HCV Guidance Panel. Recommendations for testing, managing, and treating hepatitis C. Published 2017. Available at: http://hcvguidelines.org. Accessed April 19, 2023.
26. Kwo PY, Poordad F, Asatryan A, et al. Glecaprevir and pibrentasvir yield high response rates in patients with HCV genotype 1-6 without cirrhosis. J Hepatol 2017;67:263–71.
27. Asselah T, Kowdley KV, Zadeikis N, et al. Efficacy of glecaprevir/pibrentasvir for 8 or 12 weeks in patients with hepatitis C virus genotype 2, 4, 5, or 6 infection without cirrhosis. Clin Gastroenterol Hepatol 2017;16:417–26.
28. Zeuzem S, Foster GR, Wang S, et al. Glecaprevir-pibrentasvir for 8 or 12 weeks in HCV genotype 1 or 3 infection. N Engl J Med 2018;378:354–69.
29. Poordad F, Felizarta F, Asatryan A, et al. Glecaprevir and pibrentasvir for 12 weeks for hepatitis C virus genotype 1 infection and prior direct-acting antiviral treatment. Hepatology 2017;66:389–97.
30. Foster GR, Afdhal N, Roberts SK, et al. ASTRAL-2 Investigators; ASTRAL-3 Investigators. Sofosbuvir and velpatasvir for HCV genotype 2 and 3 infection. N Engl J Med 2015;373(27):2608–17.
31. Feld JJ, Jacobson IM, Hézode C, et al. ASTRAL-1 Investigators. Sofosbuvir and velpatasvir for HCV genotype 1, 2, 4, 5, and 6 infection. N Engl J Med 2015; 373(27):2599–607.

32. Martini S, Sacco M, Strona S, et al. Impact of viral eradication with sofosbuvir-based therapy on the outcome of post-transplant hepatitis C with severe fibrosis. Liver Int 2017;37(1):62–70.

33. El-Sherif O, Jiang ZG, Tapper EB, et al. Baseline factors associated with improvements in decompensated cirrhosis after direct-acting antiviral therapy for hepatitis C virus infection. Gastroenterology 2018;154(8):2111–21.e8.

34. Kwong AJ, Wall A, Melcher M, et al. Liver transplantation for hepatitis C virus (HCV) non-viremic recipients with HCV viremic donors. Am J Transplant 2019; 19(5):1380–7.

35. Bethea E, Arvind A, Gustafson J, et al. Immediate administration of antiviral therapy after transplantation of hepatitis C-infected livers into uninfected recipients: implications for therapeutic planning. Am J Transplant 2020;20(6):1619–28.

36. Bohorquez H, Bugeaud E, Bzowej N, et al. Liver transplantation using hepatitis C virus–viremic donors into hepatitis C virus–aviremic recipients as standard of care. Liver Transpl 2021;27(4):548–57.

37. Terrault NA, Burton J, Ghobrial M, et al. Prospective multicenter study of early antiviral therapy in liver and kidney transplant recipients of HCV-viremic donors. Hepatology 2021;73(6):2110–23.

38. Aqel B, Wijarnpreecha K, Pungpapong S, et al. Outcomes following liver transplantation from HCV-seropositive donors to HCV-seronegative recipients. J Hepatol 2021;74(4):873–80.

39. Wong TC, Fung JY, Cui TY, et al. Liver transplantation using hepatitis B core positive grafts with antiviral monotherapy prophylaxis. J Hepatol 2019;70:1114–22.

40. Zhou K, Zhou S. Risk of disease transmission in an expanded donor population: the potential of hepatitis B virus donors. Curr Opin Organ Transplant 2020;25: 631–9.

41. Todo S, Demetris AJ, Van Thiel D, et al. Orthotopic liver transplantation for patients with hepatitis B virus-related liver disease. Hepatology 1991;13:619–26.

42. O'Grady JG, Smith HM, Davies SE, et al. Hepatitis B Virus Reinfection After Orthotopic Liver Transplantation. J Hepatol 1992;14:104–11.

43. Cholongitas E, Papatheodoridis GV, Burroughs AK. Liver grafts from antihepatitis B core positive donors: a systematic review. J Hepatol 2010;52:272–9.

44. Skagen CL, Jou JH, Said A. Risk of De Novo Hepatitis in Liver Recipients from Hepatitis-B Core Antibody-Positive Grafts – A Systemic Analysis. Clin Transplant 2011;25:E243–9.

45. Huprikar S, Dansiger-Isakov L, Ahn J, et al. Solid Organ Transplantation From Hepatitis B Virus Positive Donors: Consensus Guidelines for Recipient Management. Am J Transplant 2015;5:1162–72.

46. Ju W, Chen M, Guo Z, et al. Allografts positive for hepatitis B surface antigen in liver transplant for disease related to hepatitis B virus. Exp Clin Transplant 2013; 11:245–9.

47. Wei L, Chen D, Zhang B, et al. Long-term Outcome and Recurrence of Hepatitis B Virus Following Liver Transplantation from Hepatitis B Surface Antigen-Positive Donors in a Chinese Population. J Viral Hepat 2018;25:1576–81.

48. Saidi RF, Jabbour N, Shah SA, et al. Liver transplantation from hepatitis B surface antigen-positive donors. Transplant Proc 2013;45:279–80.

49. Li Z, Hu Z, Xiang J, et al. Use of hepatitis B surface antigen-positive grafts in liver transplantation: a matched analysis of the US National database. Liver Transpl 2014;20:35–45.

50. Yu S, Cen C, Zhang X, et al. Utilization of Hepatitis B Virus Surface Antigen Positive Grafts in Liver Transplantation: A Matched Study Based on a National Registry Cohort. J Gastroenterol Hepatol 2022;37:1052–9.

51. Delman AM, Turner KM, Safdar K, et al. Expanding the Donor Pool: First Use of Hepatitis B Virus Nat Positive Solid Organ Allografts Into Seronegative Recipients. Ann Surg 2021;274:556–64.

52. Terrault NA, Lok ASF, McMahon BJ, et al. Update on Prevention, Diagnosis, and Treatment of Chronic Hepatitis B: AASLD 2018 Hepatitis B Guidance. Hepatology 2018;67(4):1560–99.

53. Croome KP, Lee DD, Pungpapong S, et al. What are the outcomes of declining a public health service increased risk liver donor for patients on the liver transplant waiting list? Liver Transpl 2018;24(4):497–504.

Outcomes of Living Donor Liver Transplantation Compared with Deceased Donor Liver Transplantation

Kiara A. Tulla, MD[a], Francis J. Tinney Jr, MD[a],
Andrew M. Cameron, MD, PhD[b],*

KEYWORDS

- Living donor liver transplant outcomes • Decease donor liver transplant outcomes
- MELD strata • Hepatocellular carcinoma

KEY POINTS

- Living donor liver transplant (LDLT) remains challenging, demonstrating more biliary and vascular complications, likely due to anatomic factors.
- After the first 30 days following liver trasplantation, according to data from the United States and abroad, graft and patient survival, show that LT is noninferior from LDLT, donation after brain death-deceased donor liver transplant (DDLT), and donation after circulatory death-DDLT.
- LDLT has been proven to be beneficial for a model for end-stage liver disease (MELD) score greater than 11 in most recent literature, and should be considered following careful review of donor and recipient factors, so as to maximize survival benefit.
- Complex high-MELD patients without access to DDLT will also have expeditious access to LDLT due to the survival benefit it provides and the comparable outcomes it has to DDLT.

INTRODUCTION

Transplantation remains the most effective and durable therapy for end-stage liver disease. The demand for liver transplantation is rising due to improvements in long-term results, owing to improved surgical techniques and revolutionary immunosuppressive agents. In 2021, 13,165 additional candidates, more than in any previous year, were added to the waitlist, joining the 11,771 individuals who were already listed at the

Funding/support: No funding sources were used for this study.
[a] Department of Surgery, Division of Transplant Surgery, John Hopkins Medicine;
[b] Department of Surgery, Johns Hopkins University School of Medicine, John Hopkins Medicine, 720 Rutland Avenue, Ross 765, Baltimore, MD 21205, USA
* Corresponding author.
E-mail address: Acamero5@jhmi.edu

Surg Clin N Am 104 (2024) 79–88
https://doi.org/10.1016/j.suc.2023.08.007
0039-6109/24/© 2023 Elsevier Inc. All rights reserved.

surgical.theclinics.com

beginning of the year.[1] According to their model for end-stage liver disease (MELD) score,[2] the patients who were listed for transplantation were sicker than in years past, with more than 25% having an MELD score > 25, and 10% > 35. In 2021, a record 9,234 liver transplants were performed in the United States, with 93.8% representing deceased donor liver transplant (DDLT) and 6.2% living donor liver transplant (LDLT). This corresponded with shorter waiting times and an overall increase in total transplant rates, with 37.7% receiving a DDLT within 3 months, 43.8% within 6 months, and 53.3% within 1 year. Fortunately, results have remained positive, with overall posttransplant mortality rates of 13.3% after 3 years, 18.6% at 5 years, and 35.9% at 10 years.[1]

In order to solve the issue of ciritical organ scacity in adults, LDLT was developed as one alternative to DDLT. It continues to support the rising need for liver transplantation. The first LDLT was performed in United States in 1998,[3] with 49 centers currently performing at least one LDLT. After rapid growth of the technique for three years, the death of a donor in 2002 lead to a drop in the number of LDLTs performed. Furthermore, adoption was impeded by the availability of deceased donors, worries about donor morbidity and mortality, and early studies showing inferious results.[4] This forced centers in the United States to reintroduce the practice with caution, and in a deliberate, gradual manner.[5] LDLT has been adopted faster in places where DDLT has remained relatively underdeveloped. Recently, the technique is becoming more prevalent in the United States,[6] as a number of single-center,[7,8] national data,[9] and multi-center investigations[10] have suggested superior results in LDLT, particularly once a center has passed its learning curve.[11] Despite this, not all centers have adopted the technique, and it is still only used by a small number of programs in selective situations, primarily in patients with lower acuity of illness.

Fortunately, since 2018, more than 400 LDLT (**Fig. 1**) have been performed annually in the United States, and the numbers have continued to rise, reflecting the need for more donors to replace the 20% to 25% of patients awaiting a liver transplant (LT) in the United States who die or become too sick for the transplantation.[2]

The argument for growing the donor pool with live donors has limitations, as other methods of expansion have been developed that demonstrate minimal impact on a live donor patient. For example, increasing the use of extended criteria donors (ECD), including the use of older donors beyond the age of 60 to 70 years of age. Additional strategies include donation after cardiac death (DCD), normothermic regional

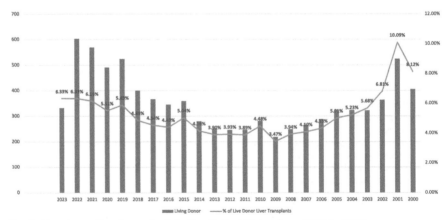

Fig. 1. Live donor liver transplants in the United States from 2000 to 2023.

perfusion,[12] machine perfusion technology,[13] and use of livers with steatosis or infection with Hepatitis B or C.

The Adult-to-Adult Living Donor Liver Transplantation Cohort Study (A2ALL), funded by the National Institutes of Health (NIH), demonstrated a survival benefit in LDLT.[11,14] One of the methods by which LDLT affects the overall decrease in waitlist mortality is with planned, elective and timely operations.[15] Additionally, receiving an allograft froma living donor on a voluntary basis enables recipient optimization at the time of transplantation, reducing post-transplant complications. These hypothetical advantages must be weighed against the fact that a partial graft requires more complexity.[11]

In this review, we will compare the existing data surrounding LDLT, with the intention of identifying areas where the use of LDLT may be supported beyond traditional DDLT in patients seeking liver transplantation.

How Low of a MELD Score Should Be Used to Identify Patients for Liver Transplantation in General and Specifically LDLT?

The introduction of MELD score in the allocation schema, together with 1-year posttransplant survival data, it has become easier to determine when in concert has helped delineate when the benefit of transplantation outweighs the risk of the surgery.[16] By comparing how the waitlist mortality according to MELD score stratified by the quality of the donor graft assessed with the donor risk index (DRI)[17] allowed for a more nuanced consideration of transplant timing. All candidates prefer a lower risk organ; however, what if an offer of a higher risk organ is provided for a candidate that is clinically able to tolerate the insult before a clinical deterioration? Results from Schaubel and colleagues[16] shows that high-MELD patients experienced a significant survival benefit even when they received a high-DRI organ. However, patients with low-MELD patients (and their correspondingly low waiting list mortality risk) have limited survival benefit from transplantation. The current informal practice of inverse matching of recipient MELD score and liver DRI (occurring, presumably, through turndowns of high-DRI liver offers for high-MELD candidates) should be discouraged, as 3 years of posttransplant follow-up data found that patients transplanted in the MELD 6 to 11 categories experienced significantly higher mortality with transplant, as a function of their relatively low waiting list mortality rates and their greater propensity to receive higher DRI livers. Overall, patients with an MELD score of 15 or greater experienced a significant mortality reduction via liver transplantation, a finding consistent with the results from prior studies with Markov simulation.[18–20] This information provided a framework to reexamine the survival benefit of LDLT.[14]

The A2ALL corhot study further demonstrated the survival benefit for MELD scores < 15 and the survival advantage of LDLT.[21] Mortality for LDLT recipients was compared with mortality for patients who remained on the waiting list or received DDLT according to MELD score (<15 or ≥15) and diagnosis of hepatocellular carcinoma (HCC). Of 868 potential LDLT recipients (half high and low MELD at entry), 712 underwent transplantation (406 LDLT; 306 DDLT), 83 died without transplant, and 73 were alive without transplant at last follow-up. Overall, LDLT recipients had 56% lower mortality. Among candidates without HCC, mortality benefit was seen both candidates with an MELD score of less than 15 and candidates with an MELD score of 15 or greater. In the MELD liver allocation era, LDLT offers a significant survival advantage over waiting for DDLT, supporting the practices adoption.

Waitlist Mortality as the Primary Endpoint

Rates of transplantation are higher when a potential live donor is identified for candidates.[22] With LDLT, patients with lower MELD scores who can, in theory, tolerate a partial graft will also benefit from transplantation sooner. Jackson and colleagues[23] looked at the life-years saved as a result of receiving an LDLT, as well as 1-year relative mortability and risk, when compared to patients who stayed on the wait list. Furhter, they evaluated the MELD-Na score, a score developed to evaluate mortality among those placed on the liver transplant waitlist, at which that survival benefit was achieved for individuals who received an LDLT c. A significant survival benefit for patients receiving a LDLT who had a MELD-Na score of 11 or higher (adjusted hazard ratio, 0.64;95% CI, 0.47–0.88; $P = .006$) was found. LDLT recipients gained an additional 15 life-years compared with patients who never received an LDLT. Given that the hazards to living donors are high, as we further embrace LDLT, It is helpful to assess the value that transplantation offers and to provide guidance in continuing to extend the necessity for transplantation early.[23]

Utility in Patients with Hepatocellular Carcinoma

It is promising to employ LDLT for HCC patients because of the traditionally low MELD scores of this patient population, but it must be done carefully. According to data from the Organ and Procurement Transplantation Network (OPTN), 17.4% of adult LDLT recipients between 2003 and 2019 had a diagnosis of HCC. After liver transplantation, the 1-, 5-, and 10-year overall survival rates for DDLT and LDLT groups were comparable.[24] A higher likelihood of death was associated with older donors and recipient age. In comparison to HCV, alcohol liver disease, hepatitis B virus, nonalcoholic fatty liver disease, and autoimmune liver disease were associated with lower risk of death . Further, worse outcomes were correlated with unfavorable tumor features. A wait time of less than 6-months on the LT list was associated with better patient outcomes. Concerns have been raised about the United States A2ALL cohort's report of grater 5-year recurrence with LDLT (38%) compared with DDLT (11%; $P = .0004$).[25] In a comparable study, Vakili and colleagues found a substantial correlation between tumor grade and 5-year survival of 81% and a recurrence rate of 28.6%, in recipients with LDLT for HCC.[26] Potential explanations for higher tumor recurrence in the LDLT group may be due to the shorter wait times, insufficient time to test tumor biology and allowing for selective patient dropout.

Using data from the United Network of Organ Sharing (UNOS), a total of 239 LDLT patients, 13,873 donation after brain death (DBD)-DDLT, and 1,132 donation after circulatory death (DCD)-DDLT patients with HCC were each assessed independently. 158 (66.1%) of the 239 LDLT patients, 158 had an HCC MELD exception score. All DDLT patients included had HCC MELD exception scores. Days spent on the waiting list were considerably reduced in the LDLT group compared to the DCD-DDLT or DBD-DDLT groups, as was expected. The 1-year graft survival and adjusted Hazard Ratio's were significantly better in DBD-DDLT, with similar outcomes for LDLT and DCD-DDLT groups. In comparison to DBD-DDLT and DCD-DDLT, the incidence of graft loss attributed to vascular thrombosis and hepatic artery thrombosis (HAT) was significantly higher in the LDLT group. The incidence of biliary complication within 1 year was significantly higher in the DCD-DDLT and LDLT groups than in the DBD-DDLT group.

Markov models have suggested a benefit of LDLT in comparison to waiting for DDLT, particularly for patients with HCC.[27] The data from Berg and colleagues[21] that demonstrated no benefit to transplantation when the MELD score was < 15 and a survival benefit when patients with HCC have an MELD > 15, offereing greater context to when LDLT should be utilized for HCC patients, has been used to partially refute this claim.

Comparing Living Donor Liver Transplant to Donation After Circulatory Death-Deceased Donor Liver Transplant

As DCD grafts are used more widely, we might learn more about how DBD, DCD, and LDLT grafts effect patient outcomes. Using OPTN/UNOS data, the Detroit group sought to evaluate and contrast various various liver transplant (LT) types and to identify the variables influencing outcomes in recipients with MELD scores < 30.[28] The significantly lower risk of graft loss in DBD-DDLT was especially apparent in the mid-MELD (15–29) score group, when assessing the risk of graft loss by MELD score category. The probability of 30-day graft loss in in the mid-MELD score group was considerably reduced in the DCD-DDLT group compared to the LDLT, group, although it was comparable in the lower-MELD score group. The risks of 1-year graft loss were comparable between the LDLT and DCD-DDLT groups regardless of MELD score category (lower-MELD: adjusted Hazard Ratio, 0.73; 95% CI, 0.34-1.56; P = .42; mid-MELD: adjusted Hazard Ratio, 0.88; 95% CI, 0.67-1.15; P = .33). The higher risk of graft loss in the LDLT group was more prominent in patients with a mid-MELD score. Furthermore, the presence of significant ascites was associated with worse outcomes in the LDLT group but not in the DDLT group. Notably, the negative effect of ascites in the LDLT group was not seen in the lower MELD score group. Retransplant was performed in 80 of 174 patients who lost their LDLT grafts within a year, which may have contributed to the similar patient survival rates between the LDLT and DDLT groups. In this study, 30-day graft loss associated with vascular thrombosis and HAT was significantly higher in LDLTs than in DCD-DDLTs or DBD-DDLTs. When compared to DBD-DDLTs and DCD-DDLTs, LDLTs exhibited significantly greater occurrences of graft loss due to biliary complications.

The A2ALL consortium showed that reported a significantly higher incidence of HAT (6% vs 4%) and bile leak (31.8% vs 10.2%) in LDLT patients.[29] Vascular and biliary reconstructions in LDLTs are technically more demanding than in DDLTs.[30] Although the incidence of biliary and vascular complications was lower than in previous A2ALL studies,[29] the UNOS registry may not fully capture all of these complications, and inferior graft survival in the early period after LDLT might be partially attributable to technical difficulties. Graft loss associated with biliary complications was higher in DCD-DDLTs than in DBD-DDLTs, consistent with previous studies.[31]

A more recent study compared the outcomes of DBD-DDLT to LDLT utilizing a similar OPTN/UNOS data set including transplants up to 2021 and a similar MELD classification methodology, but included MELD > 30 patient results.[32] During the study period, the annual number of LDLTs increased from 282 to 569, and the proportion of high-MELD LDLTs increased from 3.9% to 7.7%. Graft survival was greater in low-MELD recipients compared to high-MELD LDLT recipients (adjusted Hazard Ratio = 1.36, 95%CI: 1.03–1.79); however, the 5-year survival rate was above 70% in both groups, leaving room for higher MELD patients to be considered for LDLT. There was no significant difference in observed graft survival between high-MELD LDLT and high-MELD DBD-DDLT recipients, with 5-year survival of 71.5% and 77.3%, respectively.

Further support is found in the literature from a single-center study outside of the United States, including patients with MELD greater than 30, supporting utilization of LDLT for patients with comparable outcomes.[33] Patients' characteristics and a lack of center experience were associated with poorer graft outcomes in high-MELD LDLT recipients.[32] So, in prder to ensure optimal outcomes, LDLT requires both medical and surgical expertise, and center experience is also crucial. However, it should be stressed nevertheless, recipient and donor selection remain critical even at experienced centers. In order to aid with the donor shortage, future practice guidance should take into account expanding the LDLT recommendations to include high-MELD patients in centers with expertise.

Living Donor Liver Transplant with Complex Liver Failure and Comorbidities: Ascites and Hepatorenal Syndrome

Worse post-tranplant outcomes are observed with increased portal hypertension (PHT) in LDLT.[34,35] Patients who received partial left grafts and had mid-MELD scores had worse results in LDLT patients with severe ascites. The findings are consistent with less tolerance of PHT in these LDLT recipients. These results emphasize the importance of careful recipient and donor selection. Left grafts should be used with caution in patients with ascites and especially in those with mid-MELD scores.[36] Attention should be paid to an optimal graft to donor weight ratios, appropriate portal vein inflow modulation, and hepatic vein reconstruction technique. The UNOS registry does not include data on graft size or weight, small-for-size graft syndrome, or techniques to optimize vascular flow. The MELD score, the presence of ascites, and the size of the liver transplant will all be crucial factors for continued definition of the role of LDLT, allowing for the anticipation and implementation of strategies to maximize portal flow and hepatic vein reconstruction in patients with severe PHT.[34]

In trying to assess who is the most ill patient who may benefit from LDLT evaluation of patients with hepatorenal syndrome (HRS) and liver failure is a subgroup that has been assessed nationally and internationally. Evidence supporting the use of LDLT to treat critically ill patients suffering from HRS is scarce and predominately published from the Asian experience.[37,38] With the known particularly poor prognosis with a median survival that ranges between 2 weeks and 6 months without LT,[39] it is group of patients who were seeing if LDLT outcomes equaling DDLT outcomes brings another avenue of providing hope and access to transplantation. Survival benefits of intention to treat (ITT)-LDLT occurred within the first month after listing.[40] This group often becomes dialysis dependent and since renal recovery posttransplant is inversely proportional to the time waiting for a transplant, rapid transplantation is key. The increased MELD score of HRS patient results in a better chance of DDLT but also these patients have higher risk to further deteriorate and drop out from the waiting list. In this scenario, LDLT is an attractive option for this patient population. The University of Toronto group[41] queried their patient population where they analyzed their LDLT cohort of 30 patients with HRS and MELD score of 20 or greater. The LDLT group (n = 30) was compared with a matched (1:3) control group of 90 patients with HRS that received a DDLT (DDLT group). Subgroup analysis of HRS types 1 and 2 did not show any difference between DDLT and LDLT groups in the number of patients developing chronic kidney disease of 3 or greater after LT, or in graft and patient survival (60%–80% in all cohorts and timepoints).

In 2012, Chok and colleagues[38] analyzed the outcome of 33 patients who received LDLT for acute hepatic decompensation with HRS. In the investigation, the study group was compared to 71 patients suffering from acute hepatic decompensation in the absence of HRS. They observed that the HRS group had a higher ICU stay, postoperative complications, higher need of postoperative hemodialysis, poorer kidney function, and poorer overall survival. However, the results of the study may not be generalizable to most practices in the modern MELD era because the recipients tended to have low-MELD scores and a low rate of preoperative hemodialysis. In the same year, Lee and colleagues[37] published a series of 48 patients with HRS undergoing LDLT. The study compared this group against 23 HRS patients receiving DDLT and reported a higher survival rate in the LDLT recipients when compared to patients receiving DDLT. In a multivariate Cox regression analysis, they found that LDLT was associated with a significantly improved recipient survival. However, these favorable results could have been influenced by the small sample size of the DDLT group.

Wong and colleagues[40] group in Hong Kong demonstrateed that LDLT had similar outcome to full graft DDLT in recipients with HRS. A 325 patients were listed (ITT-LDLT n = 212, ITT-DDLT n = 113). In multivariable analysis on mortality from the time of listing, patients with higher BMI and in the ITT-LDLT group had a lower risk of mortality, whereas a higher MELD score at listing predicted poorer survival. It is significant to note that there was no live donor mortality in the current study, and overall donor complication rate was 17.4% with an exceedingly low risk of grade 3 complications. When comparing LDLT to DDLT for recipients with MELD > 25 and recipients with both MELD > 25 and HRS, there were no patient survival differences at 1-year, 3-years, and 5-years after transplant. In this study, waiting list mortality for patients with high MELD and HRS was decreased, and LDLT consistently improved survival outcomes with ITT analysis. These advantages were consistently seen across different MELD categories. For improved patient outcomes, it would be advantageous to consider LDLT as an option early given the increased risk of mortality within 1 month of listing.

In the discussion of the subject, it is also interesting to note that research by Piano and colleagues[42] demonstrated that patients who responded to terlipressin for the treatment of HRS have improved 30-day survival, longer waiting list times, and lower MELD scores at the time of liver transplantation. This leads us to question if LDLT could be used on this particular population if DDLT is unable to be completed in a timely manner due to an improvement in their chemical MELD.

As comfort with LDLT increases, the utilization of it for high-MELD patients, retransplants, elderly patients, acute liver failure patients, and those with tumors outside of criteria acceptable for a transplant with a DDLT will increase as well. The Pittsburg team in their early experience showed that the results have generally been equivalent. Retransplant recipients, high-MELD recipients, and recipients with HCC all experienced similar outcomes after LDLT compared to DDLT (P = ns), while elderly patients (aged ≥71 years) fared better after LDLT compared to DDLT (1 year survival of 93% vs 79%, P = .03).[36]

SUMMARY

Liver transplantation is life saving and serving the greatest number of candidates in a timely manner is important. LDLT is more technically challenging given the anatomical factors, leading to more biliary and vascular complications. However, the majority of internation and domestic data demonstrate that LDLT is non-inferior to DBD-DDLT and DCD-DDLT after 30 days of graft and patient survival. Although currently, many centers with less experience, favor LDLT in lower MELD patients, we must provide the best care possible for all of our patients. Therefore, LDLT has been used in patients with MELD greater than 11 with careful consideration for donor and recipient factors to maximize their survival benefit. Over time, we hope that complex high-MELD patients without access to DDLT, will eventually be given quick access to LDLT when safe.

CLINICS CARE POINTS

- LDLT should be considered for all transplant candidates, especially if their success of obtaining DDLT is unlikely within the first month after listing for high-MELD patients (>25).

- Candidates with hepatocellular carcinoma and other patients with cancer who meet the requirements for DDLT are listed and considered heavily for transplantation; howevere, if LDLT is used as a tool to transplant this population, careful selection and appropriate waitlist time and restaging assessment should be completed before LDLT.
- Safety and efficacy of using live donors for transplantations is proven; careful assessment and frequent utilization of the technique will help to continue growing success in numbers and outcomes.

CONFLICT OF INTEREST DISCLOSURES

Dr A.M. Cameron is PI on grant P50AA027054 from the National Institutes of Health, United States. For the remaining authors none were declared.

ACKNOWLEDGMENTS

None.

REFERENCES

1. Kwong AJ, Ebel NH, Kim WR, et al. OPTN/SRTR 2021 Annual Data Report: Liver. Am J Transplant 2023;23(2 Suppl 1):S178–263.
2. Kamath PS, Wiesner RH, Malinchoc M, et al. A model to predict survival in patients with end-stage liver disease. Hepatology 2001;33(2):464–70.
3. Wachs ME, Bak TE, Karrer FM, et al. Adult living donor liver transplantation using a right hepatic lobe. Transplantation 1998;66(10):1313–6.
4. Abt PL, Mange KC, Olthoff KM, et al. Allograft survival following adult-to-adult living donor liver transplantation. Am J Transplant 2004;4(8):1302–7.
5. Brown RS Jr. Live donors in liver transplantation. Gastroenterology 2008;134(6): 1802–13.
6. Chen CL, Cheng YF, Yu CY, et al. Living donor liver transplantation: the Asian perspective. Transplantation 2014;97(Suppl 8):S3.
7. Maluf DG, Stravitz RT, Cotterell AH, et al. Adult living donor versus deceased donor liver transplantation: a 6-year single center experience. Am J Transplant 2005;5(1):149–56.
8. Pomposelli JJ, Verbesey J, Simpson MA, et al. Improved survival after live donor adult liver transplantation (LDALT) using right lobe grafts: program experience and lessons learned. Am J Transplant 2006;6(3):589–98.
9. Hoehn RS, Wilson GC, Wima K, et al. Comparing living donor and deceased donor liver transplantation: A matched national analysis from 2007 to 2012. Liver Transpl 2014;20(11):1347–55.
10. Olthoff KM, Smith AR, Abecassis M, et al. Defining long-term outcomes with living donor liver transplantation in North America. Ann Surg 2015;262(3):465–75 ; discussion 473-5.
11. Olthoff KM, Merion RM, Ghobrial RM, et al. Outcomes of 385 adult-to-adult living donor liver transplant recipients: a report from the A2ALL Consortium. Ann Surg 2005;242(3):314–23, discussion 323-5.
12. Bekki Y, Croome KP, Myers B, et al. Normothermic Regional Perfusion Can Improve Both Utilization and Outcomes in DCD Liver, Kidney, and Pancreas Transplantation. Transplant Direct 2023;9(3):e1450.
13. Sousa Da Silva RX, Weber A, Dutkowski P, et al. Machine perfusion in liver transplantation. Hepatology 2022;76(5):1531–49.

14. Berg CL, Gillespie BW, Merion RM, et al. Improvement in survival associated with adult-to-adult living donor liver transplantation. Gastroenterology 2007;133(6): 1806–13.

15. Brown RS Jr, Russo MW, Lai M, et al. A survey of liver transplantation from living adult donors in the United States. N Engl J Med 2003;348(9):818–25.

16. Schaubel DE, Sima CS, Goodrich NP, et al. The survival benefit of deceased donor liver transplantation as a function of candidate disease severity and donor quality. Am J Transplant. Feb 2008;8(2):419–25.

17. Feng S, Goodrich NP, Bragg-Gresham JL, et al. Characteristics associated with liver graft failure: the concept of a donor risk index. Am J Transplant 2006;6(4): 783–90.

18. Merion RM, Schaubel DE, Dykstra DM, et al. The survival benefit of liver transplantation. Am J Transplant 2005;5(2):307–13.

19. Amin MG, Wolf MP, TenBrook JA Jr, et al. Expanded criteria donor grafts for deceased donor liver transplantation under the MELD system: a decision analysis. Liver Transpl 2004;10(12):1468–75.

20. RM M. Doc, should I accept this offer or not? Liver Transpl. Liver Transpl 2004;10.

21. Berg CL, Merion RM, Shearon TH, et al. Liver transplant recipient survival benefit with living donation in the model for endstage liver disease allocation era. Hepatology 2011;54(4):1313–21.

22. Russo MW, LaPointe-Rudow D, Kinkhabwala M, et al. Impact of adult living donor liver transplantation on waiting time survival in candidates listed for liver transplantation. Am J Transplant 2004;4(3):427–31.

23. Jackson WE, Malamon JS, Kaplan B, et al. Survival Benefit of Living-Donor Liver Transplant. JAMA Surg 2022;157(10):926–32.

24. Muhammad H, Gurakar M, Ting PS, et al. Long-Term Outcomes of Living Donor Versus Deceased Donor Liver Transplant for Hepatocellular Carcinoma in the United States. Exp Clin Transplant 2022;20(3):279–84.

25. Kulik LM, Fisher RA, Rodrigo DR, et al. Outcomes of living and deceased donor liver transplant recipients with hepatocellular carcinoma: results of the A2ALL cohort. Am J Transplant 2012;12(11):2997–3007.

26. Vakili K, Pomposelli JJ, Cheah YL, et al. Living donor liver transplantation for hepatocellular carcinoma: Increased recurrence but improved survival. Liver Transpl 2009;15(12):1861–6.

27. Cheng SJ, Pratt DS, Freeman RB Jr, et al. Living-donor versus cadaveric liver transplantation for non-resectable small hepatocellular carcinoma and compensated cirrhosis: a decision analysis. Transplantation 2001;72(5):861–8.

28. Kitajima T, Moonka D, Yeddula S, et al. Outcomes in Living Donor Compared With Deceased Donor Primary Liver Transplantation in Lower Acuity Patients With Model for End-Stage Liver Disease Scores <30. Liver Transpl 2021;27(7):971–83.

29. Samstein BSA, Freise CE, Zimmerman MA, et al. Complications and their resolution in recipients of deceased and living donor liver transplants: findings from the A2ALL Cohort study. Am J Transplant 2016;16.

30. Uchiyama H, Harada N, Sanefuji K, et al. Dual hepatic artery reconstruction in living donor liver transplantation using a left hepatic graft with 2 hepatic arterial stumps. Surgery 2010;147(6):878–86.

31. Jay CL, Lyuksemburg V, Ladner DP, et al. Ischemic cholangiopathy after controlled donation after cardiac death liver transplantation: a meta-analysis. Ann Surg 2011;253(2):259–64.

32. Anouti A, Patel MS, VanWagner LB, et al. Increasing practice and acceptable outcomes of High-MELD Living-Donor liver transplantation in the USA. Liver Transpl 2023. https://doi.org/10.1097/LVT.0000000000000228.

33. Matoba D, Noda T, Kobayashi S, et al. Analysis of Short-Term and Long-Term Outcomes of Living Donor Liver Transplantation for Patients with a High Model for End-Stage Liver Disease Score. Transplant Proc 2023;55(4):893–7.

34. Ogura Y, Hori T, El Moghazy WM, et al. Portal pressure <15 mm Hg is a key for successful adult living donor liver transplantation utilizing smaller grafts than before. Liver Transpl 2010;16(6):718–28.

35. Ito T, Kiuchi T, Yamamoto H, et al. Changes in portal venous pressure in the early phase after living donor liver transplantation: pathogenesis and clinical implications. Transplantation 2003;75(8):1313–7.

36. Humar A, Ganesh S, Jorgensen D, et al. Adult Living Donor Versus Deceased Donor Liver Transplant (LDLT Versus DDLT) at a Single Center: Time to Change Our Paradigm for Liver Transplant. Ann Surg 2019;270(3):444–51.

37. Lee JP, Kwon HY, Park JI, et al. Clinical outcomes of patients with hepatorenal syndrome after living donor liver transplantation. Liver Transpl 2012;18(10): 1237–44.

38. Chok KS, Fung JY, Chan SC, et al. Outcomes of living donor liver transplantation for patients with preoperative type 1 hepatorenal syndrome and acute hepatic decompensation. Liver Transpl 2012;18(7):779–85.

39. Gine' s PGM, Arroyo V, Rode's J, et al. Hepatorenal syndrome. Lancet 2003;362: 1819–27.

40. Wong TC, Fung JY, Pang HH, et al. Analysis of Survival Benefits of Living Versus Deceased Donor Liver Transplant in High Model for End-Stage Liver Disease and Hepatorenal Syndrome. Hepatology 2021;73(6):2441–54.

41. Goldaracena N, Marquez M, Selzner N, et al. Living vs. deceased donor liver transplantation provides comparable recovery of renal function in patients with hepatorenal syndrome: a matched case-control study. Am J Transplant 2014; 14(12):2788–95.

42. Piano S, Gambino C, Vettore E, et al. Response to Terlipressin and Albumin Is Associated With Improved Liver Transplant Outcomes in Patients With Hepatorenal Syndrome. Hepatology 2021;73(5):1909–19.

Living Donor Liver Transplantation
Left Lobe or Right Lobe

J. Michael Cullen, MD[a], Kendra D. Conzen, MD[a],*,
Elizabeth A. Pomfret, MD, PhD[b]

KEYWORDS

- Liver transplantation • Living donor liver transplantation • Transplant oncology
- Liver anatomy • Living donor hepatectomy • Graft-recipient weight ratio
- Portal inflow modulation

KEY POINTS

- Living liver donation offers an alternative allograft source for liver transplant candidates with limited access to deceased donor organs.
- Successful living donor liver transplantation requires appropriate donor-recipient pairing and graft selection.
- Graft selection (left versus right lobe) is influenced by donor vasculobiliary anatomy, graft size relative to recipient, and other recipient factors (eg, severity of illness).
- Smaller grafts may be used in select patients with inflow/outflow optimization.
- Donor mortality risk is similar for left and right living donor hepatectomy and must be minimized.

INTRODUCTION

The era of living donor liver transplantation (LDLT) began in 1988, with the first successful case reported by Dr Russell Strong in Australia and the first series published by Dr Christoph Broelsch in 1991.[1,2] Living donation was proposed as an option for pediatric patients with minimal access to appropriately sized deceased donor allografts. The first living donor transplants were performed using left lateral section grafts

[a] Colorado Center for Transplantation Care, Research and Education (CCTCARE), University of Colorado Anschutz, University of Colorado Anschutz Medical Campus, 1635 Aurora Ct, AOP 7th Fl, C-318, Aurora, CO 80045, USA; [b] Division of Transplant Surgery, Igal Kam, MD Endowed Chair in Transplantation Surgery, Colorado Center for Transplantation Care, Research and Education (CCTCARE), University of Colorado Anschutz Medical Campus, 1635 Aurora Ct, AOP 7th Fl, C-318, Aurora, CO 80045, USA
* Corresponding author.
E-mail address: Kendra.conzen@cuanschutz.edu

Surg Clin N Am 104 (2024) 89–102
https://doi.org/10.1016/j.suc.2023.07.003
0039-6109/24/© 2023 Elsevier Inc. All rights reserved.
surgical.theclinics.com

from adults to children.[2,3] Early utilization of left lateral section grafts for adult recipients provided inadequate liver mass and resulted in poor outcomes.[2,4] Concerns for donor safety restricted the use of major hepatectomy for transplantation, as initial experience established a correlation between hepatectomy volume and overall donor risk.[5–7] With time, adult-to-adult LDLT with larger volume grafts became more prevalent as experience with LDLT improved and living donation received greater acceptance in the medical community.

In 1997, Wachs and colleagues[8] performed the first successful adult LDLT with a right lobe graft in North America. The right lobe subsequently became the most common graft type used in adult LDLT.[9] Recent studies demonstrate improvement in morbidity associated with donor right hepatectomy and some suggest similar mortality rates between right and left lobe donation.[9–11] However, overall morbidity with donor right hepatectomy remains high despite modern advances in perioperative care. Consequently, left lobe donation is again becoming more popular.[12]

This article explores the nuances of living donor hepatectomy and considerations in left versus right lobe graft selection. The complexities of LDLT mandate rigorous preoperative evaluation of the donor and the recipient. Careful assessment of donor liver anatomy and recipient factors is crucial to appropriate allograft selection and operative planning. Minimization of risk and harm to donors remains paramount in LDLT.

DONOR EVALUATION

The living donor liver evaluation requires a comprehensive assessment of medical, anatomic, psychological, and social factors. A prospective donor is educated about the evaluation process and completes a detailed history and physical examination. Laboratory evaluation and cross-sectional imaging are performed. The potential donor and health providers discuss the operation, anticipated postoperative course, surgical risks, long-term risks, and possible recipient outcomes. Prospective donors should be informed that living donor hepatectomy outcomes are well documented, with reported morbidity rates of 10% to 40% and mortality rates of less than 0.5%.[13,14] A multidisciplinary approach to donor evaluation and adherence to institutional protocols are critical.[15]

Potential donors should be healthy and sufficiently physically fit to undergo a major hepatectomy. Candidates are typically aged between 18 and 65 years, depending on national laws.[16] Prospective donors ideally have no comorbidities. However, select persons with well-controlled, mild comorbidities may be considered for living donation, including those with obesity, prediabetes, or hypertension.[17] Body mass index (BMI) greater than 30 has not been associated with inferior outcomes.[18] Cardiac disease, pulmonary disease, and history of cancer are usually considered to be contraindications to living donation.

A psychological evaluation of a potential donor should be completed by a psychiatrist or licensed mental health provider to determine psychological fitness for donation. The intent is to assess emotional wellness, motivation for donation, and ability to tolerate postoperative recovery and complications. Potential donors may be declined for donation if there is underlying mental illness or evidence of primary or secondary gain. In addition, an Independent Living Donor Advocate (ILDA) is required by the Organ Procurement and Transplantation Network (OPTN) to participate in the evaluation. Per OPTN guidelines, the ILDA must document that the donor has completed appropriate medical and psychosocial evaluation, received information about the surgery and expected follow-up, and has provided informed consent.[15]

GRAFT SELECTION
Imaging

Preoperative imaging is necessary for all prospective donors. Cross-sectional imaging permits assessment of liver size, vascular and biliary anatomy, and parenchymal abnormalities (eg, presence of steatosis or masses). This information guides graft selection and serves as a roadmap for surgery, contributing to risk reduction for donor and recipient.[19] Most centers use triple-phase contrast computed tomography (CT) scan and/or magnetic resonance cholangiopancreatography (MRCP). Contrast CT and/or MRI demonstrates the hepatic arterial, portal venous, and hepatic venous vascular anatomy in addition to volumetric assessment of the liver. MRCP is the gold standard for evaluating biliary anatomy, and it offers superior fat quantification compared with CT. Advanced MRI techniques, such as proton density fat fraction scanning, are being increasingly used.[20] However, histological examination with core needle biopsy remains the gold standard for steatosis assessment and is generally recommended when greater than 10% steatosis is detected on imaging. Acceptable fat content varies by center and ranges from 10% to 30%.[21] Additional indications for liver biopsy include abnormal liver enzymes, positive genetic markers, family history, or other atypical imaging features based on individual center protocol.[22]

Many centers supplement preoperative imaging by obtaining 3-dimensional and interactive virtual reconstructions of the liver anatomy (**Fig. 1**). Benefits of this software include visualization of the relationship of the vascular and biliary anatomy as well as the planned transection plane relative to major segmental vascular and biliary branches and volume estimations of major vascular territories (eg, volume of liver parenchyma drained by a segmental or accessory hepatic venous branch). Such information aids in preoperative planning for the recipient operation (see **Fig. 1**).

Graft Size

Volume analysis is performed using CT with dedicated volumetric software.[23] Total liver, predicted graft, and predicted remnant liver volumes are determined (see **Fig. 1**). Volumetry provides critical information regarding the adequacy of the remnant liver for the donor and the predicted graft for the recipient; this is an important aspect of the feasibility and safety of the proposed LDLT. It is generally accepted that the donor's remnant liver volume should be greater than 30% of the total liver volume to minimize risk of posthepatectomy liver failure.[24] Right lobe grafts generally constitute

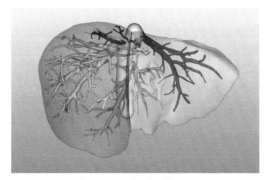

Fig. 1. MeVis Liver Suite Software (MeVis Medical Solutions AG, Bremen, Germany) 3-dimensional reconstruction of prospective donor liver demonstrating segmental venous outflow with right hepatic lobe colored red and left hepatic lobe colored green. (*With permission from* MeVis Medical Solutions AG software.)

about 60% of total liver volume and remain the most commonly used graft in LDLT.[25] A minimum graft-to-recipient weight ratio (GRWR = predicted graft weight [kg]/recipient weight [kg] x 100%) of 0.8% is considered optimal, although this remains contested.[26,27] A GRWR less than 0.8% is associated with increased risk of portal hyperperfusion, early allograft dysfunction, and small-for-size syndrome (SFSS). A small liver graft might be inadequate to support the recipient's metabolic needs, resulting in ascites, hyperbilirubinemia, coagulopathy, and possibly hepatic encephalopathy.[28] A graft with GRWR 0.6% to 0.8% can be tolerated in younger, healthier recipients with lower Model for End-Stage Liver Disease (MELD) scores and without significant portal hypertension.[29,30] For grafts with GRWR less than 0.8%, it has been suggested that a minimum liver graft weight of 650 grams reduces risk of early allograft dysfunction and death.[31] Technical maneuvers exist that can modulate portal inflow and augment outflow to optimize a smaller graft (see "Volume and Recipient Considerations: Right versus Left").[32,33]

ANATOMIC CONSIDERATIONS
Hepatic Artery Anatomy

Variations in hepatic artery anatomy are common and can influence the selection of a right versus left lobe graft (**Table 1**).[34] Conventional anatomy consists of the proper hepatic artery bifurcating into the left hepatic artery (LHA) and a right hepatic artery (RHA), with the segment IV arterial branch arising from the LHA.[35] The presence of a completely replaced RHA from the superior mesenteric artery or a replaced LHA from the left gastric artery can provide a longer length of artery to the allograft, which is favorable for implantation. However, presence of an accessory hepatic artery can require reconstruction of 2 allograft arteries; this is not necessarily a contraindication but does increase the technical difficulty of the recipient operation.

Segment IV artery

The segment IV artery perfuses the left medial sector of the left lobe and a portion of the left bile duct. When performing a donor right hepatectomy, it is important to preserve the segment IV artery in the donor to maximize remnant liver perfusion. Consequently, the RHA to the right lobe graft will be shorter if the segment IV branch arises from the RHA, potentially increasing difficulty with implantation in the recipient. Test

Table 1
Hepatic artery anatomy

Hepatic Arterial Anatomy	Percent Within Population
Conventional Anatomy	~60%
Replaced LHA	~7.5%
Replaced RHA	~10%
Replaced LHA and replaced RHA	~1%
Accessory LHA	~10%
Accessory RHA	~5%
Accessory LHA and accessory RHA	~1%
CHA replaced to SMA	~3%
CHA branch from aorta	~2%

Abbreviations: CHA, common hepatic artery; LHA, left hepatic artery; RHA, right hepatic artery; SMA, superior mesenteric artery.

clamping the segment IV artery with forceps and confirming adequate perfusion of segment IV with intraoperative ultrasound can be performed if ligation of the segment IV artery is being considered. The presence of arterial flow with a good diastolic wave form in the left medial sector provides evidence that left medial sector perfusion is reconstituted from the segment II and III arterial system; this suggests that the segment IV branch can be ligated to provide a longer RHA for the recipient operation.

Multiple graft arteries

Other arterial variations exist, including segmental perfusion from individual arteries. These variations require either back-table reconstruction or multiple anastomoses to optimize arterial inflow to the graft. If multiple anastomoses are anticipated, arterial branches in the recipient (left hepatic, right hepatic, and cystic artery branches) should be preserved during hepatectomy. If there is evidence of collateral arterial flow (demonstrated by brisk back bleeding through the smaller accessory artery after reconstruction of the main artery), then ligation of the accessory artery can be considered. The presence of multiple arteries to a potential graft, especially those with small caliber, is a relative contraindication due to higher risk of thrombotic and biliary complications.[2]

Portal Vein Anatomy

Portal vein (PV) anatomy has fewer variants than arterial anatomy (**Fig. 2**). The main PV typically bifurcates into the left and right PV branches. For technical simplicity, it is advantageous to select the lobe that requires just one anastomosis. A true trifurcation, in which the main PV divides into the left, right anterior, and right posterior PV branches, occurs in approximately 7% of the population. Right lobe grafts with this anatomy require either a back-table venoplasty, extension graft reconstruction, or 2 separate anastomoses with the right anterior and posterior PV branches (**Fig. 3**).[36] An early right posterior PV branch requires similar consideration.[37]

A relative contraindication to right or left donor hepatectomy is the origin of a dominant right anterior PV branch from the left PV within the liver parenchyma (see **Fig. 2**).[38] The presence of more than one PV branch to the left lobe is rare.[39]

Hepatic Vein Anatomy

Venous outflow from the liver varies significantly. The left, middle, and right hepatic veins constitute most of the outflow. Inferior accessory hepatic veins and segmental branches draining into the middle hepatic vein (MHV) can provide significant segmental outflow and may require reconstruction for outflow optimization. The middle hepatic vein serves as a landmark for the transection plane in right or left donor

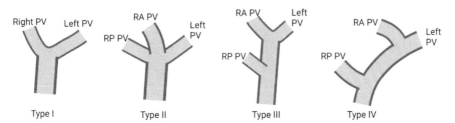

Fig. 2. Variations in portal venous anatomy. Although much less complex compared with the arterial anatomy, anatomic variants and contraindications for transplant should be discerned. PV, portal vein; RA, right anterior; RP, right posterior (Created with BioRender.com).

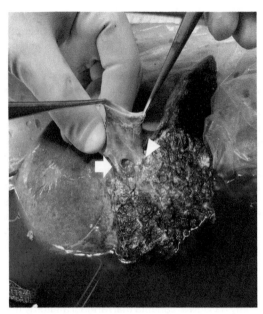

Fig. 3. Reconstruction of graft right posterior (*arrow*) and right anterior (*arrowhead*) portal branches using recipient portal vein bifurcation.

hepatectomy. The significance of segment 5 and 8 veins is discussed further in "Outflow Optimization."

Bile Duct Anatomy

Biliary anatomy is highly variable (**Fig. 4**). Conventional anatomy occurs in only 60% of individuals.[40] With conventional anatomy, the right posterior sector duct courses posterior to the right anterior duct and then joins the medial aspect of the right anterior duct forming the right hepatic duct (see **Fig. 4**A).[40] The most common variant of biliary anatomy to the right lobe (approximately 16% of patients) involves the right posterior

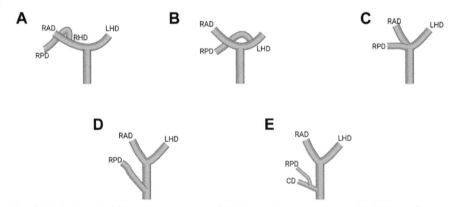

Fig. 4. Variations in biliary tree anatomy. (*A*) Conventional anatomy, (*B*) RPD confluence with LHD, (*C*) Trifurcation, (*D*), Low insertion of the RPD into main duct, and (*E*) Aberrant RPD inserting into CD. CD, cystic duct; LHD, left hepatic duct; RAD, right anterior duct; RHD, right hepatic duct; RPD, right posterior duct (Created with BioRender.com).

duct draining directly into the left hepatic duct (see **Fig. 4**B). A true trifurcation occurs in approximately 12% of the population (see **Fig. 4**C).[40] Another variant seen in about 6% of patients involves a low insertion of the right posterior duct that drains directly into the common hepatic duct (see **Fig. 4**D). An aberrant right posterior duct draining into the cystic duct is rare but has been described (see **Fig. 4**E).[41,42] The segmental ducts of the left lobe typically converge to form a single duct requiring reconstruction for left lobe grafts.

The biliary anastomosis in the recipient remains the "Achilles heel" of living donor liver transplantation, and simplicity is preferred. With 3-dimensional imaging reconstruction demonstrating the proposed transection plane, the recipient surgical team can predict and plan the appropriate recipient biliary reconstruction (**Fig. 5**). A single bile duct is preferred to minimize risk of biliary complications in the recipient and may be reconstructed with a standard choledochocholedochostomy, Roux-en-Y hepaticojejunostomy, or hepaticoduodenostomy. If 2 ducts are present, options for reconstruction include side-to-side ductoplasty to create a single duct, duct-to-duct anastomosis, duct-to-cystic duct reconstruction, and bilioenteric reconstruction, or a combination thereof. The bilioenteric anastomosis can be performed with the duodenum or a Roux limb, depending on surgeon preference and anatomic considerations. To minimize donor risk, the donor surgeon should preserve the donor's common bile duct intact and avoid bilioenteric reconstruction of the remnant liver.[43]

RECIPIENT CONSIDERATIONS: RIGHT VERSUS LEFT

The clinical equipoise of removing the least amount of liver parenchyma from the donor while providing adequate graft volume for the recipient remains challenging to navigate. A right lobe graft should be considered in the following scenarios: when the recipient has a high BMI requiring more volume for adequate GRWR, recipient MELD greater than 20, recipient age greater than 45 years and older donor age, and/or severe portal hypertension.[44–47] Recipients with evidence of severe portal hypertension (eg, severe splenomegaly, large portosystemic shunts) have increased risk of dysfunction with small grafts, and a larger graft is preferred; likewise sicker patients require good early postoperative function, and a larger graft is preferred. The

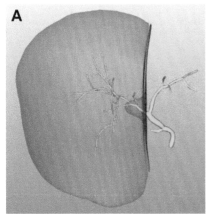
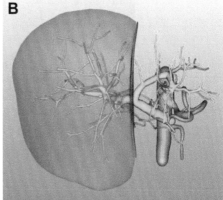

Fig. 5. (*A*) MeVis Liver Suite Software (MeVis Medical Solutions AG, Bremen, Germany) reconstruction of the transection plane for the right lobe graft in relation to the biliary anatomy and (*B*) hepatic arterial and portal vein anatomy. (*With permission from* MeVis Medical Solutions AG software.)

investigators also prefer a larger graft for LDLT with female donor to male recipient as a result of experience with hyperperfusion of smaller female grafts in male recipients with significant portal hypertension.[48] Similarly, recipients with risk factors for complicated hepatectomy (eg, prior operations, redo liver transplant, and severe portal hypertension) also benefit from a larger graft with good early function.

In situations where both the right lobe and the left lobe will provide adequate GRWR, the lobe with the most favorable anatomy should generally be used for greater donor safety and optimal recipient outcome. When the GRWR will be sufficient with a left lobe graft, anatomy is favorable, and the recipient is of a lower MELD and age, then the left lobe will be used.

Portal Inflow Modulation

As discussed earlier in this text, SFSS most commonly occurs with portal hyperperfusion, low GRWR graft, or with inadequate outflow. Left lobe grafts are more prone to this complication, as they provide recipients with a smaller GRWR. As a result, left lobe grafts are typically paired with smaller recipients and MELD scores less than 19.[49] However, with inflow modulation and outflow optimization strategies, these grafts can be augmented for good results even with GRWR as low as 0.6%. Inflow modulation strategies include shunting,[50] splenectomy,[32] and splenic artery ligation.[51] Inflow modulation for the graft is recommended when there is evidence of portal hyperperfusion: absolute portal pressure greater than 20 mm Hg, PV-to-cava gradient greater than 12 to 15 mm Hg, hepatic artery flow less than 100 mL/min, poor arterial diastolic flow within the graft on intraoperative ultrasound, and portal flow more than 2.5 cc/gram graft weight.

As an alternative option, surgeons at Asan Medical Center, Seoul, Korea introduced dual graft LDLT.[52] Dual graft LDLT involves transplantation of 2 donor grafts, typically 2 left lateral sections, into a single recipient; this allows for a smaller, safer operation for each donor but optimizes liver parenchyma volume for the recipient to overcome inadequate donor volumes or inadequate GRWR from each individual donor (**Fig. 6**).

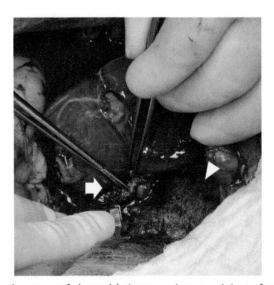

Fig. 6. A left lateral sector graft (*arrow*) being sewn into a recipient after a left lobe graft (*arrow*) has been implanted. (*Courtesy of* Trevor Nydam MD.)

Outflow Optimization

In the early days of LDLT, the MHV was preserved with the right lobe graft to optimize venous outflow and reduce risk of graft congestion.[53] Currently, most centers do not include the MHV with the right lobe graft in an effort to preserve more remnant liver volume with the donor. If the MHV is not included, optimizing the venous outflow of the right lobe graft, especially the anterior sector with potential reimplantation of large (≥5 mm) segment V and/or VIII veins, can be critical for achieving ideal outcomes in the recipient.[5] Segmental or accessory veins with a diameter greater than or equal to 5 mm or drain greater than or equal to 10% of liver parenchyma should be reconstructed.[54] Drainage territories can be estimated using the 3-dimensional reconstruction software and are a useful adjunct when planning outflow modification for the recipient operation and accurately assessing the "functional volume" of the graft. These segments can be reimplanted individually into the inferior vena cava (IVC) or can be reconstructed creating a "neo-middle hepatic vein" using autologous or synthetic material.[55,56] This neo-middle hepatic vein can then be implanted directly into the IVC, to the left/middle hepatic vein confluence of the recipient, or anastomosed to the right hepatic vein to create a single lumen for anastomosis with the vena cava (**Fig. 7**).[56] Convention dictates that this outflow reconstruction is necessary in the early posttransplant period to avoid venous congestion of the graft during recovery and hypertrophy.[51] Alternatively, a double vena cava technique can be used to enlarge outflow with 2 large hepatic veins that are widely spaced as described by Kishi and colleagues.[57]

In donor left hepatectomy, the middle hepatic vein is preserved with the graft. The left and middle hepatic veins commonly join before drainage into IVC. If concerns exist for inadequate outflow, the septum between the left and middle hepatic veins can be opened and a venoplasty performed before anastomosis with the vena cava.[58] Absence of the MHV in the donor's remnant right lobe may be associated with mild, but temporary, congestion of the right medial sector.

OUTCOMES

Donor and recipient outcomes after LDLT have been well documented and heavily scrutinized. Risks to living liver donors include bleeding, bile leak, remnant liver insufficiency and failure, venous thromboembolism, surgical site infection, incisional hernia, cerebrovascular and cardiovascular events, respiratory complications, and death. A comprehensive review of the literature over the past 2 decades shows complications

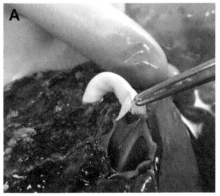
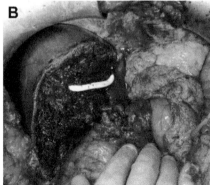

Fig. 7. Right lobe graft after reconstruction of (*A*) segment 8 and (*B*) segment 5.

occurring in 8% to 40% of donors.[59] Biliary complications, including biloma and stricture, continue to be the most common, comprising approximately 6% overall.[59]

Early experience showed right hepatectomy for donation to be associated with greater overall mortality and donor complications compared with left lobe donation, and this was thought to be due to the amount of liver tissue removed.[10,60,61] Right lobe donors continue to have significant risk in the contemporary era, with statistically higher rates of bile leak and stricture, cardiopulmonary complications, and longer lengths of stay.[14,44,45,50,60–62] The largest North American series found a significantly higher rate of postoperative liver dysfunction with elevated postoperative bilirubin and international normalized ratio.[45] Mortality continues to be greatest among right lobe donors, with a reported 23 donor deaths worldwide from 1999 to 2017.[61] As a result, the International Liver Transplantation Society consensus conference on enhanced recovery recommends left donor hepatectomy when possible due to the improved short-term outcomes in the donor.[63]

However, some studies have challenged the notion that right hepatectomy is associated with greater donor risk.[9,62,64] A meta-analysis of 33 studies evaluating donor complications based on right or left hepatectomy showed an equivalent morbidity profile to the donor, and no difference was seen in Clavien-Dindo classification III or greater complications.[62] Furthermore, an analysis of survival data from 4111 living liver donors from the United States found that mortality risk did not vary with left or right lobe donation.[64]

Minimally invasive techniques for donor hepatectomy are being adopted rapidly but remain controversial due to an absence of large studies. However, several recent multiinstitutional studies demonstrated robotic-assisted donor hepatectomy to be as safe as the open operation at experienced centers.[65,66] Importantly, morbidity and mortality did not vary with robotic-assisted left versus right donor hepatectomy.[66]

In regard to recipient outcomes, with careful graft selection in the modern era, recipients receiving left lobe grafts have no difference in vascular or biliary complications compared with recipients with right lobe grafts.[44,45] However, it has been shown that patients receiving left lobe grafts have higher rates of SFSS and postoperative mortality compared with patients receiving right lobe grafts.[46,49,67] Despite this increased risk of SFSS and mortality, left lobe recipients do not have lower rates of overall or graft survival.[44,46]

SUMMARY

In the modern era, surgical techniques and advances have helped improve the risks of right versus left lobe donation and equilibrated the outcomes in recipients as seen in large series.[44] However, careful consideration is still required in the balance of donor risk with recipient risk and the clinical equipoise of sufficient remnant liver volume and adequate graft size. In addition, the complexity of these operations has increased dramatically over the past decades, and now some centers routinely perform LDLT with multiple ducts, arteries, and veins. Although this increases the risk of the donor operation, it especially increases the risk to the recipient. Higher complexity cases should be performed at higher volume centers with commensurate level of experience.

CLINICS CARE POINTS

Right lobe graft should be considered in the following scenarios:
- Larger recipient requiring more volume for adequate GRWR

- Recipient MELD greater than 20
- Recipient age greater than 45 years
- High recipient BMI greater than 30
- Older donor age and/or severe portal hypertension

Inflow modification for the graft is typically performed in the following scenarios:
- When absolute portal pressure is greater than 20 mm Hg
- PV-to-cava gradient is greater than 12 to 15 mm Hg
- Hepatic artery flow is less than 100 mL/min
- Poor arterial diastolic flow within the graft on intraoperative ultrasound
- Portal flow greater than 2.5 cc/gram graft weight.

DISCLOSURE

The authors have nothing to disclose.

REFERENCES

1. Strong R, Lynch S, Ong TH, et al. Successful liver transplantation from a living donor to her son. N Engl J Med 1990;322:1505–7.
2. Broelsch CE, Whitington PF, Emond JC, et al. Liver transplantation in children from living related donors. Ann Surg 1991;214(4):428–37.
3. Raia S, Nery J, Mies S. Liver transplantation from live donors. Lancet 1989; 334:497.
4. Emond JC, Renz JF, Ferrell LD, et al. Functional analysis of grafts from living donors: implications for the treatment of older recipients. Ann Surg 1996;224: 544–54.
5. Chan SC, Fan ST. Historical perspective of living donor liver transplantation. WJG 2008;14:15–21.
6. Habib N, Tanaka K. Living-related liver transplantation in adult recipients: a hypothesis. Clin Transplant 1995;9:31–4.
7. Abecassis MM, Fisher RA, Olthoff KM, et al. Complications of living donor hepatic lobectomy—a comprehensive report. Am J Transplant 2012;12:1208–17.
8. Wachs ME, Bak T, Karrer F, et al. Adult living donor liver transplantation using a right hepatic lobe. Transplantation 1998;66:1313–6.
9. Vargas PA, Goldaracena N. Right vs left hepatectomy for LDLT, safety and regional preference. Curr Transpl Rep 2022;9:240–9.
10. Emond JC. Right versus left: progress but no conclusion in selecting donors for live donor liver transplantation. Transplantation 2022;106:2293–4.
11. Roll GR, Parekh JR, Parker WF, et al. Left hepatectomy versus right hepatectomy for living donor liver transplantation: shifting the risk from the donor to the recipient: shifting the risk from the donor to the recipient. Liver Transpl 2013;19: 472–81.
12. Rammohan A, Reddy MS, Narasimhan G, et al. Live liver donors: is right still right? World J Surg 2020;44:2385–93.
13. Lee JG, Lee K, Kwon CHD, et al. Donor safety in living donor liver transplantation: the Korean organ transplantation registry study. Liver Transpl 2017;23:999–1006.
14. Rössler F, Sapisochin G, Song G, et al. Defining benchmarks for major liver surgery: a multicenter analysis of 5202 living liver donors. Ann Surg 2016;264: 492–500.

15. Organ Procurement and Transplantation Network. OPTN Policies Statement: *Policy 14:* LivingDonation. OPTN, 2023. OPTN Policies Effective as of Aug 1 2023 [NOOC] (hrsa.gov).
16. Campbell M, Wright L, Greenberg RA, et al. How young is too young to be a living donor? Am J Transplant 2013;13:1643–9.
17. Chung JH, Ryu JH, Yang KH, et al. Efficacy and safety of weight reduction of the donor in hepatic steatosis for living donor liver transplantation. Ann Transplant 2020;25:e923211.
18. Knaak M, Goldaracena N, Doyle A, et al. Donor BMI >30 is not a contraindication for live liver donation. Am J Transplant 2017;17:756–62.
19. Vernuccio F, Whitney SA, Ravindra K, et al. CT and MR imaging evaluation of living liver donors. Abdom Radiol 2021;46:17–28.
20. Zheng D, Guo Z, Schroder PM, et al. Accuracy of MR imaging and MR spectroscopy for detection and quantification of hepatic steatosis in living liver donors: a meta-analysis. Radiology 2017;282:92–102.
21. Lee SG. A complete treatment of adult living donor liver transplantation: a review of surgical technique and current challenges to expand indication of patients. Am J Transplant 2015;15:17–38.
22. Jackson WE, Kaplan A, Saben JL, et al. Practice patterns of the medical evaluation of living liver donors in the United States. Liver Transplant 2023;29:164–71.
23. Hecht EM, Wang ZJ, Kambadakone A, et al. Living donor liver transplantation: preoperative planning and postoperative complications. Am J Roentgenol 2019;213:65–76.
24. Testa G, Nadalin S, Klair T, et al. Optimal surgical workup to ensure safe recovery of the donor after living liver donation – a systematic review of the literature and expert panel recommendations. Clin Transplant 2022;36:1–12.
25. Goldaracena N, Barbas AS. Living donor liver transplantation. Curr Opin Organ Transplant 2019;24:131–7.
26. Sugawara Y, Makuuchi M, Takayama T, et al. Small-for-size grafts in living-related liver transplantation. J Am Coll Surg 2001;192:510–3.
27. Kiuchi T, Tanaka K, Ito T, et al. Small-for-size graft in living donor liver transplantation: how far should we go? Liver Transpl 2003;9:S29–35.
28. Hernandez-Alejandro R, Sharma H. Small-for-size syndrome in liver transplantation: new horizons to cover with a good launchpad. Liver Transpl 2016;22:33–6.
29. Alim A, Erdogan Y, Yuzer Y, et al. Graft-to-recipient weight ratio threshold adjusted to the model for end-stage liver disease score for living donor liver transplantation. Liver Transpl 2016;22:1643–8.
30. Patel MS, Egawa H, Kwon YK, et al. The role of graft to recipient weight ratio on enhanced recovery of the recipient after living donor liver transplantation – A systematic review of the literature and expert panel recommendations. Clin Transplant 2022;36:e14630.
31. Agarwal S, Selvakumar N, Rajasekhar K, et al. Minimum absolute graft weight of 650 g predicts a good outcome in living donor liver transplant despite a graft recipient body weight ratio of less than 0.8. Clin Transplant 2019;33:e13705.
32. Fujiki M, Hashimoto K, Quintini C, et al. Living donor liver transplantation with augmented venous outflow and splenectomy: a promised land for small left lobe grafts. Ann Surg 2022;276:838–45.
33. Jo HS, Yu YD, Choi YJ, et al. Left liver graft in adult-to-adult living donor liver transplantation with an optimal portal flow modulation strategy to overcome the small-for-size syndrome – A retrospective cohort study. Int J Surg 2022;106:106953.

34. Michels NA. Blood supply and anatomy of the upper abdominal organs, with a descriptive atlas. Philadelphia: Lippincott; 1955.
35. Michels NA. Newer anatomy of the liver and its variant blood supply and collateral circulation. Am J Surg 1966;112:337–47.
36. Sureka B, Patidar Y, Bansal K, et al. Portal vein variations in 1000 patients: surgical and radiological importance. BJR 2015;88:20150326.
37. Kishi Y, Sugawara Y, Kaneko J, et al. Classification of portal vein anatomy for partial liver transplantation. Transplant Proc 2004;36:3075–6.
38. Lee SG, Hwang S, Kim KH, et al. Approach to anatomic variations of the graft portal vein in right lobe living-donor liver transplantation. Transplantation 2003;75: S28–32.
39. Carneiro C, Brito J, Bilreiro C, et al. All about portal vein: a pictorial display to anatomy, variants and physiopathology. Insights Imaging 2019;10:38.
40. Castaing D. Surgical anatomy of the biliary tract. HPB 2008;10:72–6.
41. Oyama K, Nakahira S, Ogawa H, et al. Successful management of aberrant right hepatic duct during laparoscopic cholecystectomy: a rare case report. Surg Case Rep 2019;5:74.
42. Sofi AA, Alaradi OH, Abouljoud M, et al. Aberrant right hepatic duct draining into the cystic duct: clinical outcomes and management. Gastroenterology Research and Practice 2011;2011:458915.
43. Baker TB, Zimmerman MA, Goodrich NP, et al. Biliary reconstructive techniques and associated anatomic variants in adult living donor liver transplantations: The adult-to-adult living donor liver transplantation cohort study experience. Liver Transpl 2017;23:1519–30.
44. Acuna S, Zhang W, Yoon P, et al. Right lobe versus left love living donor liver transplnatation: a systematic review and meta-analysis of donor and recipient outcomes. Transplantation 2022;106:2370–8.
45. Halazun KJ, Przybyszewski EM, Griesemer AD, et al. Leaning to the left: increasing the donor pool by using the left lobe, outcomes of the largest single-center north american experience of left lobe adult-to-adult living donor liver transplantation. Ann Surg 2016;264:448–56.
46. Soejima Y, Shirabe K, Taketomi A, et al. Left lobe living donor liver transplantation in adults. Am J Transplant 2012;12:1877–85.
47. Sánchez-Cabús S, Cherqui D, Rashidian N, et al. Left-liver adult-to-adult living donor liver transplantation: can it be improved? A retrospective multicenter European study. Ann Surg 2018;268:876–84.
48. Kelly DM, Miller C. Understanding the splenic contribution to portal flow: the role of splenic artery ligation as inflow modification in living donor liver transplantation. Liver Transpl 2006;12:1186–8.
49. Ikegami T, Yoshizumi T, Sakata K, et al. Left lobe living donor liver transplantation in adults: what is the safety limit? Liver Transpl 2016;22:1666–75.
50. Braun HJ, Roberts JP. Current status of left lobe adult to adult living donor liver transplantation. Curr Opin Organ Transplant 2021;26:139–45.
51. Emond JC, Goodrich NP, Pomposelli JJ, et al. Hepatic hemodynamics and portal flow modulation: the A2ALL experience. Transplantation 2017;101:2375–84.
52. Song GW, Lee SG, Moon DB, et al. Dual-graft adult living donor liver transplantation: an innovative surgical procedure for live liver donor pool expansion. Ann Surg 2017;266:10–8.
53. Fan ST, Lo CM, Liu CL, et al. Safety and Necessity of including the middle hepatic vein in the right lobe graft in adult-to-adult live donor liver transplantation. Ann Surg 2003;238:137–48.

54. Gyu Lee S, Min Park K, Hwang S, et al. Modified right liver graft from a living donor to prevent congestion1. Transplantation 2002;74:54–9.
55. Guo HJ, Wang K, Chen KC, et al. Middle hepatic vein reconstruction in adult right lobe living donor liver transplantation improves recipient survival. Hepatobiliary Pancreat Dis Int 2019;18:125–31.
56. Pomposelli JJ, Akoad M, Khwaja K, et al. Evolution of anterior segment reconstruction after live donor adult liver transplantation: a single-center experience: middle hepatic vein reconstruction after live donor liver transplantation. Clin Transplant 2012;26:470–5.
57. Kishi Y, Sugawara Y, Matsui Y, et al. Alternatives to the double vena cava method in partial liver transplantation. Liver Transpl 2005;11:101–3.
58. Takemura N, Sugawara Y, Hashimoto T, et al. New hepatic vein reconstruction in left liver graft. Liver Transpl 2005;11:356–60.
59. Braun HJ, Ascher NL, Roll GR, et al. Biliary complications following living donor hepatectomy. Transplant Rev 2016;30:247–52.
60. Iwasaki J, Iida T, Mizumoto M, et al. Donor morbidity in right and left hemiliver living donor liver transplantation: the impact of graft selection and surgical innovation on donor safety. Transpl Int 2014;27:1205–13.
61. Brige P, Hery G, Chopinet S, et al. Morbidity and mortality of hepatic right lobe living donors: systematic review and perspectives. JGLD 2018;27:169–78.
62. Vargas PA, McCracken EKE, Mallawaarachchi I, et al. Donor morbidity is equivalent between right and left hepatectomy for living liver donation: a meta-analysis. Liver Transpl 2021;27:1412–23.
63. Pollok JM, Tinguely P, Berenguer M, et al. Enhanced recovery for liver transplantation: recommendations from the 2022 International Liver Transplantation Society consensus conference. The Lancet Gastroenterology & Hepatology 2023;8: 81–94.
64. Muzaale AD, Dagher NN, Montgomery RA, et al. Estimates of early death, acute liver failure, and long-term mortality among live liver donors. Gastroenterology 2012;142:273–80.
65. Cherqui D, Ciria R, Kwon CHD, et al. Expert consensus guidelines on minimally invasive donor hepatectomy for living donor liver transplantation from innovation to implementation: a joint initiative from the international laparoscopic liver society (ILLS) and the Asian-Pacific Hepato-Pancreato-Biliary Association (A-PHPBA). Ann Surg 2021;273:96–108.
66. Soubrane O, Eguchi S, Uemoto S, et al. Minimally invasive donor hepatectomy for adult living donor liver transplantation: an international, multi-institutional evaluation of safety, efficacy and early outcomes. Ann Surg 2022;275:166–74.
67. Chan SC, Fan ST, Lo CM, et al. Effect of side and size of graft on surgical outcomes of adult-to-adult live donor liver transplantation. Liver Transpl 2007; 13:91–8.

Transplantation for Hepatocellular Carcinoma

Angela Hill, MD, MPHS[a,1], Franklin Olumba, MD, MPHS[a,1], William Chapman, MD[b,*]

KEYWORDS

- Liver transplant • Transplantation • HCC • Hepatocellular carcinoma • Liver cancer

KEY POINTS

- Hepatocellular carcinoma (HCC) is the most common primary liver cancer, with increasing incidence worldwide and in the United States.
- Liver transplantation is a primary treatment for early-stage HCC, requiring careful evaluation by a multidisciplinary team.
- Downstaging of HCC tumors using neoadjuvant therapies offers the best survival for patients waiting for liver transplant as well as the best post-transplant survival.
- Immunosuppression after transplant for HCC put patients at risk for cancer recurrence. They must undergo surveillance during their period of highest risk, which is the first 2 to 3 years post-transplant.
- Research is ongoing to find the upper limits of HCC tumors that can be transplanted. Recurrence-free survival must be balanced with organ availability.

INTRODUCTION/BACKGROUND

Since Dr Vincenzo Mazzaferro's landmark 1996 paper entitled "Liver Transplantation for the Treatment of Small Hepatocellular Carcinoma in Patients with Cirrhosis," liver transplantation (LT) has become standardized as a curative treatment for hepatocellular carcinoma (HCC).[1] Before this, resection had been the primary operative treatment of patients, with a less than 50% survival rate; furthermore, resection was not available for patients with cirrhosis with insufficient functional reserve.[2] In Dr Mazzaferro's initial paper, his group outlined tumor characteristics amenable to transplant or what became termed the Milan criteria (MC): a single tumor less than 5 cm or up to three tumors, none larger than 3 cm, with no evidence of extrahepatic disease or

[a] Division of General Surgery, Washington University School of Medicine, MSC 8109-05-06, 660 South Euclid Avenue, St Louis, MO 63110, USA; [b] Division of General Surgery, Washington University School of Medicine, Section of Transplantation, MSC 8109-05-06, 660 South Euclid Avenue, St Louis, MO 63110, USA
[1] Both authors are co-first authors.
* Corresponding author.
E-mail address: chapmanw@wustl.edu

Surg Clin N Am 104 (2024) 103–111
https://doi.org/10.1016/j.suc.2023.09.002
0039-6109/24/© 2023 Elsevier Inc. All rights reserved.
surgical.theclinics.com

macrovascular invasion. The initial cohort of patients who met this criteria had a 4-year overall survival rate of 75% and recurrence-free survival rate of 83%.[1]

Presently, transplant offers a definitive curative option for either (1) patients with HCC and cirrhosis who do not have sufficient hepatic reserve to tolerate other therapies such as resection or (2) patients with unresectable HCC. Since the development of MC, many centers have demonstrated comparable postoperative survival results using broadened LT criteria for HCC. For example, in 2001, the University of California in San Francisco (UCSF) published institutional guidelines defined by tumors measuring 6.5 cm or less, three lesions with the largest lesion measuring less than or equal to 4.5 cm, and total tumor diameter measuring less than 8 cm. Five-year overall survival was 75.2%, akin to MC results.[3] Since the publication of the UCSF criteria, transplant for HCC has expanded by approximately 5% to 20%.[4]

In this article, the authors briefly review the history and epidemiology of transplant for HCC, evolving criteria for transplantation, and management of recurrent disease.

HISTORY/EPIDEMIOLOGY

Globally, HCC is the most common primary liver malignancy, and its incidence continues to increase over time. Approximately 14 million HCC cases existed in 2012, a number projected to increase to 22 million by 2032. It is the seventh most common cause of death in the United States. Although most commonly caused by the hepatitis B virus globally, its most common etiology is hepatitis C in the United States.[5]

HCC remains a common indication for liver transplant, representing 10.9% of all liver transplants in 2021 (**Fig. 1**). The number of patients transplanted for HCC has varied not only with the prevalence of disease but also policy changes in waitlisting for HCC. Given that patients who undergo transplant for HCC typically do not have as high Model End-Stage Liver Disease (MELD) scores as other patients transplanted for other indications, such as end-stage liver disease (ESLD) secondary to nonalcoholic steatohepatitis or cirrhosis, the Organ Procurement and Transplantation Network (OPTN) has awarded exception points to patients with HCC to increase waitlist priority, to avoid disease progression obviating the benefit of transplant. Since the institution of MELD-based listing in February 2002, the proportion of patients transplanted for HCC increased dramatically, by approximately sixfold. Initially, patients with stage 1 HCC (or with a single tumor measuring <2 cm in size) were given 24 points, and patients with stage 2 (single tumor measuring 2–5 cm or 2–3 nodules each measuring

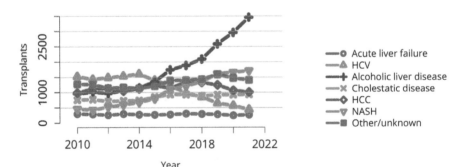

Fig. 1. All liver transplants by diagnosis, 2010 to 2021. (*Data from* Kwong AJ, Ebel NH, Kim WR, Lake JR, Smith JM, Schladt DP, Schnellinger EM, Handarova D, Weiss S, Cafarella M, Snyder JJ. OPTN/SRTR 2021 Annual Data Report: Liver. American Journal of Transplantation. 2023 Feb 1;23(2):S178-263.)

3 cm or less) were given 29 points. In April 2003, this was modified so that patients with stage 1 were given 20 points and stage 2, 24 points. In March 2005, this was adjusted so that stage 1 was not awarded any points and stage 2, 22 points.[6] In October 2015, waitlisted patients were transitioned to a time-based point allocation system, with a calculated score for the first 3 months, 28 points at 6 months and 29 points at 9 months. This policy change was found to improve allocation equity between patients listed for HCC and non-HCC etiologies, without significant changes in waitlist mortality and dropout among patients with HCC.[7]

As of 2019, patients with T2 HCC are awarded exception points after having been observed with stable disease for 6 months, with a cap of 34 exception points.[8] The goal is to facilitate just and expedient transplant before tumor progression that would render transplant unsafe. In 2021, given the most recent policy changes, transplant rates for patients with HCC with versus without exception points were comparable between the two groups. Five-year graft survival was noted to be similar between the two groups at approximately 79.4%.[9]

Patient Evaluation Overview

Preoperative evaluation of patients with HCC begins with careful preoperative staging by either CT or MRI. Imaging remains the cornerstone of diagnosis and staging, as most of the patients do not have tissue diagnosis at the time of transplant.[10] Unfortunately, previous studies comparing imaging and explant pathologies have suggested that a quarter of cases underestimate disease burden and approximately 30% overestimate, with an overall staging accuracy of 50%.[11] The role of biopsy remains controversial, however, as biopsies have been associated with a high false negative rate.

Presently, patients may be listed and be awarded exception points after 6 months if they either have stable T2 disease or if they have been downstaged to T2 disease and have no evidence of metastatic disease, macrovascular invasion or have a serum alpha-fetoprotein (AFP) of greater than 1000. Patients who have had more aggressive disease but underwent complete resection and developed T1 or T2 disease recurrence may also be awarded points after 6 months. Per OPTN guidelines, macrovascular invasion of the main portal or hepatic vein, extrahepatic disease, ruptured HCC, and T1 disease are all contraindications to transplant.

The question remains whether more aggressive disease may warrant transplantation in the future. As previously discussed, the criteria for transplant eligibility for HCC have continued to evolve since the development of the MC (**Table 1**).[12] Following the publication of UCSF criteria, several Canadian centers proposed using total tumor volume (TTV) with a cutoff of 115 cm³ with equivalent patient outcomes to MC and UCSF criteria.[13] In 2009, Mazzaferro published the "Up to Seven Criteria," which limited the total number of tumors to 7 and the total sum of tumor sizes to be less than 7 cm. Tumors could not demonstrate any microvascular invasion to be included. Post-transplant 5-year survival was comparable to patients transplanted under the MC.[14]

Increasingly, tumor biology has been investigated as a potential preoperative indicator of post-transplant outcomes. AFP has been the most studied prognostic marker. Although a universal cutoff has not been established, previous studies using cutoffs of 400, 500, and 1000 IU/mL are associated with poorer postoperative survival.[12] When considered in combination with imaging characteristics, several algorithms have been developed, such as the New York/California (NYCA) score. This scoring system recategorized the majority of patients outside of MC has having low to acceptable risk and demonstrated an improved discrimination ability relative to MC.[15]

Table 1
Expanded criteria for liver transplantation for hepatocellular carcinoma

| System | Year | Sample Size | | Parameters | OS (%) | RFS (%) |
		DDLT	LDLT			
UCSF[2]	2001	70	0	Tumor ≤6.5 cm or ≤3 nodule < s with largest ≤4.5 cm and a total tumor ≤8 cm	75.2	None
Asan[4]	2008	0	221	Tumor ≤5 cm, ≤6 nodule, no gross vascular invasion	81.6	None
Total tumor volume (TTV)[12]	2008	0	288	Total tumor volume <115 cm^3	74	78
UP-to-7[10]	2009	1404	121	Sum of the tumor number and size of the largest tumor ≤7	71.2	None

Abbreviations: DDLT, deceased donor liver transplant; LDLT, living donor liver transplant; OS, overall survival; RFS, recurrence-free survival.

Data from Halazun KJ, Sapisochin G, von Ahrens D, Agopian VG, Tabrizian P. Predictors of outcome after liver transplantation for hepatocellular carcinoma (HCC) beyond Milan criteria. International Journal of Surgery. 2020 Oct 1;82:61-9.

Beyond tumor staging, transplant evaluation of patients with HCC is largely akin to that of patient presenting with ESLD of other etiologies. Consideration for transplant requires multidisciplinary evaluation, including transplant surgeons, hepatologists, psychiatrists, social work, and pharmacist involvement. Absolute contraindications to transplant include conditions that would prevent a patient from tolerating transplant, including uncontrolled sepsis and severe cardiopulmonary comorbidities. Relative contraindications to transplant are institution-specific and may include older age, extensive portal vein thromboses, and poor psychosocial support that may interfere with postoperative immunosuppression medication adherence.[16]

Downstaging Therapies

For patients who present with tumors beyond the MC, neoadjuvant downstaging therapies are traditionally recommended. Although there is no clear upper limit for downstaging, extrahepatic disease and macrovascular invasion are typically considered to be contraindications.[17]

Downstaging treatments can include radiofrequency ablation (RFA), transarterial chemoembolization (TACE), transarterial radioembolization, and resection. Previously, the rate of successful downstaging has been reported at 48%, and post-transplant survival outcomes between patients who present with transplant-eligible disease burden versus downstaged disease have been comparable at 88% and 90%, respectively.[18]

Details regarding downstaging methodology, in isolation and combination, are outlined here but described in further detail in *Chapter 7: Downstaging Techniques for HCC for Liver Transplant.*

Treatment Complications

Transplantation remains a remarkable therapy for patients with HCC, with excellent outcomes, but treatment resistance still occurs in the form of cancer recurrence. As previously discussed, current guidelines attempt to balance the risk of this recurrence due primarily to immunosuppression with the benefit of post-transplant survival compared with survival with HCC progression. In the MC investigators' first report, recurrence at 4 years was noted around 8%.[1] More recent systematic reviews report the recurrence of HCC around 16% with mean time to recurrence of 13 months.[19,20] This problem has created an urgent need for recurrence prediction with tools such as the previously mentioned NYCA pre-transplant as well as post-transplant risk prediction with models such as RETREAT (recently externally validated) and post-MORAL, which use histology and biomarkers like AFP to make risk predictions.[21–23]

Patients must be followed closely and at regular intervals with surveillance. Unfortunately, no high quality evidence exists to standardize the best laboratory and imaging testing to perform. It is known that recurrence tends to happen within 2 to 3 years of transplant, with earlier recurrence having the poorest survival. Often, recurrence sites will spread from hepatic to extrahepatic with metastases going to lungs and bones.[20] Surveillance strategies vary by transplant center but most perform cross-sectional imaging (computed tomography of the chest, abdomen, and pelvis or MRI) every 6 month for up to 5 years with or without AFP level every 6 months for similar duration. Models such as the previously mentioned RETREAT score can be used as well to guide surveillance planning.

In the transplant evaluation of all patients with HCC, multidisciplinary discussion is focused on reducing tumor burden and slowing progression. The main therapies used are the previously mentioned locoregional therapies (LRTs) such as TACE, Yttrium-90 radioembolization, RFA, microwave ablation, percutaneous ethanol injections, cryoablation, and recently stereotactic body radiation therapy (SBRT). Whether outside or within MC, before transplant, most patients receive therapy to provide the best survival post-transplant. The updated Barcelona Clinic Liver Cancer (BCLC) prognosis and treatment strategy outlines the HCC stages and their first-line treatments with a special section for treatment stage migration, an unfortunate but not uncommon complication of LRTs (**Fig. 2**).[24]

Depending on their BCLC stage, which accounts for tumor burden-related performance status and preserved liver function as given by albumin–bilirubin score, tumor

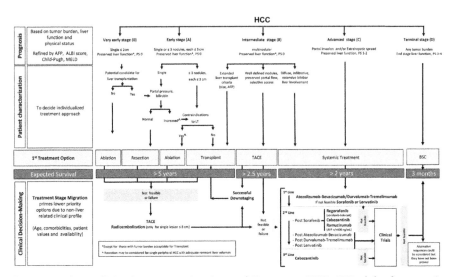

Fig. 2. Barcelona Clinic Liver Cancer Staging and Treatment 2022. AFP, alpha-fetoprotein; ALBI, albumin–bilirubin; BCLC, Barcelona Clinic Liver Cancer; BSC, best supportive care; ECOG PS, Eastern Cooperative Oncology Group Performance Status; LT, liver transplantation; MELD, Model of End-Stage Liver Disease; TACE, transarterial chemoembolization.

ablation (radiofrequency), resection, or TACE will be done first.[24] Sometimes, treatment fails to shrink the tumors or there is radiological progression that does not reclassify the patient into a new BCLC stage. In these cases, treatment proceeds to that of the next BCLC stage especially if the first-line therapy is not felt to be effective or safe to repeat. For tumors not responding to ablation or resection, TACE is typically indicated, or if unsuccessful, migration to advanced stage systemic therapies will be warranted.

There are several complications to be aware of when patients undergo LRTs ahead of transplant. These will be briefly mentioned here, but are discussed in greater detail in further detail in *Chapter 7: Downstaging Techniques for HCC for Liver Transplant.* TACE, for example, has many ischemic-related complications such as hepatic abscess, splenic abscess, cholecystitis, and biliary stenoses. It can also result in upper gastrointestinal (GI) bleeding from gastroduodenal ulcers, acute kidney injury or, rarely, hepatic failure.[25] The most common complications are liver abscess across all the modalities. Complications specific to RFA include incomplete treatment due to convective heat sink effect for tumors close to large vessels and biliary stenosis for those close to bile ducts.[26] Ethanol injection and radioembolization are techniques that can minimize these complications but they are not proven as effective as TACE and RFA which are better studied.

New Developments

Not all patients can undergo traditional LRTs for downstaging before transplant, and new techniques are being developed to help these patients. SBRT is a noninvasive therapy for HCC originally adapted from lung cancer treatment. It works by precisely delivering external beam radiation to a single target (liver) in either a single dose or several small high doses. It has not yet been incorporated into widely used HCC treatment protocols like the latest version of the BCLC prognosis and treatment strategy.[24] This is because it has generally been reserved for higher stage and higher risk patients who have contraindications for traditional percutaneous LRTs, resection, or upfront transplantation.[27] For this reason, it has not yet been compared in randomized control trials to LRT for downstaging before transplant. There are, however, a few small single-center studies evaluating the use of SBRT as a bridge to transplant with promising results.[28,29] The liver transplant waiting list drop out among treated patients is comparable to those receiving traditional bridging therapy like LRT for similar stage.[29] It has become attractive due to potential to treat and bridge patients with worse underlying liver function and complications like ascites, as many of these patients cannot undergo resection or LRT even with smaller tumors. There are notable side effects to SBRT however such as radiation toxicity which would be more common than even Yttrium-90 (Y-90) embolization. More studies, including randomized trials, are needed to truly assess the benefits of SBRT, which seems to have some role in bridging patients but only in circumstances traditional therapies have higher risk of complication.

The use of extended criteria grafts and declined grafts for HCC transplant is covered previously in chapters 14 and 16, but will be briefly discussed here. Many HCC liver waitlist candidates will have mild or no underlying liver disease and may have no exception points for timely transplant. Select programs in the United States have begun to accept extended criteria and even declined offers for such patients due to the use of novel machine perfusion devices (normothermic machine perfusion and Hypothermic Oxygenated machine PErfusion), which can recover such organs for transplant into lower morbidity/mortality risk candidates who would otherwise not receive organs.[30,31] More studies are needed to establish safety and efficacy of this practice, however.

Evaluation of Long-Term Outcomes

LT for HCC has good long-term outcomes. Recent 10-year multicenter analysis of more than 2600 HCC transplants revealed that at 10 years, probability of HCC recurrence was around 16.4%. Median time to recurrence in this large cohort was 158 months. Of note, patients with tumors outside of the MC at diagnosis but downstaged to within MC had a 10-year overall survival rate of 52.1% with a recurrence rate of 20.6% at this same end point demonstrating the importance of neoadjuvant therapies for HCC as part of downstaging.[32] Data such as these make clear two things: transplantation for HCC is an effective treatment strategy and treatment of the patients' tumors leads to improved overall and recurrence-free survival.

Summary and Future Directions

Transplantation for HCC is a broad and complex topic due to the many fold considerations of both donor organ selection and recipient. Although it is known that tumor size is negatively associated with post-transplant outcome, the exact cutoff is difficult to determine. Much progress has been made in this field trying to strike the proper balance between good post-transplant survival, longer recurrence-free survival and fair allocation of livers, but more work is necessary. Tumor downstaging has allowed far more HCC transplants to occur and further advances in liver-directed therapy will likely increase this number. The use of new technologies such as SBRT for downstaging will increase the number of transplant candidate and machine perfusion promises to make more organs available to them. The progress of transplantation for HCC is a model for transplantation of other liver tumors such as cholangiocarcinoma and isolated colorectal liver metastases.

CLINICS CARE POINTS

- Multiple criteria exist for the selection of proper transplant candidates diagnosed with HCC, with the Milan criteria frequently serving as the standard of care and extended criteria, such as University of California in San Francisco criteria, increasingly coming into practice.

- Multidisciplinary transplant, hepatology, and oncology discussions are necessary for every patient to undergo downstaging of the tumor as appropriate before transplant.

- Evaluation of patients must account for underlying liver disease and other comorbidities to ensure success of bridging and downstaging therapies. Barcelona Clinic Liver Cancer staging and prognosis provides useful guide to treatment.

- Post-transplant surveillance of HCC patients is critical and should be most frequent during the first 2 to 3 years after transplantation when most recurrences are likely to happen.

FUNDING

Angela is funded via the T32: Research reported in this publication was supported by the Washington University School of Medicine Surgical Oncology Basic Science and Translational Research Training Program grant T32CA009621, from the National Cancer Institute (NCI).

DISCLOSURE

The authors have nothing to disclose.

REFERENCES

1. Mazzaferro V, Regalia E, Doci R, et al. Liver transplantation for the treatment of small hepatocellular carcinomas in patients with cirrhosis. N Engl J Med 1996; 334(11):693–700.
2. Murray KF, Carithers RL Jr. AASLD practice guidelines: evaluation of the patient for liver transplantation. Hepatology 2005;41(6):1407–32.
3. Yao FY, Ferrell L, Bass NM, et al. Liver transplantation for hepatocellular carcinoma: expansion of the tumor size limits does not adversely impact survival. Hepatology 2001;33(6):1394–403.
4. Elshamy M, Aucejo F, Menon KVN, et al. Hepatocellular carcinoma beyond Milan criteria: Management and transplant selection criteria. World J Hepatol 2016; 8(21):874.
5. Ghouri YA, Mian I, Rowe JH. Review of hepatocellular carcinoma: Epidemiology, etiology, and carcinogenesis. J Carcinog 2017;16.
6. Ioannou GN, Perkins JD, Carithers RL Jr. Liver transplantation for hepatocellular carcinoma: impact of the MELD allocation system and predictors of survival. Gastroenterology 2008;134(5):1342–51.
7. Ishaque T, Massie AB, Bowring MG, et al. Liver transplantation and waitlist mortality for HCC and non-HCC candidates following the 2015 HCC exception policy change. Am J Transplant 2019;19(2):564–72.
8. Rich NE, Parikh ND, Singal AG. Hepatocellular carcinoma and liver transplantation: changing patterns and practices. Curr Treat Options Gastroenterol 2017;15: 296–304.
9. Kwong AJ, Ebel NH, Kim WR, et al. OPTN/SRTR 2021 Annual Data Report: Liver. Am J Transplant 2023;23(2):S178–263.
10. Zimmerman MA, Ghobrial RM, Tong MJ, et al. Recurrence of hepatocellular carcinoma following liver transplantation: a review of preoperative and postoperative prognostic indicators. Arch Surg 2008;143(2):182–8.
11. Silva MF, Sherman M. Criteria for liver transplantation for HCC: what should the limits be? J Hepatol 2011;55(5):1137–47.
12. Halazun KJ, Sapisochin G, von Ahrens D, et al. Predictors of outcome after liver transplantation for hepatocellular carcinoma (HCC) beyond Milan criteria. Int J Surg 2020;82:61–9.
13. Toso C, Trotter J, Wei A, et al. Total tumor volume predicts risk of recurrence following liver transplantation in patients with hepatocellular carcinoma. Liver Transplant 2008;14(8):1107–15.
14. Mazzaferro V, Llovet JM, Miceli R, et al. Predicting survival after liver transplantation in patients with hepatocellular carcinoma beyond the Milan criteria: a retrospective, exploratory analysis. The lancet oncology 2009;10(1):35–43.
15. Halazun KJ, Tabrizian P, Najjar M, et al. Is it time to abandon the Milan criteria?: Results of a bicoastal US collaboration to redefine hepatocellular carcinoma liver transplantation selection policies. Annals of surgery 2018;268(4):690–9.
16. Mahmud N. Selection for liver transplantation: indications and evaluation. Current hepatology reports 2020;19:203–12.
17. Clavien P-A, Lesurtel M, Bossuyt PMM, et al. Recommendations for liver transplantation for hepatocellular carcinoma: an international consensus conference report. The lancet oncology 2012;13(1):e11–22.
18. Kulik L, El-Serag HB. Epidemiology and management of hepatocellular carcinoma. Gastroenterology 2019;156(2):477–91.

19. de'Angelis N, Landi F, Carra MC, et al. Managements of recurrent hepatocellular carcinoma after liver transplantation: A systematic review. World J Gastroenterol 2015;21(39):11185–98.
20. Verna EC, Patel YA, Aggarwal A, et al. Liver transplantation for hepatocellular carcinoma: Management after the transplant. Am J Transplant 2020;20(2):333–47.
21. Mehta N, Heimbach J, Harnois DM, et al. Validation of a Risk Estimation of Tumor Recurrence After Transplant (RETREAT) Score for Hepatocellular Carcinoma Recurrence After Liver Transplant. JAMA Oncol 2017;3(4):493–500.
22. Halazun KJ, Najjar M, Abdelmessih RM, et al. Recurrence After Liver Transplantation for Hepatocellular Carcinoma: A New MORAL to the Story. Ann Surg 2017; 265(3):557–64.
23. van Hooff MC, Sonneveld MJ, Ijzermans JN, et al. External Validation of the RETREAT Score for Prediction of Hepatocellular Carcinoma Recurrence after Liver Transplantation. Cancers 2022;14(3). https://doi.org/10.3390/cancers14030630.
24. Reig M, Forner A, Rimola J, et al. BCLC strategy for prognosis prediction and treatment recommendation: The 2022 update. J Hepatol 2022;76(3):681–93.
25. Boteon A, Boteon YL, Vinuela EF, et al. The impact of transarterial chemoembolization induced complications on outcomes after liver transplantation: A propensity-matched study. Clin Transplant 2018;32(5):e13255.
26. Llovet JM, De Baere T, Kulik L, et al. Locoregional therapies in the era of molecular and immune treatments for hepatocellular carcinoma. Nat Rev Gastroenterol Hepatol 2021;18(5):293–313.
27. Mathew AS, Atenafu EG, Owen D, et al. Long term outcomes of stereotactic body radiation therapy for hepatocellular carcinoma without macrovascular invasion. Eur J Cancer 2020;134:41–51.
28. Walter F, Fuchs F, Gerum S, et al. HDR Brachytherapy and SBRT as Bridging Therapy to Liver Transplantation in HCC Patients: A Single-Center Experience. Front Oncol 2021;11:717792.
29. Sapisochin G, Barry A, Doherty M, et al. Stereotactic body radiotherapy vs. TACE or RFA as a bridge to transplant in patients with hepatocellular carcinoma. An intention-to-treat analysis. J Hepatol 2017;67(1):92–9.
30. Olumba FC, Zhou F, Park Y, et al. Normothermic Machine Perfusion for Declined Livers: A Strategy to Rescue Marginal Livers for Transplantation. J Am Coll Surg 2023;236(4):614–25.
31. Mergental H, Laing RW, Kirkham AJ, et al. Transplantation of discarded livers following viability testing with normothermic machine perfusion. Nat Commun 2020;11(1):2939.
32. Tabrizian P, Holzner ML, Mehta N, et al. Ten-Year Outcomes of Liver Transplant and Downstaging for Hepatocellular Carcinoma. JAMA Surg 2022;157(9):779–88.

Resection Versus Transplant for Hepatocellular Carcinoma: How to Offer the Best Modality

Ioannis A. Ziogas, MD, MPH, Ana L. Gleisner, MD, PhD*

KEYWORDS

- Hepatocellular carcinoma • Liver resection • Liver transplantation • Patient selection

KEY POINTS

- Liver resection and liver transplantation are the mainstay of treatment for the management of hepatocellular carcinoma with a curative intent.
- An accurate assessment of the perioperative risk associated with liver resection is essential when deciding between liver resection and liver transplantation in patients with hepatocellular carcinoma.
- Patients with hepatocellular carcinoma and high risk of disease recurrence such as those with multifocal disease should preferably undergo liver transplantation if eligible.

INTRODUCTION

Hepatocellular carcinoma (HCC), the most common primary liver cancer, ranks as the fifth most prevalent malignancy and the third leading cause of cancer-related deaths worldwide.[1-3] In most cases, HCC originates from chronic liver disease, specifically, hepatitis B (HBV) and C (HCV) virus infections and nonalcoholic steatohepatitis.[4] Although HCC can develop without cirrhosis, particularly in HBV patients, cirrhosis significantly increases the risk of HCC.[5]

The treatment approach for HCC is multifaceted and may involve liver resection, liver transplantation, and regional therapies such as thermal ablation, chemoembolization, and radioembolization, in addition to systemic treatments.[6] A multidisciplinary team, comprising of surgeons, medical oncologists, hepatologists, pathologists, interventional radiologists, radiation oncologists, and social workers, is crucial to strategize the best treatment plan. The ultimate plan takes into account patient factors, such as

Department of Surgery, University of Colorado Anschutz Medical Campus, 12631 East 17th Avenue, Aurora, CO 80045, USA
* Corresponding author. 12631 East 17th Avenue, Aurora, CO 80045.
E-mail address: ana.gleisner@cuanschutz.edu
Twitter: @IA_Ziogas (I.A.Z.); @AnaGleisner (A.L.G.)

Surg Clin N Am 104 (2024) 113–127
https://doi.org/10.1016/j.suc.2023.08.005
0039-6109/24/© 2023 Elsevier Inc. All rights reserved.
surgical.theclinics.com

the presence of comorbidities, frailty, and social status, oncologic factors like tumor extension and vascular invasion, and the status of the underlying liver function. Additional considerations including local expertise, the availability of different treatment modalities, and the supply of grafts for transplantation from deceased and living donors also play a key role in clinical decision-making.

In the absence of metastasis, liver resection, ablation, and transplantation are prioritized, as these treatment modalities are potentially curative. Although liver resection is favored for patients without underlying liver disease, liver transplantation is ideal for those with impaired liver function (**Fig. 1**). Ablation is a suitable option for patients with lesions up to 2 cm, especially if they are not viable candidates for surgical resection or transplantation.yu

For patients with underlying liver disease but preserved liver function, and no obvious contraindications for either liver resection or transplantation, the choice between these 2 treatments options presents one of the biggest controversies in the treatment of patients with HCC. Because liver transplantation addresses occult intrahepatic metastasis as well as the underlying liver disease and, thus, the risk of de novo tumors, patients with HCC treated with liver transplantation have improved disease-free survival compared with those treated with liver resection.[7,8] The risk of recurrence after surgical resection is approximately 3 times higher than after liver transplantation,[9] with recurrence rates up to 80% in 5 years.[10] However, liver transplantation relies on donor availability and requires long-term immunosuppression. Moreover, the improved disease-free survival seen with liver transplantation has not consistently

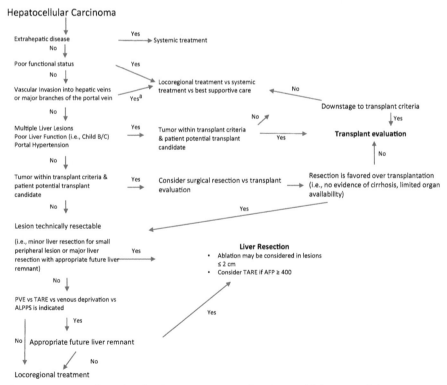

Fig. 1. Treatment algorithm for the management of patients with hepatocellular carcinoma. [a]Surgical resection and liver transplantation may be rarely considered in selected cases.

translated into improved overall survival rates. Although some observational studies have documented improved overall survival for patients with HCC undergoing liver transplantation, both from living donors and deceased donors, compared with surgical resection,[8,11] other studies found no significant difference in overall survival between these treatments.[7,12] In a recent meta-analysis including patients with HCC within the Milan criteria, there was no difference in overall survival between liver resection and liver transplantation for patients with solitary lesions and when the analysis was restricted to studies published in 2010 and beyond.[9] In the absence of data from randomized trials, the survival benefit of liver transplantation over surgical resection in patients with HCC remains uncertain.

Therefore, when choosing between transplantation and resection for patients eligible for either treatment, a comprehensive evaluation of the associated risks is required. This includes the risks related to resection, specifically the threat of post-hepatectomy liver failure (PHLF), as well as the risk of tumor recurrence, all within the context of local donor availability.

RISK OF SURGICAL RESECTION

The risk of surgical resection depends on the patients' performance status and comorbidities, the scope of the liver resection, and the function of the remaining liver. Most of the morbidity and mortality related to liver resection in patients with HCC and underlying liver disease are attributed to the size and function of the remaining liver and the ensuing development of PHLF.[13] The extent of the resection is based on the size and location of the lesion, especially related to the proximity to main vascular and biliary structures. Peripheral lesions, even larger ones, are often easily surgically resected. Deeper lesions near the liver inflow or outflow often require a major hepatectomy for surgical resection with negative margins. Ideally, the lesions should be resected with at least 1 cm margins, as narrower margins have been associated with increased recurrence rates after resection.[14] Nonetheless, the impact of surgical margins and recurrence may be at least partially mediated by the frequent association between narrow margins and other features associated with increased risk of recurrence, such as vascular invasion and/or presence of satellite lesions.[10] Early intrahepatic recurrences are often thought to be intrahepatic metastasis, something that cannot be prevented with wider margins. When planning a liver resection for a patient with HCC, the surgeon needs to balance the potential benefit of wider margins with the risk of PHLF.

For patients with cirrhosis-induced portal hypertension, the risk of PHLF and death is typically considered too high to justify surgical resection.[15] The diagnosis of portal hypertension relies on several findings, including thrombocytopenia (platelets < 100×10^9/L), splenomegaly, ascites, and/or a history of variceal bleeding. Of note, the function of the liver might not correspond with the degree of portal hypertension. If the presence of portal hypertension is suspected but not obvious, a direct measurement of the hepatic venous wedge pressure and gradient can be pursued. Patients with a hepatic venous pressure gradient equal to or exceeding 10 mm Hg are usually deemed to be at excessive risk for liver decompensation and death after surgical resection.[16] For these patients, liver transplantation is a better option. If no other alternatives are available, resection can be considered in selected cases.[17]

In patients with cirrhosis, liver function is typically evaluated using several scoring systems, including the Child-Pugh (CP) classification,[18] the Model for End-stage Liver Disease (MELD) score,[19,20] and the Albumin-Bilirubin (ALBI) score[21] (**Table 1**). The CP classification has traditionally been employed to assess the feasibility of liver resection in patients with cirrhosis. Generally, patients with CP class A cirrhosis without portal

Table 1
Liver function scoring systems

Child-Pugh Classification[18]	1 point	2 points	3 points
Albumin, g/dL	> 3.5	3.0–3.5	< 3.0
Bilirubin, mg/dL	< 2.0	2.0–3.0	> 3.0
INR	< 1.7	1.7–2.3	> 2.3
Ascites	Absent	Slight	Moderate
Encephalopathy	None	Grade I–II (mild to moderate)	Grade III–IV (severe)

Class A: 5–6 points; Class B: 7–9 points; Class C: 10–15 points

MELD score[19,20]

MELD score = $0.957 \times \ln(Cr) + 0.378 \times \ln(bilirubin) + 1.120 \times \ln(INR) + 0.643$

MELD 3.0 = $1.33*(Female) + 4.56*\ln(Serum\ bilirubin) + 0.82*(137 - Sodium) - 0.24*(137 - Sodium)*\ln(Serum\ bilirubin) + 9.09*\ln(INR) + 11.14*\ln(Serum\ creatinine) + 1.85*(3.5 - Serum\ albumin) - 1.83*(3.5 - Serum\ albumin)*\ln(Serum\ creatinine) + 6$

ALBI score[21]

ALBI = $(\log_{10} bilirubin \times 0.66) + (albumin \times -0.085)$, where bilirubin is in μmol/L and albumin in g/L

Score	Grade	Median survival
≤ −2.60	1	18.5–85.6 mo
> −2.60 to ≤ −1.39	2	5.3–46.5 mo
> −1.39	3	2.3–15.5 mo

hypertension are seen as potential candidates for liver resection,[22–24] whereas CP class B or C cirrhosis is generally deemed a contraindication for liver resection.[25,26] The MELD score can also be used to determine hepatic reserve and suitability for liver resection.[6] However, while some authors have found that the MELD score was better than the CP class to predict perioperative morbidity and mortality in patients undergoing liver resection,[27] others have found that the MELD score tends to cluster in the lower range in this patient population and it was not helpful at predicting outcomes.[28] In fact, the main shortcoming of both the CP classification and the MELD score in this scenario seems to derive from the fact that these classification systems were developed in patients with end-stage liver disease. And while some patients with HCC being evaluated for liver resection have cirrhosis, others may have mild liver abnormalities and some degree of fibrosis but no established cirrhosis. The ALBI score was specifically developed in patients with HCC in all stages to address these limitations, using only the albumin and total bilirubin levels.[21] The ALBI score has since been shown to predict PHLF in patients undergoing liver resection for a variety of diagnosis,[19–21,29] and better at predicting perioperative outcomes compared with the MELD score.[13,29] In a recent study analyzing 13,783 patients who underwent liver resection from 2014 to 2017 extracted from the American College of Surgeons National Surgical Quality Improvement Program (NSQIP), the ALBI score was a stronger predictor than the MELD score for PHLF and survival. In addition, in patients who underwent liver resection for HCC, the ALBI score had better discrimination than the MELD score for severe PHLF (area under the curve 0.67 vs 0.60) and for mortality (area under the curve 0.70 vs 0.58).[29] Differently than the MELD score, the ALBI seems sufficiently sensitive to detect early deterioration of liver function.[30] Nevertheless, the utility of the ALBI score to appropriately select patients for liver resection remains to be determine. In the aforementioned study, even though 30-day mortality was significantly higher for patients with ALBI grade 3 (9.2% vs 0.8% for ALBI grade 1% and 2.5% for ALBI grade 2), only 3% of the patients included in the study had an ALBI grade 3.

A more dynamic assessment of the liver function can be performed through the indocyanine green clearance test.[31] Although this test is not frequently used in North America, it is standard for preoperative risk assessment in major hepatectomies in many institutions worldwide. Results from the indocyanine green clearance test can be combined to the extent of liver resection to select appropriate patients for surgical resection. Using this strategy, Imamura and colleagues[32] reported only one postoperative death among 1429 consecutive hepatectomies in a single center.

For a major hepatectomy, liver volumetry should be performed to calculate the volume of the future liver remnant (FLR). In the absence of cirrhosis, liver resection is well tolerated if the FLR is at least 25% to 30% of the predicted liver volume.[33,34] In patients with cirrhosis, the size of the liver remnant should be at least 40%.[35] In patients with an inadequate FLR, different methods can be used to optimize postoperative outcomes, including preoperative portal vein embolization (PVE),[36] transarterial radioembolization (TARE),[37] liver venous deprivation (simultaneous portal and hepatic vein embolization),[38] and associating liver partition with portal vein ligation (ALPPS).[39] ALPPS is associated with faster and increased hypertrophy of the FLR compared with the other techniques. In a recent meta-analyses, the pooled estimate of mean percent FLR hypertrophy was 30.9% over 40.3 ± 26.3 days for PVE, 29.0% over 138.5 ± 56.5 days for TARE, and 54.9% over 11.1 ± 3.1 days for ALPPS.[40] Because up to a third of the patients who undergo PVE will end up foregoing liver resection due to inadequate FLR growth or tumor progression on follow-up,[41–43] ALPPS has been associated with increased rates of successful liver resection. However, that comes with increased morbidity and mortality risks compared with the other modalities.[40,44,45] A recent meta-analysis suggests that liver venous deprivation may lead to FLR hypertrophy equivalent to that of ALPPS with lower morbidity and mortality, yet after a longer waiting time interval.[38]

Emerging approaches strive to evaluate both the volume and function of the FLR, including after PVE and ALPPS. For instance, (^{99m}) Tc-labeled mebrofenin hepatobiliary scintigraphy (HS) has shown superior sensitivity, specificity, and positive and negative predictive values for predicting PHLF compared with liver volumetry.[46,47] Gadoxetic acid-enhanced MRI can also be used to assess the liver's volumetric and functional capacity,[48] with results akin to those obtained with HS.[49] In a recent systematic review, the sensitivity of gadoxetic acid-enhanced MRI parameter varied from 75% to 100%, whereas the specificity varied from 54% to 93%.[50] However, the studies were limited by a significant heterogeneity in regard to the MRI parameters used as well as the indication and extent of liver resection. Despite their promising capabilities, both HS and gadoxetic acid-enhanced MRI are yet to be widely adopted in the selection of candidates for liver resection. In North America, decisions regarding liver resection for patients with HCC are still primarily based on liver volumetrics and function as determined by the CP classification and signs of portal hypertension.

Minimally invasive approaches have gradually emerged in the field of liver surgery.[51–53] This approach has consistently been associated with improved perioperative outcomes in multiple observational studies,[54–57] as well as in recent randomized trials in patients with colorectal liver metastasis,[58–60] with long-term results that are at least comparable to open surgery. In patients with HCC and chronic liver disease, the minimally invasive approach has been associated with decreased rates of liver failure and ascites compared with open surgery,[61] including in selected patients with portal hypertension[17] and CP class B cirrhosis.[62] Importantly, minimally invasive approaches could also offer an additional advantage for patients that may eventually require a liver transplant, as it may simplify this procedure.

RISK OF RECURRENCE

The risk of tumor recurrence is a critical factor in deciding the suitability of both liver resection and transplantation. Several factors have been shown to be associated with higher risk of tumor recurrence (**Box 1**).[63–67]

When considering liver transplantation for patients with HCC, the risk of tumor recurrence is mainly based on the size and number of lesions. These parameters dictate transplant eligibility and organ allocation. In a groundbreaking paper published in 1996, Mazzaferro and colleagues[68] showed that patients with a single HCC less than 5 cm in diameter or with up to 3 lesions, none larger than less than 3 cm in diameter, universally known as the Milan criteria, experienced excellent outcomes following liver transplantation, with a 4 year survival rate of 75% and a recurrence-free survival rate of 83%. This led to the wide adoption of the Milan criteria and the inclusion of liver transplantation as a pivotal treatment option for patients with HCC. However, concerns regarding the restrictive nature of the Milan criteria prompted several groups to attempt to broaden the liver transplant indications for HCC.[69] Most notably, the University College of San Francisco (UCSF) established the UCSF criteria in 2001; these criteria include a single HCC lesion less than 6.5 cm in diameter or fewer than 3 lesions with the largest less than 4.5 cm in diameter and total tumor diameter less than 8 cm, which resulted in a 5 year survival rate of 75.2%.[70] The most commonly used criteria to liver transplantation eligibility in patients with HCC are summarized in **Table 2**.[68–74]

Predictably, tumor size is also one of the main risk factors of recurrence following liver resection, with tumors greater than 5 cm in diameter having a specially high risk of recurrence, both intrahepatic and extrahepatic.[75] However, the association between size and risk of recurrence may be at least partially mediated by the frequent prevalence of vascular invasion and poor histologic grade in patients with larger tumor.[76] Some studies have shown that, in the absence of vascular invasion, size is not prognostic factor after liver resection for HCC.[77] In fact, even patients with tumors greater than 10 cm can have favorable outcomes after surgical resection so long there is no evidence of vascular invasion.[78] Likewise, although presence of vascular invasion, either gross or microscopic, is a strong predictor of recurrence and survival,[79,80]

Box 1
Factors associated with disease recurrence in patients with hepatocellular carcinoma

Number of lesions

Tumor size

Alpha-fetoprotein level

Satellite nodules

Vascular invasion

Histologic grade

Tumor rupture

Nodal disease status

Underlying cirrhosis

Resection margin

Table 2
Criteria used to select patients with hepatocellular carcinoma for liver transplantation

Criteria	Description	Survival
Milan (1996)[68]	Single lesion < 5 cm in diameter or no more than 3 lesions with the largest < 3 cm in diameter	4 year actuarial survival: 75% 4 year recurrence-free survival: 83%
UCSF (2001)[70]	Single lesion < 6.5 cm in diameter or less than 3 lesions with the largest < 4.5 cm in diameter and total tumor diameter < 8 cm	5 year overall survival: 75.2%
Tokyo (2007)[71]	Up to 5 lesions < 5 cm in diameter	5 year overall survival: 75% 5 year recurrence-free survival: 90%
Kyoto (2007)[72]	Up to 10 tumors all of which $\leq$ 5 cm in diameter and serum protein induced by vitamin K absence or antagonist-II $\leq$ 400 mAU/mL	5 year overall survival: 86.7%
Up-to-seven (2009)[73]	Seven as the sum of the size of the largest lesion (in cm) and the number of lesions	5 year overall survival: 71.2%
Extended Toronto (2016)[74]	Any size or number of tumors, no systemic cancer-related symptoms, extrahepatic disease, vascular invasion, or poorly differentiated tumors	5 year overall survival: 78% (within Milan) vs 68% (beyond Milan)

its prognostic significance is questionable in patients with tumors less than or equal to 2 cm.[81] Because of that, both solitary tumors of any size without vascular invasion and solitary tumors less than or equal to 2 cm with or without microvascular invasion are considered T1 tumors in the most recent American Joint Committee on Cancer (AJCC) staging system (**Table 3**). Yet, because presence of microvascular invasion cannot be determined until the tumor is resected, this classification is not useful when deciding between liver resection and liver transplantation.

For patients harboring tumors larger than 2 cm, presence of microvascular invasion is a strong predictor of recurrence.[82] Therefore, liver transplantation often yields superior long-term outcomes compared with surgery in these patients, assuming they fall within the aforementioned transplant criteria. However, since diagnosing microvascular invasion requires removal of the specimen, its presence cannot be used as a determining factor when deciding between resection and transplantation for a patient who qualifies for either treatment. In some centers, liver transplantation is recommended for patients who, upon resection, exhibit microvascular invasion in their final pathology. Sala and colleagues[83] demonstrated the effectiveness of salvage liver transplant to resected patients in whom pathology evidenced high recurrence risk even in the absence of proven residual disease. This ab initio liver transplantation approach was prospectively validated with a minimum of 6 months before enlistment to prevent patients with more aggressive tumors from undergoing liver transplantation.[84]

In comparison to microvascular invasion, gross macrovascular invasion can often be diagnosed on imaging. Portal vein thrombosis must be differentiated from a bland thrombus in the portal system. The latter exhibits neither enhancement nor continuity

Table 3
Hepatocellular carcinoma TNM staging from the American Joint Committee on Cancer, 8th edition

Primary Tumor (T)	
T Category	**T Criteria**
TX	Primary tumor cannot be assessed
T0	No evidence of primary tumor
T1	Solitary tumor ≤ 2 cm, or > 2 cm without vascular invasion
T1a	Solitary tumor ≤ 2 cm
T1b	Solitary tumor > 2 cm without vascular invasion
T2	Solitary tumor > 2 cm with vascular invasion, or multiple tumors, none > 5 cm
T3	Multiple tumors, at least one of which is > 5 cm
T4	Single tumor or multiple tumors of any size involving a major branch of the portal vein or hepatic vein or tumor(s) with direct invasion of adjacent organs other than the gallbladder or with perforation of visceral peritoneum

with the primary tumor. The presence of portal vein tumor thrombosis or hepatic vein tumor thrombosis is considered a marker of poor tumor biology. Liver resection or transplantation is rarely considered for these patients.[85–87]

Multifocal disease is also associated with an elevated risk of recurrence—the greater the number of lesions, the higher the recurrence risk.[88] If eligible, patients with multifocal disease should undergo liver transplantation.[89] For those who do not qualify for transplantation, surgical resection may be considered in a case-by-case basis. However, it remains unclear which subset of patients, if any, are more likely to benefit from surgery over less invasive regional treatments.[90] For instance, a recent study showed that liver resection is likely futile in patients with HBV/HCV, more than 3 liver lesions, and alpha-fetoprotein levels greater than 200 ng/mL.[91]

Elevated alpha-fetoprotein levels have been associated with tumor recurrence, regardless of the size and number of lesions.[91,92] New models to determine transplant eligibility in patients with HCC have incorporated alpha-fetoprotein levels alongside the number and size of liver lesions to improve patient selection, such as the French alpha-fetoprotein model[93] and Metroticket 2.0 model.[94] In line with this approach, our team occasionally opts for TARE in patients presenting a large tumor coupled with heightened alpha-fetoprotein levels, employing it as a "bridge to resection". Using this approach, not only does the FLR experience hypertrophy, but potential extrahepatic disease may also be revealed, potentially sparing the patient the risks associated with a surgical procedure that would not yield any benefit.[95]

Finally, tumor histologic grade is strong predictor of tumor recurrence in patients with HCC who undergo both liver resection[96] and liver transplantation.[97,98] Patients with large solitary tumors exhibiting well or moderately differentiated histologic grades have a favorable long-term prognosis after surgical resection compared with those with poorly differentiated tumors.[99] However, the histologic grade cannot be accurately determined via a biopsy, which limits the utility of grade in patient selection for surgical resection or liver transplantation.[100]

SUMMARY

When considering surgical resection in a patient with HCC and underlying liver disease who is also within transplant criteria, it is imperative to precisely estimate the risks associated with surgical resection in addition to the risk of long-term recurrence. Patients with portal hypertension are at high risk of PHLF and are best served by liver transplantation. Similarly, patients with CP class B or C cirrhosis or a high ALBI or MELD score should preferably undergo liver transplantation over resection. For patients without cirrhosis or those with CP class A cirrhosis and no portal hypertension, liver resection should be considered if the size and function of the FLR are appropriate, especially if organ availability is a concern. Peripheral lesions that require a limited resection of the liver can typically be safely performed. When a major liver resection is required, liver volumetry must be performed, and different strategies can be applied to assure the FLR is adequate. Emerging methods to evaluate both the size and function of the FLR may be useful for the selection of patients for whom liver resection can be performed safely. Liver resection should be performed through the minimally invasive approach when possible as this approach may be associated with decrease perioperative complications, including PHLF. For patients with high risk of intrahepatic recurrence, such as those with multifocal disease, liver transplantation should be favored over resection, as liver transplantation addresses both occult intrahepatic metastasis and the underlying liver disease.

CLINICS CARE POINTS

- For patients without cirrhosis or those with CP class A cirrhosis and no portal hypertension, liver resection should be considered if the size and function of the FLR are appropriate, especially if organ availability is a concern.
- For patients with high risk of intrahepatic recurrence, such as those with multifocal disease, liver transplantation should be favored over resection, as liver transplantation addresses both occult intrahepatic metastasis and the underlying liver disease.

DISCLOSURE

The authors have nothing to disclose.

REFERENCES

1. Global Burden of Disease Liver Cancer C, Akinyemiju T, Abera S, et al. The burden of primary liver cancer and underlying etiologies from 1990 to 2015 at the global, regional, and national level: results from the global burden of disease study 2015. JAMA Oncol 2017;3(12):1683–91.
2. European Association for the Study of the Liver. Electronic address eee, European Association for the Study of the L. EASL Clinical Practice Guidelines: Management of hepatocellular carcinoma. J Hepatol 2018;69(1):182–236.
3. Siegel RL, Miller KD, Jemal A. Cancer statistics. CA A Cancer J Clin 2020; 70(1):7–30.
4. Forner A, Llovet JM, Bruix J. Hepatocellular carcinoma. Lancet 2012;379(9822): 1245–55.
5. Tarao K, Nozaki A, Ikeda T, et al. Real impact of liver cirrhosis on the development of hepatocellular carcinoma in various liver diseases-meta-analytic assessment. Cancer Med 2019;8(3):1054–65.
6. Reig M, Forner A, Rimola J, et al. BCLC strategy for prognosis prediction and treatment recommendation: The 2022 update. J Hepatol 2022;76(3):681–93.

7. Menahem B, Lubrano J, Duvoux C, et al. Liver transplantation versus liver resection for hepatocellular carcinoma in intention to treat: An attempt to perform an ideal meta-analysis. Liver Transplant 2017;23(6):836–44.

8. Li W, Li L, Han J, et al. Liver transplantation vs liver resection in patients with HBV-related hepatocellular carcinoma beyond Milan criterion: A meta-analysis. Clin Transplant 2018;32(3):e13193.

9. Koh JH, Tan DJH, Ong Y, et al. Liver resection versus liver transplantation for hepatocellular carcinoma within Milan criteria: a meta-analysis of 18,421 patients. Hepatobiliary Surg Nutr 2022;11(1):78–93.

10. Poon RT, Fan ST, Ng IO, et al. Significance of resection margin in hepatectomy for hepatocellular carcinoma: A critical reappraisal. Ann Surg 2000;231(4): 544–51.

11. Li W, Xiao H, Wu H, et al. Liver Transplantation Versus Liver Resection for Stage I and II Hepatocellular Carcinoma: Results of an Instrumental Variable Analysis. Front Oncol 2021;11:592835.

12. Karakas S, Yilmaz S, Ince V, et al. Comparison of liver resection and living donor liver transplantation in patients with hepatocellular carcinoma within Milan criteria and well-preserved liver function. Hepatol Forum 2023;4(2):47–52.

13. Morandi A, Risaliti M, Montori M, et al. Predicting Post-Hepatectomy Liver Failure in HCC Patients: A Review of Liver Function Assessment Based on Laboratory Tests Scores. Medicina (Kaunas) 2023;(6):59.

14. Tsilimigras DI, Sahara K, Moris D, et al. Effect of Surgical Margin Width on Patterns of Recurrence among Patients Undergoing R0 Hepatectomy for T1 Hepatocellular Carcinoma: An International Multi-Institutional Analysis. J Gastrointest Surg 2020;24(7):1552–60.

15. Berzigotti A, Reig M, Abraldes JG, et al. Portal hypertension and the outcome of surgery for hepatocellular carcinoma in compensated cirrhosis: a systematic review and meta-analysis. Hepatology 2015;61(2):526–36.

16. Bruix J, Castells A, Bosch J, et al. Surgical resection of hepatocellular carcinoma in cirrhotic patients: prognostic value of preoperative portal pressure. Gastroenterology 1996;111(4):1018–22.

17. Azoulay D, Ramos E, Casellas-Robert M, et al. Liver resection for hepatocellular carcinoma in patients with clinically significant portal hypertension. JHEP Rep 2021;3(1):100190.

18. Pugh RN, Murray-Lyon IM, Dawson JL, et al. Transection of the oesophagus for bleeding oesophageal varices. Br J Surg 1973;60(8):646–9.

19. Kamath PS, Wiesner RH, Malinchoc M, et al. A model to predict survival in patients with end-stage liver disease. Hepatology 2001;33(2):464–70.

20. Kim WR, Mannalithara A, Heimbach JK, et al. MELD 3.0: The Model for End-Stage Liver Disease Updated for the Modern Era. Gastroenterology 2021; 161(6):1887–95.e4.

21. Johnson PJ, Berhane S, Kagebayashi C, et al. Assessment of liver function in patients with hepatocellular carcinoma: a new evidence-based approach-the ALBI grade. J Clin Oncol 2015;33(6):550–8.

22. Kusano T, Sasaki A, Kai S, et al. Predictors and prognostic significance of operative complications in patients with hepatocellular carcinoma who underwent hepatic resection. Eur J Surg Oncol 2009;35(11):1179–85.

23. Giuliante F, Ardito F, Pinna AD, et al. Liver resection for hepatocellular carcinoma </=3 cm: results of an Italian multicenter study on 588 patients. J Am Coll Surg 2012;215(2):244–54.

24. Kabir T, Syn NL, Tan ZZX, et al. Predictors of post-operative complications after surgical resection of hepatocellular carcinoma and their prognostic effects on outcome and survival: A propensity-score matched and structural equation modelling study. Eur J Surg Oncol 2020;46(9):1756–65.
25. Berardi G, Morise Z, Sposito C, et al. Development of a nomogram to predict outcome after liver resection for hepatocellular carcinoma in Child-Pugh B cirrhosis. J Hepatol 2020;72(1):75–84.
26. Tanaka S, Noda T, Komeda K, et al. Surgical Outcomes for Hepatocellular Carcinoma in Patients with Child-Pugh Class B: a Retrospective Multicenter Study. J Gastrointest Surg 2023;27(2):283–95.
27. Teh SH, Christein J, Donohue J, et al. Hepatic resection of hepatocellular carcinoma in patients with cirrhosis: Model of End-Stage Liver Disease (MELD) score predicts perioperative mortality. J Gastrointest Surg 2005;9(9):1207–15 [discussion: 1215].
28. Schroeder RA, Marroquin CE, Bute BP, et al. Predictive indices of morbidity and mortality after liver resection. Ann Surg 2006;243(3):373–9.
29. Fagenson AM, Gleeson EM, Pitt HA, et al. Albumin-Bilirubin Score vs Model for End-Stage Liver Disease in Predicting Post-Hepatectomy Outcomes. J Am Coll Surg 2020;230(4):637–45.
30. Toyoda H, Johnson PJ. The ALBI score: From liver function in patients with HCC to a general measure of liver function. JHEP Rep 2022;4(10):100557.
31. Hoekstra LT, de Graaf W, Nibourg GA, et al. Physiological and biochemical basis of clinical liver function tests: a review. Ann Surg 2013;257(1):27–36.
32. Imamura H, Sano K, Sugawara Y, et al. Assessment of hepatic reserve for indication of hepatic resection: decision tree incorporating indocyanine green test. J Hepatobiliary Pancreat Surg 2005;12(1):16–22.
33. Vauthey JN, Chaoui A, Do KA, et al. Standardized measurement of the future liver remnant prior to extended liver resection: methodology and clinical associations. Surgery 2000;127(5):512–9.
34. Shoup M, Gonen M, D'Angelica M, et al. Volumetric analysis predicts hepatic dysfunction in patients undergoing major liver resection. J Gastrointest Surg 2003;7(3):325–30.
35. Ribero D, Chun YS, Vauthey JN. Standardized liver volumetry for portal vein embolization. Semin Intervent Radiol 2008;25(2):104–9.
36. Kinoshita H, Sakai K, Hirohashi K, et al. Preoperative portal vein embolization for hepatocellular carcinoma. World J Surg 1986;10(5):803–8.
37. Vouche M, Lewandowski RJ, Atassi R, et al. Radiation lobectomy: time-dependent analysis of future liver remnant volume in unresectable liver cancer as a bridge to resection. J Hepatol 2013;59(5):1029–36.
38. Gavriilidis P, Marangoni G, Ahmad J, et al. Simultaneous portal and hepatic vein embolization is better than portal embolization or ALPPS for hypertrophy of future liver remnant before major hepatectomy: A systematic review and network meta-analysis. Hepatobiliary Pancreat Dis Int 2023;22(3):221–7.
39. Schnitzbauer AA, Lang SA, Goessmann H, et al. Right portal vein ligation combined with in situ splitting induces rapid left lateral liver lobe hypertrophy enabling 2-staged extended right hepatic resection in small-for-size settings. Ann Surg 2012;255(3):405–14.
40. Charalel RA, Sung J, Askin G, et al. Systematic Reviews and Meta-Analyses of Portal Vein Embolization, Associated Liver Partition and Portal Vein Ligation, and Radiation Lobectomy Outcomes in Hepatocellular Carcinoma Patients. Curr Oncol Rep 2021;23(11):135.

41. Broering DC, Hillert C, Krupski G, et al. Portal vein embolization vs. portal vein ligation for induction of hypertrophy of the future liver remnant. J Gastrointest Surg 2002;6(6):905–13 [discussion: 913].

42. Abulkhir A, Limongelli P, Healey AJ, et al. Preoperative portal vein embolization for major liver resection: a meta-analysis. Ann Surg 2008;247(1):49–57.

43. Shindoh J, Vauthey JN, Zimmitti G, et al. Analysis of the efficacy of portal vein embolization for patients with extensive liver malignancy and very low future liver remnant volume, including a comparison with the associating liver partition with portal vein ligation for staged hepatectomy approach. J Am Coll Surg. Jul 2013;217(1):126–33 [discussion: 133-4].

44. Schadde E, Ardiles V, Slankamenac K, et al. ALPPS offers a better chance of complete resection in patients with primarily unresectable liver tumors compared with conventional-staged hepatectomies: results of a multicenter analysis. World J Surg 2014;38(6):1510–9.

45. Chia DKA, Yeo Z, Loh SEK, et al. Greater hypertrophy can be achieved with associating liver partition with portal vein ligation for staged hepatectomy compared to conventional staged hepatectomy, but with a higher price to pay? Am J Surg 2018;215(1):131–7.

46. de Graaf W, van Lienden KP, Dinant S, et al. Assessment of future remnant liver function using hepatobiliary scintigraphy in patients undergoing major liver resection. J Gastrointest Surg 2010;14(2):369–78.

47. de Graaf W, van Lienden KP, van den Esschert JW, et al. Increase in future remnant liver function after preoperative portal vein embolization. Br J Surg 2011;98(6):825–34.

48. Yoon JH, Lee JM, Kang HJ, et al. Quantitative Assessment of Liver Function by Using Gadoxetic Acid-enhanced MRI: Hepatocyte Uptake Ratio. Radiology 2019;290(1):125–33.

49. Wang Q, Brismar TB, Gilg S, et al. Multimodal perioperative assessment of liver function and volume in patients undergoing hepatectomy for colorectal liver metastasis: a comparison of the indocyanine green retention test, (99m)Tc mebrofenin hepatobiliary scintigraphy and gadoxetic acid enhanced MRI. Br J Radiol 2022;95(1139):20220370.

50. Wang Q, Wang A, Sparrelid E, et al. Predictive value of gadoxetic acid-enhanced MRI for posthepatectomy liver failure: a systematic review. Eur Radiol 2022;32(3):1792–803.

51. Carpenter EL, Thomas KK, Adams AM, et al. Modern trends in minimally invasive versus open hepatectomy for colorectal liver metastasis: an analysis of ACS-NSQIP. Surg Endosc 2023;37(7):5591–602.

52. Ziogas IA, Giannis D, Esagian SM, et al. Laparoscopic versus robotic major hepatectomy: a systematic review and meta-analysis. Surg Endosc 2021; 35(2):524–35.

53. Ziogas IA, Tsoulfas G. Advances and challenges in laparoscopic surgery in the management of hepatocellular carcinoma. World J Gastrointest Surg 2017; 9(12):233–45.

54. Sotiropoulos GC, Prodromidou A, Machairas N. Meta-analysis of laparoscopic vs open liver resection for hepatocellular carcinoma: The European experience. J buon 2017;22(5):1160–71.

55. Goh EL, Chidambaram S, Ma S. Laparoscopic vs open hepatectomy for hepatocellular carcinoma in patients with cirrhosis: A meta-analysis of the long-term survival outcomes. Int J Surg 2018;50:35–42.

56. Lu Q, Zhang N, Wang F, et al. Surgical and oncological outcomes after laparoscopic vs. open major hepatectomy for hepatocellular carcinoma: a systematic review and meta-analysis. Transl Cancer Res 2020;9(5):3324–38.

57. Wang Q, Li HJ, Dai XM, et al. Laparoscopic versus open liver resection for hepatocellular carcinoma in elderly patients: Systematic review and meta-analysis of propensity-score matched studies. Int J Surg 2022;105:106821.

58. Fretland A, Dagenborg VJ, Bjørnelv GMW, et al. Laparoscopic Versus Open Resection for Colorectal Liver Metastases: The OSLO-COMET Randomized Controlled Trial. Ann Surg 2018;267(2):199–207.

59. Aghayan DL, Kazaryan AM, Dagenborg VJ, et al. Long-Term Oncologic Outcomes After Laparoscopic Versus Open Resection for Colorectal Liver Metastases : A Randomized Trial. Ann Intern Med 2021;174(2):175–82.

60. Robles-Campos R, Lopez-Lopez V, Brusadin R, et al. Open versus minimally invasive liver surgery for colorectal liver metastases (LapOpHuva): a prospective randomized controlled trial. Surg Endosc 2019;33(12):3926–36.

61. Morise Z, Ciria R, Cherqui D, et al. Can we expand the indications for laparoscopic liver resection? A systematic review and meta-analysis of laparoscopic liver resection for patients with hepatocellular carcinoma and chronic liver disease. J Hepatobiliary Pancreat Sci 2015;22(5):342–52.

62. Troisi RI, Berardi G, Morise Z, et al. Laparoscopic and open liver resection for hepatocellular carcinoma with Child-Pugh B cirrhosis: multicentre propensity score-matched study. Br J Surg 2021;108(2):196–204.

63. Li J, Wang WQ, Zhu RH, et al. Postoperative adjuvant tyrosine kinase inhibitors combined with anti-PD-1 antibodies improves surgical outcomes for hepatocellular carcinoma with high-risk recurrent factors. Front Immunol 2023;14:1202039.

64. Kim BW, Kim YB, Wang HJ, et al. Risk factors for immediate post-operative fatal recurrence after curative resection of hepatocellular carcinoma. World J Gastroenterol 2006;12(1):99–104.

65. Tung-Ping Poon R, Fan ST, Wong J. Risk factors, prevention, and management of postoperative recurrence after resection of hepatocellular carcinoma. Ann Surg 2000;232(1):10–24.

66. Shinkawa H, Tanaka S, Takemura S, et al. Nomograms predicting extra- and early intrahepatic recurrence after hepatic resection of hepatocellular carcinoma. Surgery 2021;169(4):922–8.

67. Shah SA, Cleary SP, Wei AC, et al. Recurrence after liver resection for hepatocellular carcinoma: risk factors, treatment, and outcomes. Surgery 2007;141(3):330–9.

68. Mazzaferro V, Regalia E, Doci R, et al. Liver transplantation for the treatment of small hepatocellular carcinomas in patients with cirrhosis. N Engl J Med 1996;334(11):693–9.

69. Ziogas IA, Tsoulfas G. The evolution of criteria for liver transplantation for hepatocellular carcinoma: from milan to san francisco and all around the world. Revista de la Facultad de Medicina Humana 2017;17(3).

70. Yao FY, Ferrell L, Bass NM, et al. Liver transplantation for hepatocellular carcinoma: expansion of the tumor size limits does not adversely impact survival. Hepatology 2001;33(6):1394–403.

71. Sugawara Y, Tamura S, Makuuchi M. Living donor liver transplantation for hepatocellular carcinoma: Tokyo University series. Dig Dis 2007;25(4):310–2.

72. Ito T, Takada Y, Ueda M, et al. Expansion of selection criteria for patients with hepatocellular carcinoma in living donor liver transplantation. Liver Transplant 2007;13(12):1637–44.

73. Mazzaferro V, Llovet JM, Miceli R, et al. Predicting survival after liver transplantation in patients with hepatocellular carcinoma beyond the Milan criteria: a retrospective, exploratory analysis. Lancet Oncol 2009;10(1):35–43.

74. Sapisochin G, Goldaracena N, Laurence JM, et al. The extended Toronto criteria for liver transplantation in patients with hepatocellular carcinoma: A prospective validation study. Hepatology 2016;64(6):2077–88.

75. Liang BY, Gu J, Xiong M, et al. Tumor size may influence the prognosis of solitary hepatocellular carcinoma patients with cirrhosis and without macrovascular invasion after hepatectomy. Sci Rep 2021;11(1):16343.

76. Pawlik TM, Delman KA, Vauthey JN, et al. Tumor size predicts vascular invasion and histologic grade: Implications for selection of surgical treatment for hepatocellular carcinoma. Liver Transplant 2005;11(9):1086–92.

77. Shah SA, Wei AC, Cleary SP, et al. Prognosis and results after resection of very large (>or=10 cm) hepatocellular carcinoma. J Gastrointest Surg 2007;11(5): 589–95.

78. Poon RT, Fan ST, Wong J. Selection criteria for hepatic resection in patients with large hepatocellular carcinoma larger than 10 cm in diameter. J Am Coll Surg 2002;194(5):592–602.

79. Nathan H, Schulick RD, Choti MA, et al. Predictors of survival after resection of early hepatocellular carcinoma. Ann Surg 2009;249(5):799–805.

80. Cha C, Fong Y, Jarnagin WR, et al. Predictors and patterns of recurrence after resection of hepatocellular carcinoma. J Am Coll Surg 2003;197(5):753–8.

81. Shindoh J, Andreou A, Aloia TA, et al. Microvascular invasion does not predict long-term survival in hepatocellular carcinoma up to 2 cm: reappraisal of the staging system for solitary tumors. Ann Surg Oncol 2013;20(4):1223–9.

82. Shindoh J, Kobayashi Y, Kawamura Y, et al. Microvascular Invasion and a Size Cutoff Value of 2 cm Predict Long-Term Oncological Outcome in Multiple Hepatocellular Carcinoma: Reappraisal of the American Joint Committee on Cancer Staging System and Validation Using the Surveillance, Epidemiology, and End-Results Database. Liver Cancer 2020;9(2):156–66.

83. Sala M, Fuster J, Llovet JM, et al. High pathological risk of recurrence after surgical resection for hepatocellular carcinoma: an indication for salvage liver transplantation. Liver Transplant 2004;10(10):1294–300.

84. Ferrer-Fàbrega J, Forner A, Liccioni A, et al. Prospective validation of ab initio liver transplantation in hepatocellular carcinoma upon detection of risk factors for recurrence after resection. Hepatology 2016;63(3):839–49.

85. Wang YC, Lee JC, Wu TH, et al. Improving outcomes of liver resection for hepatocellular carcinoma associated with portal vein tumor thrombosis over the evolving eras of treatment. World J Surg Oncol 2021;19(1):313.

86. Khan AR, Wei X, Xu X. Portal Vein Tumor Thrombosis and Hepatocellular Carcinoma - The Changing Tides. J Hepatocell Carcinoma 2021;8:1089–115.

87. Ghabril M, Agarwal S, Lacerda M, et al. Portal Vein Thrombosis Is a Risk Factor for Poor Early Outcomes After Liver Transplantation. Transplantation 2016; 100(1):126–33.

88. Agopian VG, Harlander-Locke M, Zarrinpar A, et al. A novel prognostic nomogram accurately predicts hepatocellular carcinoma recurrence after liver transplantation: analysis of 865 consecutive liver transplant recipients. J Am Coll Surg 2015;220(4):416–27.

89. Wong LL, Landsittel DP, Kwee SA. Liver Transplantation vs Partial Hepatectomy for Stage T2 Multifocal Hepatocellular Carcinoma <3 cm without Vascular Invasion: A Propensity-Score Matched Survival Analysis. J Am Coll Surg 2023. https://doi.org/10.1097/xcs.0000000000000725.

90. Risaliti M, Bartolini I, Campani C, et al. Evaluating the best treatment for multifocal hepatocellular carcinoma: A propensity score-matched analysis. World J Gastroenterol 2022;28(29):3981–93.

91. Guo Y, Linn YL, Koh YX, et al. Preoperative Predictors of Early Recurrence After Liver Resection for Multifocal Hepatocellular Carcinoma. J Gastrointest Surg 2023;27(6):1106–12.

92. Yao LQ, Chen ZL, Feng ZH, et al. Clinical Features of Recurrence After Hepatic Resection for Early-Stage Hepatocellular Carcinoma and Long-Term Survival Outcomes of Patients with Recurrence: A Multi-institutional Analysis. Ann Surg Oncol 2022. https://doi.org/10.1245/s10434-022-11454-y.

93. Duvoux C, Roudot-Thoraval F, Decaens T, et al. Liver transplantation for hepatocellular carcinoma: a model including alpha-fetoprotein improves the performance of Milan criteria. Gastroenterology 2012;143(4):986–94, e3; quiz: e14-5.

94. Mazzaferro V, Sposito C, Zhou J, et al. Metroticket 2.0 Model for Analysis of Competing Risks of Death After Liver Transplantation for Hepatocellular Carcinoma. Gastroenterology 2018;154(1):128–39.

95. Qadan M, Fong ZV, Delman AM, et al. Review of Use of Y90 as a Bridge to Liver Resection and Transplantation in Hepatocellular Carcinoma. J Gastrointest Surg 2021;25(10):2690–9.

96. Wayne JD, Lauwers GY, Ikai I, et al. Preoperative predictors of survival after resection of small hepatocellular carcinomas. Ann Surg 2002;235(5):722–30 [discussion: 730-1].

97. Klintmalm GB. Liver transplantation for hepatocellular carcinoma: a registry report of the impact of tumor characteristics on outcome. Ann Surg 1998; 228(4):479–90.

98. Jonas S, Bechstein WO, Steinmüller T, et al. Vascular invasion and histopathologic grading determine outcome after liver transplantation for hepatocellular carcinoma in cirrhosis. Hepatology 2001;33(5):1080–6.

99. Zhou L, Rui JA, Wang SB, et al. Prognostic factors of solitary large hepatocellular carcinoma: the importance of differentiation grade. Eur J Surg Oncol 2011; 37(6):521–5.

100. Pawlik TM, Gleisner AL, Anders RA, et al. Preoperative assessment of hepatocellular carcinoma tumor grade using needle biopsy: implications for transplant eligibility. Ann Surg 2007;245(3):435–42.

Expanding the Boundaries for Liver Transplantation for Hepatocellular Carcinoma

Jessica Lindemann, MD, PhD[a],
Maria Bernadette Majella Doyle, MD, MBA[b],*

KEYWORDS

- Hepatocellular carcinoma • Liver transplantation • Milan criteria • UCSF criteria

KEY POINTS

- Liver transplantation for HCC is the treatment of choice for eligible patients with unresectable disease.
- Current evidence supports the use of local-regional therapies to downstage patients with HCC to within Milan criteria for transplantation.
- The discovery of biomarkers, neoadjuvant therapies, and new post-transplantation immunosuppression regimens are all potential avenues to broaden selection criteria for transplantation and improve overall survival in patients with HCC.

INTRODUCTION

Primary liver cancer was the third most common cause of death due to cancer worldwide in 2020, and the incidence continues to grow.[1] By 2025, it has been estimated that more than 1 million people will develop liver cancer annually.[1] As the most common type, hepatocellular carcinoma (HCC) accounts for 85% to 90% of all liver cancers.[1,2] Incidence and etiology of HCC vary across geographic regions (**Fig. 1**). The highest incidence of HCC is in East Asia, where the most common etiology is hepatitis B virus (HBV) infection. HBV continues to be the primary etiology of HCC across most of Asia, Africa, and South America, whereas hepatitis C virus (HCV) is the predominant underlying cause in North America, Western Europe, and Japan. Alcohol intake remains the main contributor to HCC in Central and Eastern Europe. However, the incidence of non-alcoholic steatohepatitis (NASH) is rapidly increasing, particularly in high-income regions, and is likely to soon become the predominant cause of HCC.[1] Despite a continued rapid increase in incidence, mortality in the United States due

[a] Department of Surgery, Division of Abdominal Organ Transplantation, Washington University School of Medicine, Saint Louis, MO, USA; [b] Section of Abdominal Transplantation, Department of Surgery, Division of Abdominal Organ Transplantation, Washington University School of Medicine, 660 South Euclid Avenue, Campus Box 8109, Saint Louis, MO 63110, USA
* Corresponding author.
E-mail address: doylem@wustl.edu

Surg Clin N Am 104 (2024) 129–143
https://doi.org/10.1016/j.suc.2023.08.006
0039-6109/24/© 2023 Elsevier Inc. All rights reserved.
surgical.theclinics.com

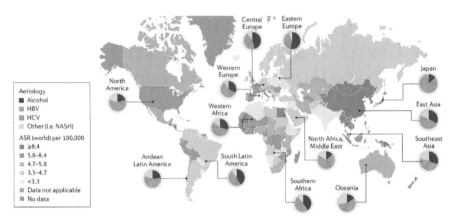

Fig. 1. The incidence of HCC according to geographic area and etiology. The pie charts represent the proportion of HCC due to varies etiologies as defined within the box in the lower left of the figure. The shades of blue represent the age-standardized incidence rate (ASR) of HCC per country with ASR categories defined within the box in the lower left of the figure. The highest incidence of HCC occurs in East Asia. Hepatitis B virus is the major etiologic factor in most of Asia (except Japan), South America, and Africa, whereas hepatitis C virus predominates in Western Europe, North America, and Japan. Alcohol intake is the most common causative factor in Central and Eastern Europe. The most common etiologic factor in the "other" category is NASH and it is expected to soon become the predominate cause of HCC in high income regions. ASR, age-standardized incidence rate, HCC, hepatocellular carcinoma; NASH, non-alcoholic steatohepatitis. (Global Cancer Observatory, World Health Organization, Estimated age-standardized incidence rates (World) in 2020, liver, both sexes, all ages, Copyright (2020) (https://gco.iarc. fr/today/online-analysis-map?v=2020&mode=population&mode_population=continents &population=900&populations=900&key=asr&sex=0&cancer=11&type=0&statistic=5&prevalence=0 &population_group=earth&color_palette=default&map_scale=quantile&map_nb_colors=5 &continent=0&rotate=%255B10%252C0%255D).)

to liver cancer has stabilized over the last 10 years, likely because of improvements in screening, treatments, and risk-factor modification.[3]

Surgical resection and liver transplantation remain the mainstay of curative treatment for HCC among patients who meet criteria for an operation. Importantly, majority of patients treated for HCC also have underlying cirrhosis, significantly increasing the risk of major hepatectomy. A series of observational studies in the 1980s to early 2000s demonstrated no statistically significant difference in post-operative mortality and long-term survival in limited resections compared to major hepatectomy for patients with small HCC.[4–6] However, limited resection leaves behind diseased liver parenchyma at risk of developing new HCCs in the future with an estimated 35% risk of recurrence at 1 year,[7] 40% to 50% recurrence at 3 years,[8–10] and up to 70% risk of recurrence at 5 years post-resection.[11–14] Therefore, transplantation is the treatment of choice for cure in patients who fall within transplant criteria.

This article describes current evidence-based practices for transplantation as the treatment for HCC. Recently published data supporting expansion of inclusion criteria for those eligible for transplant are also presented. This includes refined selection criteria, local-regional therapies for downstaging as a bridge to transplant, and the use of neoadjuvant therapies as well as new post-transplant immunosuppression regimens, all of which are helping to push the boundary on who is eligible for transplantation in the treatment of HCC.

PATIENT EVALUATION OVERVIEW
Diagnosis

Prognosis in HCC is dependent on stage and therefore earlier diagnosis generally results in longer overall survival, even after adjustment for lead time bias.[14] Current evidence-based guidelines recommend surveillance ultrasound (US) and alpha fetoprotein (AFP) levels every 6 months in high-risk patients, defined as having cirrhosis or chronic hepatitis B infection.[14,15] Several studies including randomized controlled trials (RCTs) and a meta-analysis have demonstrated a cost-effective survival benefit in high-risk patients who follow a 6-monthly surveillance program.[14,16–18] There is some debate over the use of US as it is a provider-dependent imaging modality and has been shown to be less effective in obesity and NASH.[15,19] Similarly, AFP levels can vary across ethnicities, be falsely positive or negative, particularly in acute viral hepatitis or cirrhosis due to a viral cause.[20,21] However, there is evidence to support the use of AFP in the diagnosis of HCC, particularly in patients with a liver mass and an AFP level greater than 200 ng/mL.[22] A serum AFP value of 400 ng/mL or greater is considered diagnostic of HCC, and a value greater than 1000 ng/mL is a strong predictor of vascular invasion.[23] In many transplant centers, an AFP greater than 1000 ng/mL is considered a contraindication to transplantation because of the risk of vascular involvement and poor predicted overall survival in those patients.[23] Liquid biopsy, used to detect circulating tumor DNA (ctDNA) among others, is 1 alternative modality for surveillance that is currently under investigation, although the data to support its routine use are lacking.[24–29]

The diagnosis of HCC is primarily made based on characteristic findings on imaging. Pathognomonic radiographic features include arterial enhancement with delayed washout on contrasted multiphase computed tomography (CT) imaging. When present, they represent a sensitivity of 89% and a specificity of 96% for HCC.[30] In an effort to establish a worldwide universal approach to imaging diagnosis and assessment of treatment response, the Liver Imaging Reporting and Data System (LI-RADS) was created. LI-RADS was first released in 2011 by the American College of Radiology, most recently updated in 2018, and was subsequently adopted into the American Association for the Study of Liver Diseases guidelines.[31,32] The LI-RADS system provides 4 imaging algorithms for different clinical scenarios including (1) US surveillance, (2) CT/MRI for diagnosis and staging, (3) contrast-enhanced US for diagnosis, and (4) evaluation of treatment response following local-regional therapies. In the current version, LI-RADS consists of 8 different diagnostic categories including LR-NC (non-categorizable), LR-1 through LR-5, LR-TIV (malignancy with tumor in vein), and LR-M (probably or definitely malignant, not HCC specific) (**Table 1**).[31] Treatment is guided by category with consideration of patient factors (**Fig. 2**). For patients with multiple lesions of different LI-RADS classification, treatment is guided by the highest LI-RADS category.

Preoperative Considerations

Evaluation for candidacy for liver transplantation for HCC includes clinical staging to assess tumor burden and presence of vascular invasion, as well as consideration of local liver transplant wait-list times. HCC has a predisposition to venous invasion and, less often, bile duct invasion.[12] Surrogate markers of venous involvement include tumor size, number of tumors, and AFP level, particularly AFP levels greater than 1000 ng/mL.[12] Recently proposed guidelines from the International Liver Transplantation Society include consideration of tumor biology, tumor size and number, probability of survival, transplant benefit, organ availability, wait-list composition, and allocation priorities when

Table 1
Summary of definitions of each LI-RADS category

Diagnostic Category	Description	Definition
LR-NR	Non-categorizable	Observation that cannot be meaningfully categorized because image omission or degradation prevents assessment of 1 or more major features
LR-1	Definitely benign	100% certainty that observation is non-malignant
LR-2	Probably benign	High probability but not 100% certainty observation is non-malignant
LR-3	Intermediate probability of malignancy	Non-malignant and malignant entities each have moderate probability
LR-4	Probably HCC	High probability but not 100% certainty observation is HCC
LR-5	Definitely HCC	100% certainty observation is HCC
LR-TIV	Malignancy with tumor in vein	100% certainty there is malignancy with tumor in vein
LR-M	Probably or definitely malignant, not HCC specific	High probability or 100% certainty observation is malignant but features are not HCC specific

Summarized from Chernyak V et al. Liver imaging reporting and data system (LI-RADS) version 2018. Radiology. (2018).

determining liver transplant candidacy.[33] Evidence of venous invasion on either imaging or pretransplant biopsy is a contraindication for transplantation as the risk of recurrence after transplant is unacceptably high.[12]

Long-term outcomes after liver transplantation are superior to resection with 70% 5-year and 50% 10-year survival rates and a 10% to 15% recurrence rate at 5 years[34] compared to a 15% survival rate at 10 years and a 65% recurrence rate in patients undergoing resection for HCC.[35] However, it has been shown that when transplant wait-list dropout rates exceed 20%, the probability of a cure from resection becomes similar to a cure from transplantation.[13,36] Therefore, for patients with resectable HCCs and preserved liver function in regions with long transplant wait times, consideration should be given to surgical resection to avoid disease progression and wait-list dropout.[37,38] Importantly, in a study comparing outcomes after patients with HCC underwent living liver transplant, a higher post-transplant recurrence rate was demonstrated in patients who underwent expedited transplant through living liver donation. This suggests that some time spent on the wait-list may help determine individual tumor biology and identify those patients who are perhaps more likely to recur after transplantation.[39,40] This supports the current Organ Procurement and Transplantation Network/United Network for Organ Sharing policy in the United States, which requires a 6-month waiting period on the liver transplant list before exception points are granted to patients listed for transplantation as treatment for HCC.[41]

LIVER TRANSPLANTATION IN THE MANAGEMENT OF HEPATOCELLULAR CARCINOMA

The most widely used criteria to guide management for HCC are the Barcelona Clinic Liver Cancer (BCLC) criteria.[41] The BCLC criteria not only allow for determination of

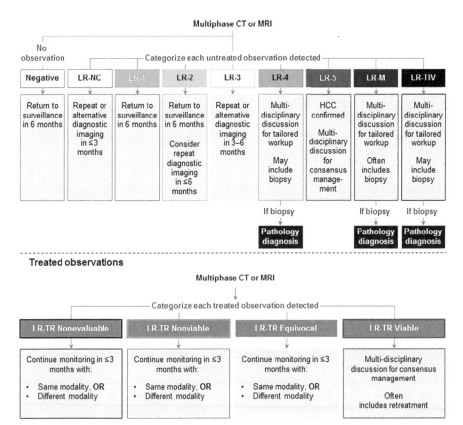

Fig. 2. Summary of CT and MRI diagnostic categories and treatment recommendations by LI-RADS classification. CT, computed tomography; LI-RADS, liver imaging reporting and data system. (Chernyak V, Fowler K J, Kamaya A, et al. Liver Imaging Reporting and Data System (LI-RADS) Version 2018: Imaging of Hepatocellular Carcinoma in At-Risk Patients. Radiology 2018;289:816-830.)

tumor stage and patient prognosis, but also guide treatment based on classification.[41] They provide an evidence-based classification system that includes patient factors such as evidence of portal hypertension and bilirubin, as well as tumor size and number to stratify patients based on prognosis with corresponding treatment schedules for each designated stage of disease. First proposed more than 20 years ago, the BCLC prognosis and treatment strategy is updated regularly and remains the primary evidence-based classification system used to guide treatment for patients with HCC today.[2,42] The current version, last updated in 2022 and shown in **Fig. 3**, demonstrates the ever-increasing complexity in medical decision-making as well as the major advances that have been made in the field over the last 2 decades.[42]

For patients with early stage, but unresectable HCC, liver transplant is the treatment of choice. Appropriate patient selection is critical to achieving overall survival comparable to survival after liver transplant for other non-malignant indications. In a landmark study published in 1996, Mazzaferro and colleagues from the University of Milan investigated the role of orthotopic liver transplantation in the treatment of otherwise unresectable HCC within what has since become known as the Milan criteria.[43] In this prospective, observational study, 48 patients with cirrhosis and unresectable

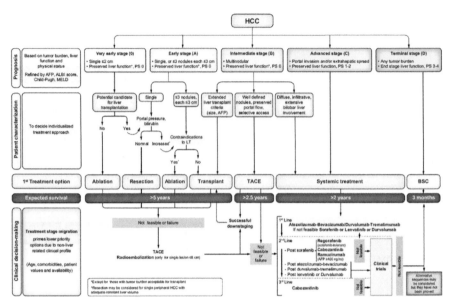

Fig. 3. Summary of CT and MRI diagnostic categories and treatment recommendations by LI-RADS classification. The top portion of the figure summarizes the diagnostic categories of HCC in patients with untreated lesions. The bottom portion of the figure summarizes the diagnostic categories of HCC in patients with treated lesions. LR-NC, LR-not categorizable, LR-M, LR-malignant (probably or definitely malignant, not specific for HCC), LR-TIV, LR-tumor in vein, LR-TR, LR-treatment response, CT, computed tomography; LI-RADS, liver imaging reporting and data system. (Reprinted with permission from: Reig M et al. BCLC strategy for prognosis prediction and treatment recommendation: The 2022 update. J Hepatol. (2022). Figure 1.)

HCC were included. Patients were followed for a median of 26 months after liver transplantation. Criteria for transplant eligibility included a single tumor 5 cm or less in diameter or no more than 3 nodules each 3 cm or less in size. The authors report a marked increase in survival with an actuarial survival rate of 75% and a recurrence-free survival rate of 83% at 4 years, compared to a 25% 3-year survival rate of untreated HCC in patients with cirrhosis.[43,44] This study clearly demonstrated the benefit of liver transplantation within a subgroup of patients with cirrhosis and HCC, and provided the field with evidence-based criteria to guide selection for transplantation in this patient population.

Twenty-five years later, the Milan criteria for liver transplantation remain the benchmark for selection of patients with HCC in the United States.[45] However, it has become clear that tumor number and size alone do not fully predict overall survival. The addition of surrogate markers for tumor biology, such as AFP, increases our ability to predict recurrence and subsequent mortality post-transplant. There have been multiple observational studies which have demonstrated a survival benefit for select patients transplanted outside of the Milan criteria.[46–51] Several other criteria have been proposed to guide patient selection for liver transplantation in HCC, which are summarized in **Table 2**, and include the University of California San Francisco (UCSF) and the up-to-seven rule among the most commonly used.[46,47] The Extended Toronto Criteria are routinely being used in Candida, and the French AFP Model has been used for liver transplant allocation since 2013.[49,50] The current US national guidelines for liver

Table 2
Summary of proposed criteria for liver transplantation for hepatocellular carcinoma

Classification System	Publication	Description	5-y Overall Survival
Milan Criteria[25]	Mazzaferro, NEJM. 1996	Single nodule < 5 cm or 3 nodules each < 3 cm	80%
UCSF Criteria[12]	Yao, Hepatol. 2001	Solitary tumor < 6.5 cm, or < 3 nodules with the largest lesion < 4.5 cm and total tumor diameter < 8 cm	77.8%
Up-to-Seven Criteria[33]	Mazzaferro, Lancet Oncol. 2009	Seven as the sum of the size of the largest tumor in cm and the number of tumors (ex: 2 tumors up to 5 cm in size, 3 up to 4 cm, 4 up to 3 cm, 5 up to 2 cm	71.2%
5-5-500[34]	Shimamura, Transplant International, 2019	Up to 5 nodules with a maximum diameter of 5 cm, AFP < 500	75.5%
Extended Toronto Criteria[35]	DuBay, Ann Surg, 2011	Any size or number of tumors, no systemic cancer-related symptoms, extrahepatic disease, vascular invasion or poorly differentiated tumors	70%
French AFP Model[36]	Duvoux, Gastroenterology, 2012	Scoring system including tumor diameter ($\leq$ 3, 3–6, >6 cm), number of nodules (1–3, $\geq$ 4), and AFP level ($\leq$ 100, 100–1000, >1000). A score of $\leq$ 2 is considered low risk	67.8%
TTV-AFP Model[13]	Toso, Hepatology, 2009	Composite score of total tumor volume < 115 cm and AFP < 400 ng/mL	60%

Abbreviations: AFP, alpha-fetoprotein; TTV-AFP, total tumor volume-alpha-fetoprotein; UCSF, University of California San Francisco.

transplantation in HCC include extent of disease falling within the Milan criteria, sustained response to local-regional therapy if downstaged to within Milan criteria, and AFP levels less than 500 ng/mL after local-regional therapy if more than 1000 ng/mL at the time of diagnosis.[32] These criteria result in an overall survival of 80% at 5-year post-liver transplant, comparable to overall survival after liver transplant for non-malignant indications.[45] The UCSF downstaging protocol for granting priority listing for liver transplant for HCC is currently the nationally adopted protocol used in the United States.[12] The initial selection criteria include 3 groups of patients, each with total tumor diameter measuring less than or equal to 8 cm: (1) 1 lesion greater than 5, but less than or equal to 8 cm, (2) 2 or 3 lesions with at least 1 greater than 3 but less than or equal to 5 cm with total tumor diameter less than or equal to 8 cm, and (3) 4 to 5 lesions each less than or equal to 3 cm with total tumor diameter less than or equal to 8 cm.[52]

TUMOR DOWNSTAGING USING LOCAL-REGIONAL THERAPIES

For patients in the United States who present outside of Milan criteria and who are expected to have a transplant wait time of greater than 6 months, local-regional therapy for downstaging tumors to within Milan criteria is often used. This strategy helps control tumor growth while on the waiting list, reducing the risk of dropout prior to transplantation. It also provides a method for assessing tumor biology, as patients who progress despite local-regional therapy have been shown to have a worse outcome post-liver transplantation.[53] Options for local-regional therapy include radiofrequency ablation and microwave ablation techniques as well as transarterial chemoembolization (TACE), transarterial radioembolization (TARE) using yttrium-90, and percutaneous ethanol injection. Of all the available local-regional therapy options, TACE is the recommended first-line treatment modality for downstaging HCC with the most evidence to support its use.[54,55] TARE has also had promising results, including potential immunomodulatory effects resulting in tumor suppression, but has not yet been widely adapted in downstaging algorithms.[56–58]

The survival benefit for patients transplanted after successful downstaging to within Milan criteria was evaluated in a recently published RCT.[59] Investigators enrolled patients across 9 Italian tertiary care and transplantation centers. The rationale for the study was based on the hypothesis that patients who undergo tumor downstaging for HCC initially outside of Milan criteria who have a good and sustained response to neoadjuvant local-regional therapy may have a survival benefit if offered liver transplantation for HCC in the setting of cirrhosis. The study was an open label, multi-center, phase 2b/3 RCT that compared liver transplantation to the best available tumor treatment. The specific aim for phase 2b was to assess the benefit of transplantation in delaying tumor recurrence in successfully downstaged patients with the primary outcome measure of 5-year tumor event-free survival. The phase 3 portion of the trial aimed to assess whether there was a long-term survival benefit following successful liver transplantation with the primary outcome measure of overall survival. There were 74 patients enrolled over a 4-year period from 2011 to 2015 with a median downstaging duration of 6 months (interquartile range 4–11). The 5-year tumor event-free survival was significantly higher in the transplantation group (76.8% vs 18.3%, hazard ratio [HR] 0.20, [95% confidence interval (CI) 0.07–0.57], P = .003). Similarly, the 5-year overall survival was significantly longer in the transplantation group (77.5% vs 31.2%, HR 0.32, [95% CI 0.11–0.92], P = .035). Unfortunately, study recruitment was ended early due to unanticipated changes in graft allocation policy and HCC priorities after the study began and was therefore underpowered. However, significant improvement in both tumor-free and overall long-term survival demonstrated in this RCT is encouraging and adds to the body of existing observational data suggesting that liver transplantation after downstaging of HCC to within Milan criteria is a viable treatment pathway for patients.[60,61]

Tabrizian and colleagues recently reported results from a multicenter observational study examining long-term outcomes after liver transplantation for patients with HCC.[62] There were 2645 patients included who underwent liver transplantation for HCC across 5 centers in the United States from January 2001 through December 2015. The study compared 10-year outcomes between 3 patient groups including patients whose disease was downstaged to within Milan criteria (n = 341), patients whose disease was always within Milan criteria (n = 2122), and patients whose disease was not successfully downstaged (n = 182). The primary outcome was overall survival and secondary outcomes included time to recurrence, recurrence-free survival, and recurrence after specific post-liver transplant therapies. The 10-year post-liver transplant survival and recurrence rates for patients successfully downstaged to within Milan criteria were 52.1% and 20.6% compared to 61.5% and 13.3% among patients transplanted who were always within Milan criteria. For those patients transplanted beyond Milan criteria, 10-year post-transplant survival and recurrence rates were 43.3% and 41.1%, respectively (all $P < .001$). Another notable finding from this large patient cohort was the significantly improved survival among patients with recurrence after transplantation treated with surgical resection compared to local-regional or systemic therapies. The results of this study strongly supported national downstaging policies for liver transplantation with excellent 10-year post-liver transplant outcomes. Additionally, the data suggest that surgical management of HCC recurrence in this patient population is associated with improved survival and should be pursued when feasible in well-selected patients.

NEW DEVELOPMENTS

As in many areas of oncology, tumor biology is the primary determinant of recurrence-free and overall survival in patients with HCC. There are several active areas of research that may allow for further expansion of transplant criteria for HCC including improved biomarkers, new neoadjuvant systemic therapies, and improved post-transplantation immunosuppression regimens.

Biomarkers to Assess Tumor Biology

AFP is currently the only approved biomarker for determining tumor biology in HCC. There are other biomarkers that have been investigated including AFP-L3 and des-γ-carboxy prothrombin.[63,64] While they did show promise in aiding in early detection of HCC, they have not yet been validated for clinical use. Liquid biopsies assessing circulating tumor cells (CTCs), cell-free DNA (cfDNA), and extracellular vesicles are also being investigated.[65,66] The use of CTCs and cfDNA may allow for gene sequencing of individual tumors and identification of favorable or unfavorable mutations which can aid in establishing an early diagnosis and determining prognosis. Similarly, extracellular vesicles, formed by budding lysosomes, cell membranes, or apoptosis and released into circulation, can be used both as targets for therapy as well as for analysis of tumor biology.[67,68] The pretransplant neutrophil to lymphocyte ratio has been suggested as a marker to aid in determining prognosis and risk of recurrence after liver transplantation.[69] Fluorodeoxyglucose (FDG)-PET avidity with AFP levels was a better predictor of recurrence compared to the Milan criteria alone in a recently published study in patients undergoing living donor liver transplantation.[70] Finally, Miltiadous and colleagues published a study on HCC patients who were transplanted beyond the Milan criteria with subsequent molecular analysis of the explanted liver looking for genomic signatures and immunohistochemical markers associated with poor outcome.[71] The group found that, in patients who did not have gene signatures of progenitor markers CK19 and S2, survival rates after transplant were similar to patients with HCC transplanted within Milan criteria.[71]

Neoadjuvant Systemic Therapies

There are several Food and Drug Administration-approved immunomodulatory agents for the systemic treatment of advanced staged HCC.[72–74] Currently, there are limited but optimistic data to support the use of neoadjuvant systemic therapies in the treatment of HCC prior to liver transplantation.[75,76] The use of immunomodulatory therapies in transplant candidates has previously been avoided due to reports of severe rejection and graft loss.[77–79] The Mount Siani group recently published a series of 9 patients who underwent liver transplantation for HCC following treatment with the programmed cell death protein-1 (PD-1) inhibitor nivolumab.[75] The authors reported no severe allograft rejection, losses, tumor recurrences, or deaths at a median follow-up of 16 months with near complete tumor necrosis observed in one-third of explanted livers. The remainder of evidence around PD-1 inhibitor use in this patient population is limited to case reports, and further investigations are required to determine whether this will be a viable treatment option in the future.

Post-Transplant Immunosuppression Regimens

Post-transplant patients are at increased risk of malignancy because of the life-long immunosuppression required to prevent organ rejection. In patients such as those transplanted for HCC, modification of immunosuppression regimens that keep organ rejection at bay but minimize the risk of recurrence is ideal. The mammalian target of rapamycin (mTOR) receptor, which plays a central role in cell proliferation, growth, and metabolism, has been implicated in the pathogenesis of HCC.[80] There is evidence to suggest that the use of mTOR inhibitors, such as everolimus for post-transplant immunosuppression, results in lower rates of recurrence and improved overall survival compared to calcineurin inhibitor regimens.[81–83]

SUMMARY

Primary liver cancer was the third most common cause of death due to cancer worldwide in 2020. As the most common type of primary liver cancer, oncologic advancements in the treatment of HCC are needed. Transplantation remains the preferred treatment for cure in otherwise unresectable HCC. There are several areas of active research that have led to the expansion of eligibility criteria for transplantation. This includes the use of local-regional therapy for downstaging patients who initially present outside of Milan criteria. Other important areas of research include identification of tumor biomarkers that can aid in the early diagnosis of HCC as well as in determining prognosis and likelihood of recurrence after transplantation. New neoadjuvant therapies as well as post-transplant immunosuppression regimens may also result in expansion of the eligibility criteria for transplantation in the treatment of HCC.

CLINICS CARE POINTS

- Liver transplantation for HCC is the treatment of choice for eligible patients with unresectable disease.
- Current evidence supports the use of local-regional therapies to downstage patients with HCC to within Milan criteria for transplantation.
- The discovery of biomarkers, neoadjuvant therapies, and new post-transplantation immunosuppression regimens are all potential avenues to broaden selection criteria for transplantation and improve overall survival in patients with HCC.

DISCLOSURE

The authors have nothing to disclose.

REFERENCES

1. International Agency for Research on Cancer. Estimated age-standardized incidence rates (World) in 2020, liver, both sexes, all ages. Available at: https://gco.iarc.fr/today/online-analysismap?v=2020&mode=population&mode_population=continents&population=900&populations=900&key=asr&sex=0&cancer=11&type=0&statistic=5&prevalence=0&population_group=0&ages_group%5B%5D=0&ages_group%5B%5D=17&nb_items=10&group_cancer=1&include_nmsc=0&include_nmsc_other=0&projection=natural-earth&color_palette=default&map_scale=''' quantile&map_nb_colors=5&continent=0&show_ranking=0&rotate=%255B10%252C0%255D. Accessed April 2, 2023.
2. Llovet JM, Kelley RK, Villaneuva A, et al. Hepatocellular carcinoma. Nat Rev Dis Primers 2021;7(6):1–28.
3. Cronin KA, Scott S, Firth AU, et al. Annual report to the nation on the status of cancer, part 1: National cancer statistics. Cancer 2022;128(24):4251–84.
4. Kanematsu T, Takenaka K, Matsumata T, et al. Limited hepatic resection effective for selected cirrhosis patients with primary liver cancer. Ann Surg 1984;199(1):51–6.
5. Shimada M, Gion T, Hamatsu T, et al. Evaluation of major hepatic resection for small hepatocellular carcinoma. Hepato-Gastroenterology 1999;46:401–6.
6. Zhou X, Tang Z, Yang B, et al. Experience of 1000 patients who underwent hepatectomy for small hepatocellular carcinoma. Cancer 2001;91(8):1479–86.
7. Lu X, Zhao H, Yang H, et al. A prospective clinical study on early recurrence of hepatocellular carcinoma after hepatectomy. J Surg Oncol 2009;100:488–93.
8. Koike Y, Shiratori Y, Sato S, et al. Risk factors for recurring hepatocellular carcinoma differ according to infected hepatitis virus - an analysis of 236 consecutive patients with a single lesion. Hepatology 2000;32:1216–23.
9. Jaeck D, Bachellier P, Oussoultzoglou E, et al. Surgical resection of hepatocellular carcinoma. Post-operative outcome and long-term results in Europe: an overview. Liver Transpl 2004;10:S58–63.
10. Sakon M, Umeshita K, Nagano H, et al. Clinical significance of hepatic resection in hepatocellular carcinoma: analysis by disease-free survival curves. Arch Surg 2000;135:1456–9.
11. Minagawa M, Makuuchi M, Takayama T, et al. Selection criteria for repeat hepatectomy in patients with recurrent hepatocellular carcinoma. Ann Surg 2003;238:703–10.
12. Bismuth H, Majno PE, Adam R. Liver transplantation for hepatocellular carcinoma. Semin Liver Dis 1999;19:311–22.

13. Llovet JM, Fuster J, Bruix J. Intention-to-treat analysis of surgical treatment for early hepatocellular carcinoma: resection versus transplantation. Hepatology 1999;30:1434–40.

14. Singal AG, Pillai A, Tiro J. Early detection, curative treatment, and survival rates for hepatocellular carcinoma surveillance in patients with cirrhosis: a meta-analysis. PLoS Med 2014;11(14):e1001624.

15. Trinchet JC, Chaffaut C, Bourcier V, et al. Ultrasonographic surveillance of hepatocellular carcinoma in cirrhosis: a randomized trial comparing 3- and 6-month periodicities. Hepatology 2011;54(6):1987–97.

16. Zhang BH, Yang BH, Tang ZY. Randomized controlled trial of screening for hepatocellular carcinoma. J Cancer Res Clin Oncol 2004;130:417–22.

17. Andersson KL, Salomon JA, Goldie SJ, et al. Cost effectiveness of alternative surveillance strategies for hepatocellular carcinoma in patients with cirrhosis. Clin Gastroenterol Hepatol 2008;6(12):P1418–24.

18. Tzartzeva K, Obi J, Rich NE, et al. Surveillance imaging and alpha fetoprotein for early detection of hepatocellular carcinoma in patients with cirrhosis: a meta-analysis. Gastroenterology 2018;154(6):P1706–18.

19. Atiq O, Tiro J, Yopp AC, et al. An assessment of benefits and harms of hepatocellular carcinoma surveillance in patients with cirrhosis. Hepatology 2017; 65(4):1196–205.

20. Soresi M, Magliarisi C, Campagna P, et al. Usefulness of alpha-fetoprotein in the diagnosis of hepatocellular carcinoma. Anticancer Res 2003;23:1747–53.

21. Nguyen MH, Garcia RT, Simpson PW, et al. Racial differences in effectiveness of alpha-fetoprotein for diagnosis of hepatocellular carcinoma in hepatitis C virus cirrhosis. Hepatology 2002;36:410–7.

22. Sherman M, Peltekian KM, Lee C. Screening for hepatocellular carcinoma in chronic carriers of hepatitis B virus: incidence and prevalence of hepatocellular carcinoma in a North American urban population. Hepatology 1995;22:432–8.

23. Hameed B, Mehta N, Sapisochin G, et al. Alpha-fetoprotein level > 1000 ng/mL as an exclusion criterion for liver transplantation in patients with hepatocellular carcinoma meeting the Milan criteria. Liver Transpl 2014;20:945–51.

24. Labgaa I, Villacorta-Martin C, D'Avola D, et al. A pilot study of ultra-deep targeted sequencing of plasma DNA identifies driver mutations in hepatocellular carcinoma. Oncogene 2018;37:3740–52.

25. Kisiel JB, Dukek BA, Kanipakam RVSR, et al. Hepatocellular carcinoma detection by plasma methylated DNA: discovery, phase I pilot, and phase II clinical validation. Hepatology 2019;69(3):1180–92.

26. Xu R, Wei W, Krawczyk M, et al. Circulating tumour DNA methylation markers for diagnosis and prognosis of hepatocellular carcinoma. Nat Mater 2017;16(11): 1155–61.

27. Qu C, Wang Y, Wang P, et al. Detection of early-stage hepatocellular carcinoma in asymptomatic HBsAg- seropositive individuals by liquid biopsy. Proc Natl Acad Sci 2019;116(13):6308–12.

28. Oh CR, Kong SY, Im HS, et al. Genome-wide copy number alteration and VEGFA amplification of circulating cell- free DNA as a biomarker in advanced hepatocellular carcinoma patients treated with Sorafenib. BMC Cancer 2019;292.

29. Torga G, Pienta KJ. Patient-paired sample congruence between 2 commercial liquid biopsy tests. JAMA Oncol 2018;4(6):868–70.

30. Marrero JA, Hussain HK, Ngheim HV, et al. Improving the prediction of hepatocellular carcinoma in cirrhotic patients with an arterially enhancing liver mass. Liver Transpl 2005;11(3):281–9.

31. Chernyak V, Fowler KJ, Kamaya A, et al. Liver Imaging Reporting and Data System (LI-RADS) Version 2018: Imaging of Hepatocellular Carcinoma in At-Risk Patients. Radiology 2018;289(3):816–30.
32. Marrero JA, Kulik LM, Sirlin C, et al. Diagnosis, staging, and management of hepatocellular carcinoma: 2018 practice guidance by the American Association for the Study of Liver Diseases. Hepatology 2018;68(2):723–50.
33. Mehta N, Bhangui P, Yao FY, et al. Liver transplantation for hepatocellular carcinoma. Working group report from the ILTS transplant oncology consensus conference. Transplantation 2020;104(6):1136–42.
34. Tabrizian P, Holzner ML, Mehta N, et al. A US multicenter analysis of 2529 HCC patients undergoing liver transplantation:10-year outcome assessing the role of down- staging to within Milan criteria. Hepatology 2019;70:10–1.
35. Franssen B, Jibara G, Tabrizian P, et al. Actual 10-year survival following hepatectomy for hepatocellular carcinoma. HPB 2014;16:830–5.
36. Cucchetti A, Zhong J, Berhane S, et al. The chances of hepatic resection curing hepatocellular carcinoma. J. Hepatol 2020;72:711–7.
37. Majno PE, Sarasin FP, Mentha G, et al. Primary liver resection and salvage transplantation or primary liver transplantation in patients with single, small hepatocellular carcinoma and preserved liver function: an outcome-oriented decision analysis. Hepatology 2000;31:899–906.
38. Sarasin FP, Giostra E, Mentha G, et al. Partial hepatectomy or orthotopic liver transplantation for the treatment of resectable hepatocellular carcinoma? A cost-effectiveness perspective. Hepatology 1998;28:436–42.
39. Kulik L, Abecassis M. Living donor liver transplantation for hepatocellular carcinoma. Gastroenterology 2004;127:S277–82.
40. Hayashi PH, Ludkowski M, Forman LM, et al. Hepatic artery chemoembolization for hepatocellular carcinoma in patients listed for liver transplantation. Am J Transplant 2004;4:782–7.
41. Llovet JM, Bru C, Bruix J. Prognosis of hepatocellular carcinoma: the BCLC staging classification. Semin Liv Dis 1999;19(3):329–38.
42. Reig M, Forner A, Rimola J, et al. BCLC strategy for prognosis prediction and treatment recommendation: the 2022 update. J Hepatol 2022;76(3):681–93.
43. Mazzaferro V, Regalie E, Doci R, et al. Liver transplantation for the treatment of small hepatocellular carcinomas in patients with cirrhosis. N Eng J Med 1996; 334(11):693–9.
44. Barbara L, Benzi G, Gaiani S, et al. Natural history of small untreated hepatocellular carcinoma in cirrhosis: a multivariate analysis of prognostic factors of tumor growth rate and patient survival. Hepatology 1992;16:132–7.
45. Mehta N. Liver transplantation criteria for hepatocellular carcinoma, including posttransplant management. Clin Liver Dis 2021;17(5):332–6.
46. Yao FY, Ferrell L, Bass NM, et al. Liver transplantation for hepatocellular carcinoma: expansion of tumor size limits does not adversely impact survival. Hepatology 2001;33(6):1347–61.
47. Mazzaferro V, Llovet JM, Miceli R, et al. Predicting survival after liver transplantation in patients with hepatocellular carcinoma beyond the Milan criteria: a retrospective, exploratory analysis. Lancet Oncol 2009;10(1):35–43.
48. Shimamura T, Akamatsu N, Fujiyoshi M, et al. Expanded living-donor liver transplantation criteria for patients with hepatocellular carcinoma based on the Japanese nationwide survey: the 5-5-500 rule - a retrospective study. Transpl Int 2019; 32(4):356–68.

49. DuBay D, Sandroussi C, Sandhu L, et al. Liver transplantation for advanced hepatocellular carcinoma using poor tumor differentiation on biopsy as an exclusion criterion. Ann Surg 2011;253(1):166–72.

50. Duvoux C, Roudot-Thoraval F, Decaens T, et al. Liver transplantation for hepatocellular carcinoma: a model including α-fetoprotein improves the performance of Milan criteria. Gastroenterology 2012;143(4):986–94.

51. Toso C, Asthana S, Bigam DL, et al. Reassessing selection criteria prior to liver transplantation for hepatocellular carcinoma utilizing the Scientific Registry of Transplant Recipients database. Hepatology 2009;832–8.

52. Yao FY, Mehta N, Flemming J, et al. Downstaging of hepatocellular cancer before liver transplant: long-term outcome compared to tumors within Milan Criteria. Hepatology 2015;61(6):1968–77.

53. Lai Q, Vitale A, Lesari S, et al. Intention-to-treat survival benefit of liver transplantation in patients with hepatocellular cancer. Hepatology 2017;66(6):1910–9.

54. Yao FY, Fidelman N. Reassessing the boundaries of liver transplantation for hepatocellular carcinoma: where do we stand with tumor down-staging? Hepatology 2016;63:1014–25.

55. Parikh ND, Waljee AK, Singal AG. Downstaging hepatocellular carcinoma: a systematic review and pooled analysis. Liver Transpl 2015;21:1142–52.

56. Lewandowski RJ, Kulik LM, Riaz A, et al. A comparative analysis of transarterial downstaging for hepatocellular carcinoma: chemoembolization versus radioembolization. Am J Transplant 2009;9:1920–8.

57. Salem R, Johnson GE, Kim E, et al. Yttrium-90 radioembolization for the treatment of solitary, unresectable HCC: the LEGACY study. Hepatology 2021;74:2242–52.

58. Chew V, Lee YH, Pan I, et al. Immune activation underlies a sustained clinical response to Yttrium-90 radioembolization in hepatocellular carcinoma. Gut 2019;68:335–46.

59. Mazzaferro V, Citterio D, Bhoori S. Liver transplantation in hepatocellular carcinoma after tumour downstaging (XXL): a randomised, controlled, phase 2b/3 trial. Lancet Oncol 2020;21(7):947–56.

60. Yao FY, Mehta N, Flemming J, et al. Downstaging of hepatocellular cancer before liver transplant: long-term outcome compared to tumors within Milan criteria. Hepatology 2015;61(6):1968–77.

61. Ravaioli M, Grazi GL, Piscaglia F, et al. Liver transplantation for hepatocellular carcinoma: results of down- staging in patients initially outside the Milan selection criteria. Am J Transplant 2008;8(12):2547–57.

62. Tabrizian P, Holzner ML, Mehta N, et al. Ten-year outcomes of Liver Transplant and Downstaging for Hepatocellular Carcinoma. JAMA Surg 2022;157(9): 779–88.

63. Marrero JA, Su GL, Wei W, et al. Des-gamma carboxyprothrombin can differentiate hepatocellular carcinoma from nonmalignant chronic liver disease in American patients. Hepatology 2003;37:1114–21.

64. Hiraoka A, Ishimaru Y, Kawasaki H, et al. Tumor markers AFP, AFP-L3, and DCP in hepatocellular carcinoma refractory to transcatheter arterial chemoembolization. Oncology 2015;89:167–74.

65. Chen VL, Xu D, Wicha MS, et al. Utility of liquid biopsy analysis in detection of hepatocellular carcinoma, determination of prognosis, and disease monitoring: a systematic review. Clin Gastroenterol Hepatol 2020;18:2879–902.

66. Wu X, Li J, Gassa A, et al. Circulating tumor DNA as an emerging liquid biopsy biomarker for early diagnosis and therapeutic monitoring in hepatocellular carcinoma. Int J Biol Sci 2020;16:1551–62.

67. Andaloussi SEL, Mager I, Breakefield XO, et al. Extracellular vesicles: biology and emerging therapeutic opportunities. Nat Rev Drug Discov 2013;12:347–57.
68. Azmi AS, Bao B, Sarkar FH. Exosomes in cancer development, metastasis, and drug resistance: a comprehensive review. Cancer Metastasis Rev 2013;32: 623–42.
69. Agopian VG, Harlander-Locke M, Zarrinpar A, et al. A novel prognostic nomogram accurately predicts hepatocellular carcinoma recurrence after liver transplantation: analysis of 865 consecutive liver transplant recipients. J Am Coll Surg 2015;220:416–27.
70. Hong G, Suh KS, Suh SW, et al. Alpha-fetoprotein and (18)F-FDG positron emission tomography predict tumor recurrence better than Milan criteria in living donor liver transplantation. J Heptol 2016;64(4):852–9.
71. Miltiadous O, Sia D, Hoshida Y, et al. Progenitor cell markers predict outcome of patients with hepatocellular carcinoma beyond Milan criteria undergoing liver transplantation. J Hepatol 2015;63:1368–77.
72. Kudo M, Finn RS, Qin S, et al. Lenvatinib versus sorafenib in first-line treatment of patients with unresectable hepatocellular carcinoma: a randomised phase 3 non-inferiority trial. Lancet 2018;391:1163–73.
73. Finn RS, Qin S, Ikeda M, et al. Atezolizumab plus bevacizumab in unresectable hepatocellular carcinoma. N Engl J Med 2020;382:1894–905.
74. AstraZeneca. Imfinzi plus tremelimumab significantly improved overall survival in HIMALAYA Phase III trial in 1st-line unresectable liver cancer. Available from: https://www.astrazeneca-us.com/media/press-releases/2021/imfinzi-plus-tremelimumab-significantly-improved-overall-survival-in-himalaya-phase-iii-trial-in-1st-line-unresectable-liver-cancer-10152021.html. Accessed 4 April 2023.
75. Tabrizian P, Florman SS, Schwartz ME. PD-1 inhibitor as bridge therapy to liver transplantation? Am J Transplant 2021;21(5):1979–80.
76. Kang E, Martinez M, Moisander-Joyce H, et al. Stable liver graft post anti-PD1 therapy as a bridge to transplantation in an adolescent with hepatocellular carcinoma. Pediatric Transplant 2022;26(3):e14209.
77. Abdel-Wahab N, Shah M, Suarez-Almazor ME, et al. Adverse events associated with immune checkpoint blockade in patients with cancer: a systematic review of case reports. PLoS One 2016;11(7):e0160221.
78. Wang DY, Johnson DB, Davis EJ. Toxicities associated with PD-1/PD-L1 blockade Cancer. J 2018;24(1):36–40.
79. Nordness MF, Hamel S, Godfrey CM, et al. Fatal hepatic necrosis after nivolumab as a bridge to liver transplant for HCC: are checkpoint inhibitors safe for the pre-transplant patient? Am J Transplant 2020;20(3):879–83.
80. El-Khoueiry AB, Sangro B, Yau T, et al. Nivolumab in patients with advanced hepatocellular carcinoma (CheckMate 040): an open-label, non-comparative, phase 1/2 dose escalation and expansion trial. Lancet 2017;389:2492–502.
81. Toso C, Merani S, Bigam DL, et al. Sirolimus-based immunosuppression is associated with increased survival after liver transplantation for hepatocellular carcinoma. Hepatology 2010;51:1237–43.
82. Grigg SE, Sarri GL, Gow PJ, et al. Systematic review with meta-analysis: sirolimus- or everolimus-based immunosuppression following liver transplantation for hepatocellular carcinoma. Aliment Pharmacol Ther 2019;49:1260–73.
83. Yan X, Huang S, Yang Y, et al. Sirolimus or everolimus improves survival after liver transplantation for hepatocellular carcinoma: a systematic review and meta-analysis. Liver Transpl 2022;28:1063–77.

Downstaging Techniques for Hepatocellular Carcinoma in Candidates Awaiting Liver Transplantation

Lauren Matevish, MD, Madhukar S. Patel, MD, MBA, ScM,
Parsia A. Vagefi, MD*

KEYWORDS

- Hepatocellular carcinoma • Downstaging • Locoregional therapies
- Immunotherapy • Liver transplant

KEY POINTS

- Interventional options for downstaging include transarterial chemoembolization, transarterial radioembolization, percutaneous ablation, and stereotactic body radiotherapy; however, in the absence of clear superiority, choice of a first-line treatment should be based on patient factors and center-specific expertise.
- Downstaging of advanced HCC for liver transplant using the UNOS-DS (or UNOS Downstaging) protocol has shown long-term survival and tumor recurrence rates equivalent to those of patients transplanted within Milan criteria
- Systemic immunotherapy lies at the forefront of novel treatment strategies; although less is known regarding patient selection and optimal treatment regimens preceding liver transplant, it remains a promising avenue for further research and discovery.

INTRODUCTION

Primary liver cancer is the sixth most common cause of cancer deaths in the United States with hepatocellular carcinoma (HCC) representing approximately 75% of cases.[1] The most definitive curative intent strategy for hepatic neoplasms is liver transplant, especially in the setting of underlying liver disease. The scarcity of liver grafts has necessitated stringent selection criteria and allocation guidelines to maintain maximal transplant survival benefit.

In the United States, more than 12,000 patients were listed for liver transplant in 2020.[2] More than 10% of new liver transplant registrations were for a primary diagnosis of HCC, and this rate has nearly doubled during the past decade. In the United States,

Division of Surgical Transplantation, Department of Surgery, University of Texas Southwestern Medical Center, Dallas, Texas, USA
* Corresponding author. 5959 Harry Hines Boulevard, HP04.102, Dallas, TX 75390-8567.
E-mail address: Parsia.Vagefi@UTSouthwestern.edu

Surg Clin N Am 104 (2024) 145–162
https://doi.org/10.1016/j.suc.2023.07.004
0039-6109/24/© 2023 Elsevier Inc. All rights reserved.

the model for end-stage liver disease score (MELD) is used for allocation, and when the calculated score does not reflect a candidate's medical urgency, an exception score can be requested. For HCC, exception points are granted for patients with greater than T1 stage disease (ie, >2 cm) that are within Milan criteria (MC; single tumor ≤5 cm or 3 tumors ≤3 cm, no macrovascular invasion or extrahepatic metastasis) or who were outside MC and successfully downstaged to within MC. When accounting for all patients on the wait list, 16.2% of those listed had HCC exception points.[2]

For patients within MC, 5-year postliver transplant overall survival typically reaches 75% to 80%.[3] Although adherence to MC keeps posttransplant survival high and recurrence low, its reliance on tumor morphology fails to consider tumor biology, the latter of which may expand favorable tumor profiles with potential for equivalent survival outcomes.[4] Newer models of posttransplant outcomes, such as the French AFP model and the Metroticket 2.0 model, have incorporated surrogates of tumor biology (eg, alpha fetoprotein [AFP]) to create more robust predictions of patient outcomes.[3]

Initially recommended in 1997,[5] tumor downstaging is the process through which locoregional therapies (LRTs) or pharmacologic therapies are used to reduce HCC tumor size so that a patient's disease fits within MC, thus meeting eligibility for exception points. The increased acceptance of downstaging has allowed for listing of patients with initially prohibitively large tumor burden and increased the number of potential transplant candidates. Given the shortage of liver grafts, this selection process has sought to identify patients with HCC with favorable tumor biology who will ultimately undergo successful liver transplant with acceptable recurrence-free survival.

PATIENT EVALUATION
Barcelona Clinic Liver Cancer Stage

For patients diagnosed with HCC, a determination of liver transplant eligibility starts with staging. The Barcelona Clinic Liver Cancer (BCLC) staging system, initially published in 1999, is one of the most well established and used. Liver cancer is staged based on the primary lesion, patient performance status, vascular invasion, and extrahepatic spread (**Table 1**).[6–8] Patient prognosis and initial treatment strategies by stage are incorporated, and the recent 2022 update offers a model for individualized clinical decision-making (**Fig. 1**).[8]

Compared with patients with BCLC-0 and BCLC-A disease who fall within MC, those comprising the heterogenous BCLC-B category were the targeted population of downstaging therapies, with multifocal disease that exceeded MC. Liver transplant has remained an option for those with well-defined HCC nodules that meet institution-dependent extended liver transplant criteria, generally including surrogates of tumor

Table 1		
Barcelona Clinic Liver Cancer staging of hepatocellular carcinoma		
Stage	**PS**	**Tumor stage**
Very early stage (0)	0	Single, <2 cm
Early stage (A)		
Solitary	0	Single, any size
Multifocal	0	≤3 nodules, each ≤3 cm
Intermediate Stage (B)	0	Multinodular
Advanced stage (C)	1–2	Portal invasion and or extrahepatic spread
Terminal stage (D)	3–4	Any tumor burden

Abbreviation: PS, performance status.

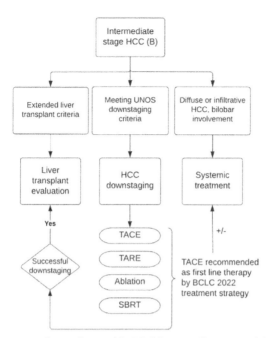

Fig. 1. Treatment strategy for patients with BCLC intermediate stage (B) HCC. Attempts at HCC downstaging may include a combination of the available LRTs as well as systemic therapies. HCC, hepatocellular carcinoma; TACE, transarterial chemoembolization; TARE, transarterial radioembolization; SBRT, stereotactic beam radiation therapy. (*Adapted from* Reig M, Forner A, Rimola J, et al. BCLC strategy for prognosis prediction and treatment recommendation: The 2022 update. J Hepatol 2022; 76(3):681–693).

biology (eg, AFP) and/or response to downstaging therapies to select patients with responsive disease. Multiple studies have shown acceptable posttransplant survival in this population.[9] Although no international consensus exists regarding expanded criteria,[10] the United States has standardized downstaging criteria for granting MELD exception points.

United Network for Organ Sharing Downstaging Protocol

In 2016, the Organ Procurement and Transplantation Network/United Network for Organ Sharing (UNOS) adopted a downstaging protocol (UNOS-DS) based on the criteria developed at the University of California, San Francisco (UCSF), creating a national pathway for patients with HCC outside of MC to become eligible for standardized MELD exception points should their posttreatment tumor burden meet the requirements for transplant. In addition to size criteria, any patient with AFP levels greater than 1000 ng/mL must demonstrate a biochemical response posttherapy, with a decrease to less than 500 ng/mL. The UNOS-DS criteria are summarized in **Box 1**. These automatic MELD exception points take effect after a mandatory 6-month waiting period during which the tumor must remain controlled within MC.

SURGICAL AND INTERVENTIONAL TREATMENT OPTIONS FOR DOWNSTAGING

Downstaging modalities for patients meeting UNOS-DS inclusion criteria are typically divided into LRTs and systemic therapies. LRTs are more frequently used and are

---

Box 1
United Network for Organ Sharing downstaging criteria with definitions of posttreatment success and failure

UNOS Downstaging Criteria

Inclusion Criteria: HCC exceeding MC but meeting ONE of the following
1. Single tumor size 5.1–8 cm
2. 2 to 3 tumors, each ≤5 cm and sum of maximal tumor diameters ≤8 cm
3. 4 to 5 tumors each ≤3 cm and sum of maximal tumor diameter ≤8 cm

AND absence of vascular invasion or extrahepatic disease on cross-sectional imaging

Successful Downstaging
 Posttreatment tumor size within MC
 Tumor burden must remain within MC for 6 months after downstaging to qualify for MELD exception points
 Only viable tumors are included in measurement, necrosis from LRTs is not
 If there are 2+ areas of enhancement in a tumor after treatment, the diameter of the entire lesion is counted toward the residual tumor burden

Downstaging Failure
1. Tumor progression beyond eligibility criteria as defined above
2. Tumor invasion of a major hepatic vessel on cross-sectional imaging
3. Lymph node involvement or extrahepatic extension
4. Infiltrative tumor growth
5. AFP level >1000 ng/mL (AFP must decrease to <500 ng/mL after LRT)

Abbreviations: HCC, hepatocellular carcinoma, MC: Milan Criteria; MELD: Model for end-stage liver disease; AFP, alpha-fetoprotein; LRT, locoregional therapy.

---

typically image-guided, liver tumor-directed therapies. Transarterial chemoembolization (TACE) is the most common modality in published reports,[11,12] although with increased experience, transarterial radioembolization (TARE) continues to gain traction. Current data are yet to provide definitive consensus regarding optimal therapy because reported efficacies of available downstaging options are highly variable.[13] Although choice of initial therapy is controversial, and algorithms such as the BCLC 2022 update have provided general guidelines, individualized clinical decision-making should be prioritized.[8] Consideration of tumor location, underlying liver function, patient functional status, as well as local expertise, are all pertinent in the decision-making process. Analyses of available data report overall downstaging rates with LRTs nearing 50%, with a posttransplant HCC recurrence rate of 16%,[11] and with the highest success rates being observed in candidates who undergo multimodal therapy.[13] The most common LRT options for downstaging are further discussed below and summarized in **Table 2**.

Transarterial Chemoembolization

First performed in the 1970s, TACE in liver cancer is the directed delivery of chemotherapy via selected hepatic artery branches feeding the targeted tumor. This technique is based off the principle that HCC recruits hepatic artery branches to promote growth, whereas the remainder of the liver parenchyma derives its dominant blood supply from the portal vein.[14] In conventional TACE, chemotherapy is delivered first along with a lipiodol contrast agent, followed by an embolization agent (eg, gelfoam) to induce a cytotoxic effect with ischemia.[15] The procedure is performed under moderate sedation, or less commonly general anesthesia. Newer techniques have used drug-eluting beads (DEB-TACE), which lodge within the artery and release a

Table 2
Summary of interventional options for hepatocellular carcinoma downstaging

Modality	Technique	Risks	Benefits
TACE	Injection of chemotherapy + lipiodol contrast agent into feeding HA, followed by embolization agent (conventional TACE); Drug-eluting bead TACE delivers chemotherapeutic and embolization effect via single injection of drug-eluting beads	PES, liver failure (especially with PVT), liver abscess/biloma	Improved OS compared with best supportive care; Downstaging rate 54%, with a 17% rate of recurrence after transplant
TARE	Similar to DEB-TACE, with injection of microspheres loaded with Y[90]	RILD, radiation-induced pneumonitis, PES, liver failure, liver abscess/biloma, GI issues	More favorable safety profile, longer time to progression than TACE but no difference in OS; potentially better tumor shrinkage effect than TACE
Ablation	Percutaneous thermal modalities, utilizing RFA alternating current (RFA) or microwaves (MWA), which cause tumor coagulation necrosis	PAS, bleeding, adjacent organ injury; RFA has a slightly better safety profile	Similar outcomes as resection for tumors <3 cm; improved tumor response of TACE + ablation vs TACE alone
SBRT	Precise direction of an external beam of ionizing radiation to target and destroy cancerous cells	Thrombocytopenia, GI bleeding or ulcer	Improved tumor response rates, OS for TACE + SBRT compared with TACE alone
Resection	Surgical removal of HCC-involved liver segments or lobe	Only 20% candidates at diagnosis; higher perioperative risks (eg, liver failure)	Typically only used as salvage therapy; able to assess high-risk features on explant

Abbreviations: HA, hepatic artery; PES, postembolization syndrome; PVT, portal vein thrombus; OS, overall survival; RILD, radiation-induced liver disease; PAS, postablation syndrome.

low and constant amount of chemotherapy during a period of 2 weeks. DEB-TACE has been shown to result in less systemic chemotherapy uptake and a more homogenous drug distribution.[16]

TACE is recommended as the initial treatment strategy in patients with unresectable HCC (BCLC-B) with Child-Pugh B disease or better in the absence of extrahepatic spread or portal vein thrombosis (PVT); this strategy was endorsed by the National Comprehensive Cancer Network (NCCN).[17,18] Although not an absolute contraindication, the presence of PVT confers a higher risk of posttreatment liver failure, especially in the setting of a main portal vein thrombus without adequate collateral flow.[19] Other relative contraindications include a large tumor burden, severe medical comorbidities, untreated esophageal varices, and elevated liver function markers. TACE is not recommended for patients with decompensated cirrhosis (ie, Child-Pugh C or equivalent), creatinine clearance less than 30 mL/min (or other contraindication to chemotherapy), or extensive bilobar tumor involvement.[18] Consideration should be given to treating biliary obstruction before therapy because TACE can precipitate worsening obstruction due to fragmented tumor necrosis.[20] Large lesions comprising greater than 50% of the liver volume have often necessitated 2 or more staged embolizations.

The most frequently used chemotherapeutic regimens are doxorubicin/epirubicin or cisplatin/miriplatin; multiple drug regimens including a combination of doxorubicin, cisplatin, and mitomycin are also described.[15] A summary of regimens and dose ranges are seen in **Table 3**.[15] Gelatin sponge has been the most commonly used embolic agent.[15] For patients undergoing DEB-TACE, doxorubicin is the most widely used agent, though rarely other anthracyclines may be substituted.[21]

Following TACE, postembolization syndrome (PES) is the most frequently encountered complication, with rates around 80%.[22] Often manifested in the first 72 hours following treatment, PES presents with symptoms of right upper quadrant abdominal pain, lethargy, fever, or nausea, and biochemically with elevated liver enzymes or bilirubin. Recovery is usually self-limited and resolves after 7 to 10 days.[23] Another major concern with TACE is liver toxicity, which may warrant superselective embolization to limit ischemic damage to noncancerous liver parenchyma. DEB-TACE may mitigate these risks through more predictable drug-delivery, with fewer systemic adverse effects and a lower incidence of toxicity.[24] However, the PRECISION-V trial found comparable 30-day adverse event incidence between patients undergoing conventional TACE and DEB-TACE,[25] which has been confirmed on meta-analysis.[26]

Imaging and laboratory testing is performed at 4 to 6 weeks after most LRT interventions to assess response. The NCCN further recommends follow-up imaging with

---

Table 3
Most common chemotherapeutic regimens and dosing for transarterial chemoembolization therapy

TACE Chemotherapeutic Regimens	Dose Ranges
Doxorubicin or epirubicin	Doxorubicin, 10–100 mg; Epirubicin, 5–120 mg
Cisplatin or miriplatin	Cisplatin, 10–100 mg; Miriplatin, 20–140 mg
Mitomycin	Mitomycin, 2–30 mg
Doxorubicin + cisplatin or mitomycin Doxorubicin + cisplatin + mitomycin	

Abbreviation: TACE, transarterial chemoembolization.
Data from Lencioni R, de Baere T, Soulen MC, et al. Lipiodol transarterial chemoembolization for hepatocellular carcinoma: A systematic review of efficacy and safety data. Hepatology 2016; 64(1):106 to 16.

computed tomography (CT) or magnetic resonance imaging (MRI) every 3 to 6 months for the first 2 years, as well as surveillance with serum AFP monitoring.[18] CT or MRI is used to evaluate treatment efficacy and confirm tumor necrosis using the modified Response Evaluation Criteria in Solid Tumors (mRECIST),[27] summarized in **Box 2**.[27]

TACE has been shown to provide therapeutic benefit for patients with HCC.[28] Successful downstaging rates with TACE are highly variable in the literature, ranging from 23.7% to 90%,[13] with transplant rates greater than 50% after being within MC.[29] A pooled analysis from Parikh and colleagues found a 48% successful downstaging rate, which increased to 54% when patients with PVT were excluded. The recurrence rate of HCC after transplant was 17%.[11] A more recent study by Yin and colleagues confirmed similar findings; 54.8% of patients with early/intermediate HCC beyond MC were downstaged using TACE, 38.8% of whom received a liver transplant. They also reported significantly higher rates of receiving liver transplant if a tumor responded to within MC after first, second, or third TACE procedure (52% vs 22%, 53% vs 11%, and 44% vs 3.7%, respectively), compared with those beyond Milan but subsequently downstaged after additional TACE.[30] No studies have shown clear superiority of the chemoembolic options,[14] although PRECISION V demonstrated significant increase in tumor complete response with DEB-TACE.[25]

Transarterial Radioembolization

TARE targets HCC through the delivery of yttrium-90 (Y^{90}) attached to radioembolic microspheres, which are injected through the hepatic artery. These spheres lodge within the arterioles and undergo beta decay, delivering continuous, low-dose radiation to the tumor during a 2-week period, damaging cell repair mechanisms and precipitating cell death.[31] TARE may be performed as an outpatient, and arteriography is performed 1 to 2 weeks before the procedure for mapping of the tumor blood supply, as well as calculation of the hepatopulmonary shunt fraction, which can increase the risk of unintended radiation damage after TARE. This mapping is done via technetium-99m-labeled macroaggregated albumin, combined with single photon emission computed tomography imaging technology (SPECT).[31] Presence of a large intrahepatic portosystemic shunt is an absolute contraindication to TARE if the lung shunting fraction is greater than 20%,[32] or if the estimated lung mean dose of a single treatment is 30 Gy or greater or cumulative dose of multiple treatments is 50 Gy or greater[33] as there is a prohibitively high risk of posttreatment radiation pneumonitis.

Box 2
Modified Response Evaluation Criteria in Solid Tumors guidelines for measuring tumor response to locoregional therapy

mRECIST Criteria for HCC
  CR: Disappearance of any intratumoral arterial enhancement in all target lesions
  PR: At least a 30% decrease in the sum of diameters of viable (enhancement in the arterial phase) target lesions, taking as reference the baseline sum of the diameters of target lesions
  SD: Any cases that do not qualify for either partial response or progressive disease
  PD: An increase of at least 20% in the sum of the diameters of viable (enhancing) target lesions, taking as reference the smallest sum of the diameters of viable (enhancing) target lesions recorded since treatment started

Abbreviations: CR, complete response; PR, partial response; SD, stable disease; PD, progressive disease.

Adapted from Lencioni R, Llovet JM. Modified RECIST (mRECIST) assessment for hepatocellular carcinoma. Semin Liver Dis 2010; 30(1):52–60.

Techniques in TARE delivery have evolved since its inception as a treatment of HCC. Radiation segmentectomy delivers a high dose of radiation (target dose of >190 Gy) to a maximum of 2 liver segments, concentrating cytotoxic effects and limiting unnecessary parenchymal damage.[34] This strategy has offered a low risk of hepatic toxicity while still maintaining adequate margins for obliteration of any satellite lesions.[35] Similar to chemoembolization, patients with Child-Pugh class C, inadequate liver reserve (ie, large tumor burden), and/or limited performance status have tradition-ally been poor candidates for TARE.[36] However, TARE may offer a better option for patients with PVT given the reduced reliance on embolization of hepatic arterial branches.

With adequate preprocedural planning, adverse effects from nontarget radiation de-livery (eg, gastrointestinal [GI] ulceration, radiation pneumonitis, cholecystitis) are rare.[34] Radiation-induced liver disease (RILD) is a unique but still uncommon compli-cation of TARE. RILD has been seen in 1% to 4% of patients, typically in those with limited hepatic reserve or in patients undergoing lobar treatment. RILD may develop acutely or as a late-onset complication, consisting of local vascular, fibroblastic, and parenchymal change due to the radiosensitivity of nonparenchymal cells, which results in hepatic fibrosis.[37] Gemcitabine can potentiate the risk of RILD, and as such is held for 4 weeks before treatment.[31] By far the most common adverse effect after TARE is PES, which is less severe than that seen after TACE, with reported rates 20% to 70%.[32]

Radiographic response to TARE is not immediate; the tumor response evolves grad-ually during a period of 3 to 6 months before the maximum effect is fully realized.[34] This delay does not indicate a less-effective therapy. In fact, segmental TARE has been shown to lead to higher complete response rate, local tumor control, and progression-free survival than segmental TACE, while maintaining similar toxicity.[38] Complete his-tologic necrosis was induced more frequently with TARE, in 89% of small lesions (1–3 cm), 65% of medium lesions (3–5 cm), and 33% of large lesions (5 cm+), compared with 35%, 42%, and 33% with TACE.[34] Even compared with DEB-TACE, TARE pro-vided superior tumor control and survival in participants with BCLC-A and BCLC-B dis-eases in a randomized controlled trial.[39] These benefits held up in meta-analysis,[40] as TARE consistently provided a significantly longer time to progression than TACE, although overall survival times were similar. As a primary downstaging therapy, TARE has also been reported in several studies to be more effective in reducing HCC from a T3 to T2 lesion, with success in 58% of patients compared with 31% using TACE.[40] Interestingly, despite their similarity as embolic interventions, patients under-going TARE reported improvements in quality of life despite a more advanced disease than the TACE cohort.[41]

Tumor Ablation

Radiofrequency (RFA) and microwave ablation (MWA) are the predominant tumor ablative therapies used for downstaging. Although other therapies such as percuta-neous ethanol injection, cryoablation, and laser ablation exist, percutaneous thermal modalities (ie, RFA and MWA) have been considered the optimal choice.[42] Both mo-dalities rely on imaging guidance and monitoring during therapy, typically with CT or ultrasound.[14]

RFA exerts its effect through delivery of an alternating electrical current in the RFA range (350–500 kHz) to the targeted lesion. The tumor is subjected to high tempera-tures from the frictional heating, resulting in coagulation necrosis and cell death. An ablative zone develops, consisting of the tumor and a surrounding 5 to 10 mm of ab-lated adjacent liver parenchyma.[42] The utility of RFA is limited by the heat sink effect because large blood vessels proximal to the tumor can disperse some of the thermal energy created; this can lead to an unpredictable ablation zone and overall efficacy of treatment. Despite this effect, it delivers less energy to nearby tracking structures, such a bile ducts.

In comparison, MWA heats tissue through an oscillating microwave field (915/ 2450 MHz), with consistently higher temperatures and faster ablation times. MWA is able to generate a larger volume of necrosis making it a valuable alternative for tumors greater than 3 cm.[42] Notably, MWA has also been shown to be less prone to inducing a heat sink effect, and thus a more appropriate treatment of tumors adjacent to large vessels.[43] Patients with multiple lesions may be better candidates for MWA as well, given the ability to perform simultaneous treatments with multiple electrodes.[42]

The most common side effect after percutaneous ablation is postablation syndrome (PAS), a flu-like illness occurring in 25% to 35% of patients, with a direct correlation to treatment volume. Cases are typically self-limiting and last around 5 days.[31] More concerning adverse effects include damage to surrounding organs, including the diaphragm, GI tract, and gallbladder; this may be seen more often with MWA due to the higher thermal efficiency. Other rare complications include tumor seeding along the needle track, biloma formation, and bleeding in superficial tumors.[44] Increased complication rates were seen with larger tumor and ablated tissue volume, presence of multiple tumors, and Child-Pugh class B or greater. The rate of major adverse events has been demonstrated less than 5% in several reviews, with RFA maintaining a slightly better safety profile.[45,46] On the whole, ablation therapies have lower morbidity rates than other discussed LRTs, with improved liver preservation and shorter hospital lengths of stay.[31]

For tumors with a median size of 2.5 cm, the utility of percutaneous ablative therapies in local tumor control has been confirmed in a study of explanted livers, with complete radiologic response in 98.9% of nodules and complete pathologic response in 97.3% of nodules.[47] A clear superiority of MWA or RFA has not been documented in terms of outcomes, with similar efficacies and trade-offs that warrant individualized treatment plans.[43,45] A meta-analysis of 7 studies comparing RFA and MWA showed equivalent rates of complete response and local recurrence.[43] Ablative therapies were not typically first line for downstaging, and as such, there lacks evidence on their efficacy as downstaging monotherapy. However, both RFA and MWA have been studied in combination with TACE.[14] Sheta and colleagues compared combination single-session treatment with RFA or MWA, followed by TACE, to TACE monotherapy. Both MWA + TACE and RFA + TACE had higher rates of tumor response, with MWA in combination outperforming RFA in combination (80% vs 70%, vs 50% with TACE alone).[48]

Radiation Therapy

Historically, external beam radiation therapy (EBRT) for the management of HCC has been avoided due to the risk of RILD; however, modern advances with the development of three-dimensional conformal radiation therapy techniques has allowed for more refined and targeted delivery. There are a variety of dose-fractionated regimens and EBRT modalities, including stereotactic body radiotherapy (SBRT), which entails using a single or limited number (3 to 6) of high-dose radiotherapy fractions that are delivered to a precisely defined target. SBRT techniques may be especially useful for patients ineligible for percutaneous ablation (eg, with superficial lesions, tumors adjacent to large vessels or the diaphragm) and has similar indications as catheter-based therapies. Of note, in scenarios where the hollow viscera are located in close proximity to the tumor, high doses of radiotherapy should be limited because these structures are more sensitive to postradiation complications.

Although SBRT was not included in the most recent BCLC update, the 2022 clinical practice guidelines released by the American Society for Radiation Oncology (ASRO) make a conditional recommendation for ultrahypofractionated or moderately hypofractionated EBRT as a downstaging strategy for HCC.[49] Fractional regimens vary based on center but those recommended by the ASRO are presented in **Table 4**.[49]

Assessing response to therapy can be more difficult with SBRT on short-interval imaging because treated HCC may have persistent arterial phase hyperenhancement and washout. mRECIST has used the single largest diameter of the arterial phase enhancing tumor component, and thus may lead to incorrect characterization of tumor as viable.[50] However, SBRT has still been shown to have similar efficacy in pathologic response and potentially decreased side effects compared with other LRTs in bridging therapy.[51–54] The most common serious side effects studied were thrombocytopenia and GI bleeding or ulcer.[55]

The use of SBRT as a bridging strategy before liver transplant has been more highly studied than its application as a downstaging tool, with the former bridging studies having demonstrated favorable safety and efficacy profiles. SBRT has been shown to have perioperative complications, patient and recurrence-free survival rates after transplant, similar to that seen with TACE. When used in combination with TACE before liver transplant, explants have shown evidence of complete histologic necrosis.[56] Indeed, several meta-analyses have demonstrated an improvement in overall survival with TACE plus EBRT compared with TACE alone,[57,58] in addition to improved tumor complete response rates.[57] In patients undergoing SBRT bridging therapy, of which almost two-thirds were beyond MC, Sapisochin and colleagues[52] reported explant tumor necrosis in 90%, with more than half of patients having greater than 50% necrosis. Five-year survival from transplant was 73%, 69%, and 75% ($P = .7$), respectively, for the RFA, TACE, and SBRT cohorts. Data are lacking regarding its use for downstaging, and no prospective data comparing SBRT to other LRTs exist. Currently, the use of SBRT in lieu of other liver-directed therapies has depended on institutional experience as well as patient preference, given that SBRT requires multiple sessions to complete. Although it has not yet firmly entrenched itself into the treatment paradigm of HCC, SBRT may be a useful adjunct for select patients and is being increasingly used.[49]

Liver Resection

Surgical resection is often the best up-front strategy for cure and control of HCC as compared with LRT; however, only about 20% of patients with HCC are candidates

Table 4
Most common stereotactic body radiation therapy doses and fractionations for primary liver cancers

Fractionation Regimen	Total Dose and Fractionation	BED$_{10}$
Ultrahypofractionation	Noncirrhotic (IHC): 4000–6000 cGy/3–5 fx	7200–18,000 cGy
	CP class A: 4000–5000 cGy/3–5 fx	7200–12,500 cGy
	CP class B7: 3000–4000 cGy/5 fx	4800–7200 cGy
Moderate hypofractionation	4500–6750 cGy/15fx	5900–9800 cGy
Standard fractionation	5040 cGy/28 fx	5947 cGy

Abbreviations: BED$_{10}$, biologically effective dose; IHC, intrahepatic cholangiocarcinoma; CP, Child-Pugh; cGy, Centigray; fx, fractionation.
Adapted from 2022 American Society for Radiation Oncology [ASTRO] Clinical Practice Guideline; with permission.[49]

for liver resection.[59] Due to perioperative risks, as well as the potential for a more difficult reoperative field during liver transplant, resection has not been commonly used as a downstaging modality.[45] When used, pathologic review of the explanted specimen permits assessment of tumor features that may portend a higher risk of recurrence (eg, undifferentiated histology, satellite lesions, microvascular invasion, or capsular invasion).[60] Several limited studies attest to the feasibility of liver transplant following liver resection.[45,61–63] Belghiti and colleagues[63] were among the first to report similar rates of complications and survival after secondary liver transplant following resection, as compared with primary liver transplant. More recently, Liu and colleagues showed that salvage liver transplant for recurrent HCC outside of MC but within University of San Francisco criteria (ie, single tumor ≤6.5 cm or ≤3 tumors with the largest tumor diameter ≤4.5 cm and total tumor diameter ≤8 cm) demonstrated similar overall survival, perioperative mortality, posttransplant complications, and recurrence rates when compared with patients with recurrences within MC.[62]

SYSTEMIC TREATMENT OPTIONS

Systemic therapy for HCC was initially indicated only for advanced disease, not otherwise amenable to resection or interventional therapies. Although this strategy was proven to prolong survival, low tumor response rates limited its use.[64] However, the development of several novel pharmacologic agents since 2017 has changed the landscape of treatment options. Currently available medications can be broadly classified into tyrosine kinase inhibitors (TKIs) and immunotherapies (eg, PD-1 and CTLA4 inhibitors). In the setting of downstaging to liver transplant, scant data exist on the utility and long-term effects of these therapies, particularly in regards to rejection after treatment[13]; however, they have offered an opportunity to change the profile of the candidate meeting criteria for transplant.

Tyrosine Kinase Inhibitors

Approved in 2008 as the first systemic treatment for HCC, sorafenib is a multitarget oral TKI with antivascular endothelial growth factor (anti-VEGF) receptor properties. Although case reports of sorafenib as a downstaging monotherapy exist,[64–66] data from large phase III randomized clinical trials showed objective response rates of 2% to 3.3%.[67,68] These rates are likely understated however, and better methods of assessment tumor response after treatment now exist (ie, mRECIST).[27] The recent phase III REFLECT trial showed that lenvatinib, a newer TKI, was noninferior to sorafenib as a first-line treatment of unresectable HCC.[69] Indeed, case series have demonstrated it may be more effective in downstaging HCC for the purpose of surgery or ablation therapy.[70] Cabozantinib and regorafenib are TKIs approved as second-line therapy.[71] Due to their mechanism of action in molecular pathways involving tissue regeneration and repair, TKIs inhibit wound healing. Because this may confer a higher risk of complications for patients undergoing liver transplant, a washout period before transplant would be ideal, although logistically challenging for deceased donor transplants.[13] The extent of the efficacy and safety of TKIs pretransplant is largely unknown given the lack of large trials, and their true utility as a downstaging therapy has yet to be fully answered.

Immunotherapy

The currently available immune checkpoint inhibitors (ICIs) for HCC may be used alone or in combination. FDA-approved ICI regimens consist of nivolumab (PD-1), pembrolizumab (PD-1), ramucirumab (VEGFR2), nivolumab/ipilimumab (CTLA-4), atezolizumab (PD-L1)/bevacizumab (VEGF), and tremelimumab (CTLA-4)/durvalumab (PD-L1).[72,73] The combination of atezolizumab and bevacizumab was recently approved as first-line HCC therapy, with a demonstrated overall and progression-free survival benefit versus sorafenib.[74,75] Other combination therapies include tremelimumab and durvalumab, which has similarly been shown to be superior to sorafenib,[71] as well as nivolumab and ipilimumab, which has been FDA-approved for previously treated HCC.[76]

With regards to downstaging, immunotherapy has the potential to treat advanced disease and yield responses that are traditionally within transplant criteria; however, the risks of severe allograft rejection and systemic treatment-related morbidity and death remain concerning.[77] Specifically, in a review by Yin and colleagues of 28 patients treated with ICIs after transplant, nearly one-third developed rejection. It is postulated that this increased risk is seen with younger age, less time between liver transplant and ICI therapy (ie, shorter washout time), and PD-1/PD-L1 expression in the graft.[78]

There have been several case reports demonstrating the use of immunotherapy as neoadjuvant treatment before liver transplantation. The largest reported series by Tabrizian and colleagues[79] is of 9 patients receiving nivolumab, with 3 of these being beyond MC during the pretransplant course. Despite 89% of patients (8/9) receiving nivolumab within 4 weeks of transplant, there was no report of severe allograft rejection, graft loss, disease recurrence, or patient death.[79] This contrasts with a subsequent institutional series wherein patients were treated with nivolumab up until 10 days to 6 months before transplant.[80] One patient in this series required retransplant due to massive hepatic necrosis and one patient required rabbit antithymocyte globulin for salvage in the setting of allograft rejection. The investigators concluded that a withdrawal time of 3 months or more did not seem to increase rejection after transplant. A separate series has similarly demonstrated successful downstaging and transplant using atezolizumab plus bevacizumab without LRT.[81] As these reports are promising, results from ongoing and newly designed trials are warranted to inform indications for neoadjuvant use, delineation of which immunotherapy (or combinations) are most efficacious, the timing of cessation before transplant, and the management of immunosuppression after transplant.

COMBINATION THERAPIES

Many of the current downstaging trials have focused on combination therapies and the effect of LRTs (typically TACE or TARE) in various combination with systemic chemotherapies. No published study has provided evidence of superiority of any combination therapy over another; however, the highest rates of downstaging success have been seen with multimodal therapy.[13] Given the sheer number of trials currently active and recruiting,[82] full discussion of available and emerging combination therapies is beyond the scope of this review.

EVALUATION OF OVERALL OUTCOMES

Downstaging of HCC for liver transplant has provided benefit for eligible patients, over LRT alone. Indeed, in a phase 2 b/3 trial, a significant survival advantage for patients undergoing HCC downstaging followed by transplant (5-year OS rate, 77.5%) compared with LRT and systemic treatment without transplant (5-year OS rate, 31.2%; $P = .04$) was demonstrated.[83] Overall downstaging success rates with LRT range from 24% to 90%, with reported variation in rates and outcomes due to differences in pre-LRT tumor burden and assessment of treatment response.[59] On systematic review, an overall downstaging success rate of 48% and a postliver transplant HCC recurrence rate of

16% have been noted.[11] In intention-to-treat analysis, these numbers were similar:[9] 55.2% of patients (45.5%–64.5%) underwent successful down-staging and 31.5% (24.0%–40.1%) received liver transplant. Among patients who received a liver transplant, the recurrence rate was 16.1% (11.8%–21.4%). This latter study also compared transplant and HCC recurrence rates in patients within the UNOS-DS criteria or beyond, noting liver transplant in 48.6% versus 28.6% of patients ($P = .03$) and recurrence in 9.1% versus 20.4% of liver transplant recipients ($P < .001$).[9]

Tabrizian and colleagues recently published highly relevant long-term data on patients undergoing liver transplant and downstaging for HCC and found 10-year survival and recurrence rates of 52% and 20.4%, respectively, in the downstaging group, as compared with 60.5% and 14.3%, respectively, for patients always within MC, and 43.3% and 41.1%, respectively, in those whose disease was not downstaged.[84] This large multicenter study validated the UNOS-DS policy and demonstrated that extension beyond Milan with intent to downstage has remained beneficial for patients and has served an equitable strategy in an organ constrained practice environment. Findings by Mehta and colleagues that AFP of 100 ng/mL or greater at liver transplant and wait time of less than 6 months were predictors for diminished postliver transplant survival for downstaged patients, further underline the need to incorporate tumor biology (ie, AFP and expected wait times) into tumor downstaging models.[85]

SUMMARY

Downstaging has been shown to be feasible for HCC within UNOS-DS criteria, with successful long-term outcomes for patients and grafts. Interventional liver-directed therapies have been the standard of care for amenable HCC lesions, and are well studied, with TACE, TARE, and ablation remaining first-line treatments for tumor control. Most recently, however, the treatment paradigm has begun to shift with the introduction of more effective systemic therapies. Immunotherapy holds promise in the downstaging setting, although further trials are warranted to assess feasibility, efficacy, and safety, as well as timing in the context of liver transplant. Until such data are produced, individual patient and center-specific expertise will likely continue to guide treatment regimens.

CLINICS CARE POINTS

- Successful HCC downstaging rates after LRT approach 50%, with posttransplant recurrence rates similar to patients always within Milan criteria.
- Validation of current downstaging protocols supports the incorporation of markers of tumor biology, such as AFP, into modern models for posttransplant outcomes.
- The choice between available LRTs should be guided by patient and tumor factors, as well as center-specific expertise.
- While a promising forefront in HCC downstaging, the utility and safety of systemic therapies (ie, TKIs and immune checkpoint inhibitors) is currently limited by a lack of data to guide neoadjuvant use and management of immunosuppression posttransplant.

DISCLOSURE

The authors have no relevant commercial or financial conflicts of interest.
Funding: No funding to disclose.

REFERENCES

1. Centers for Disease Control and Prevention. An Update on Cancer Deaths in the United States. In: Disease Control and Prevention, Division of Cancer Prevention and Control; 2022. Prevention. CfDCa. An Update on Cancer Deaths in the United States. Atlanta, GA: US Department of Health and Human Services, Centers for; 2022.
2. Kwong AJ, Ebel NH, Kim WR, et al. OPTN/SRTR 2020 Annual Data Report: Liver. Am J Transplant 2022;22(Suppl 2):204–309.
3. Mehta N. Liver Transplantation Criteria for Hepatocellular Carcinoma, Including Posttransplant Management. Clin Liver Dis 2021;17(5):332–6.
4. Seehofer D, Petrowsky H, Schneeberger S, et al. Patient Selection for Downstaging of Hepatocellular Carcinoma Prior to Liver Transplantation-Adjusting the Odds? Transpl Int 2022;35:10333.
5. Majno PE, Adam R, Bismuth H, et al. Influence of preoperative transarterial lipiodol chemoembolization on resection and transplantation for hepatocellular carcinoma in patients with cirrhosis. Ann Surg 1997;226(6):688–701 [discussion 701-3].
6. Llovet JM, Bru C, Bruix J. Prognosis of hepatocellular carcinoma: the BCLC staging classification. Semin Liver Dis 1999;19(3):329–38.
7. Llovet JM, Fuster J, Bruix J, et al. The Barcelona approach: diagnosis, staging, and treatment of hepatocellular carcinoma. Liver Transplant 2004;10(2 Suppl 1):S115–20.
8. Reig M, Forner A, Rimola J, et al. BCLC strategy for prognosis prediction and treatment recommendation: The 2022 update. J Hepatol 2022;76(3):681–93.
9. Tan D.J.H., Lim W.H., Yong J.N., et al., UNOS Down-Staging Criteria for Liver Transplantation of Hepatocellular Carcinoma: Systematic Review and Meta-Analysis of 25 Studies, Clin Gastroenterol Hepatol, 21 (6),2023, 1475-1484.
10. Mehta N, Bhangui P, Yao FY, et al. Liver Transplantation for Hepatocellular Carcinoma. Working Group Report from the ILTS Transplant Oncology Consensus Conference. Transplantation 2020;104(6):1136–42.
11. Parikh ND, Waljee AK, Singal AG. Downstaging hepatocellular carcinoma: A systematic review and pooled analysis. Liver Transplant 2015;21(9):1142–52.
12. Yao FY, Fidelman N. Reassessing the boundaries of liver transplantation for hepatocellular carcinoma: Where do we stand with tumor down-staging? Hepatology 2016;63(3):1014–25.
13. Frankul L, Frenette C. Hepatocellular Carcinoma: Downstaging to Liver Transplantation as Curative Therapy. J Clin Transl Hepatol 2021;9(2):220–6.
14. Makary MS, Khandpur U, Cloyd JM, et al. Locoregional Therapy Approaches for Hepatocellular Carcinoma: Recent Advances and Management Strategies. Cancers 2020;12(7).
15. Lencioni R, de Baere T, Soulen MC, et al. Lipiodol transarterial chemoembolization for hepatocellular carcinoma: A systematic review of efficacy and safety data. Hepatology 2016;64(1):106–16.
16. Woo HY, Heo J. Transarterial chemoembolization using drug eluting beads for the treatment of hepatocellular carcinoma: Now and future. Clin Mol Hepatol 2015; 21(4):344–8.
17. Tovoli F, Negrini G, Bolondi L. Comparative analysis of current guidelines for the treatment of hepatocellular carcinoma. Hepat Oncol 2016;3(2):119–36.
18. Benson AB, D'Angelica MI, Abbott DE, et al. Hepatobiliary Cancers, Version 2.2021, NCCN Clinical Practice Guidelines in Oncology. J Natl Compr Canc Netw 2021;19(5):541–65.

19. Silva JP, Berger NG, Tsai S, et al. Transarterial chemoembolization in hepatocellular carcinoma with portal vein tumor thrombosis: a systematic review and meta-analysis. HPB (Oxford) 2017;19(8):659–66.

20. Galle PR, Tovoli F, Foerster F, et al. The treatment of intermediate stage tumours beyond TACE: From surgery to systemic therapy. J Hepatol 2017;67(1):173–83.

21. Lu J, Zhao M, Arai Y, et al. Clinical practice of transarterial chemoembolization for hepatocellular carcinoma: consensus statement from an international expert panel of International Society of Multidisciplinary Interventional Oncology (IS-MIO). Hepatobiliary Surg Nutr 2021;10(5):661.

22. Blackburn H, West S. Management of Postembolization Syndrome Following Hepatic Transarterial Chemoembolization for Primary or Metastatic Liver Cancer. Cancer Nurs 2016;39(5):E1–18.

23. Castells A, Bruix J, Ayuso C, et al. Transarterial embolization for hepatocellular carcinoma. Antibiotic prophylaxis and clinical meaning of postembolization fever. J Hepatol 1995;22(4):410–5.

24. Melchiorre F, Patella F, Pescatori L, et al. DEB-TACE: a standard review. Future Oncol 2018;14(28):2969–84.

25. Lammer J, Malagari K, Vogl T, et al. Prospective randomized study of doxorubicin-eluting-bead embolization in the treatment of hepatocellular carcinoma: results of the PRECISION V study. Cardiovasc Intervent Radiol 2010; 33(1):41–52.

26. Chen P, Yuan P, Chen B, et al. Evaluation of drug-eluting beads versus conventional transcatheter arterial chemoembolization in patients with unresectable hepatocellular carcinoma: A systematic review and meta-analysis. Clin Res Hepatol Gastroenterol 2017;41(1):75–85.

27. Lencioni R, Llovet JM. Modified RECIST (mRECIST) assessment for hepatocellular carcinoma. Semin Liver Dis 2010;30(1):52–60.

28. Llovet JM, Bruix J. Systematic review of randomized trials for unresectable hepatocellular carcinoma: Chemoembolization improves survival. Hepatology 2003; 37(2):429–42.

29. Yao FY, Mehta N, Flemming J, et al. Downstaging of hepatocellular cancer before liver transplant: long-term outcome compared to tumors within Milan criteria. Hepatology 2015;61(6):1968–77.

30. Yin C, Armstrong S, Shin R, et al. Bridging and downstaging with TACE in early and intermediate stage hepatocellular carcinoma: Predictors of receiving a liver transplant. Ann Gastroenterol Surg 2023;7(2):295–305.

31. Makary MS, Ramsell S, Miller E, et al. Hepatocellular carcinoma locoregional therapies: Outcomes and future horizons. World J Gastroenterol 2021;27(43): 7462–79.

32. Riaz A, Awais R, Salem R. Side effects of yttrium-90 radioembolization. Front Oncol 2014;4:198.

33. Salem R, Parikh P, Atassi B, et al. Incidence of radiation pneumonitis after hepatic intra-arterial radiotherapy with yttrium-90 microspheres assuming uniform lung distribution. Am J Clin Oncol 2008;31(5):431–8.

34. Miller FH, Lopes Vendrami C, Gabr A, et al. Evolution of Radioembolization in Treatment of Hepatocellular Carcinoma: A Pictorial Review. Radiographics 2021;41(6):1802–18.

35. Lewandowski RJ, Gabr A, Abouchaleh N, et al. Radiation Segmentectomy: Potential Curative Therapy for Early Hepatocellular Carcinoma. Radiology 2018; 287(3):1050–8.

36. Kis B, El-Haddad G, Sheth RA, et al. Liver-Directed Therapies for Hepatocellular Carcinoma and Intrahepatic Cholangiocarcinoma. Cancer Control 2017;24(3). 1073274817729244.

37. Kim J, Jung Y. Radiation-induced liver disease: current understanding and future perspectives. Exp Mol Med 2017;49(7):e359.

38. Padia SA, Johnson GE, Horton KJ, et al. Segmental Yttrium-90 Radioembolization versus Segmental Chemoembolization for Localized Hepatocellular Carcinoma: Results of a Single-Center, Retrospective, Propensity Score-Matched Study. J Vasc Intervent Radiol 2017;28(6):777–785 e1.

39. Dhondt E, Lambert B, Hermie L, et al. (90)Y Radioembolization versus Drug-eluting Bead Chemoembolization for Unresectable Hepatocellular Carcinoma: Results from the TRACE Phase II Randomized Controlled Trial. Radiology 2022; 303(3):699–710.

40. Lewandowski RJ, Kulik LM, Riaz A, et al. A comparative analysis of transarterial downstaging for hepatocellular carcinoma: chemoembolization versus radioembolization. Am J Transplant 2009;9(8):1920–8.

41. Salem R, Gilbertsen M, Butt Z, et al. Increased quality of life among hepatocellular carcinoma patients treated with radioembolization, compared with chemoembolization. Clin Gastroenterol Hepatol 2013;11(10):1358–1365 e1.

42. Poulou LS, Botsa E, Thanou I, et al. Percutaneous microwave ablation vs radiofrequency ablation in the treatment of hepatocellular carcinoma. World J Hepatol 2015;7(8):1054–63.

43. Facciorusso A, Di Maso M, Muscatiello N. Microwave ablation versus radiofrequency ablation for the treatment of hepatocellular carcinoma: A systematic review and meta-analysis. Int J Hyperther 2016;32(3):339–44.

44. Martin RC, Scoggins CR, McMasters KM. Safety and efficacy of microwave ablation of hepatic tumors: a prospective review of a 5-year experience. Ann Surg Oncol 2010;17(1):171–8.

45. Pompili M, Francica G, Ponziani FR, et al. Bridging and downstaging treatments for hepatocellular carcinoma in patients on the waiting list for liver transplantation. World J Gastroenterol 2013;19(43):7515–30.

46. Bertot LC, Sato M, Tateishi R, et al. Mortality and complication rates of percutaneous ablative techniques for the treatment of liver tumors: a systematic review. Eur Radiol 2011;21(12):2584–96.

47. Bale R, Schullian P, Eberle G, et al. Stereotactic Radiofrequency Ablation of Hepatocellular Carcinoma: a Histopathological Study in Explanted Livers. Hepatology 2019;70(3):840–50.

48. Sheta E, El-Kalla F, El-Gharib M, et al. Comparison of single-session transarterial chemoembolization combined with microwave ablation or radiofrequency ablation in the treatment of hepatocellular carcinoma: a randomized-controlled study. Eur J Gastroenterol Hepatol 2016;28(10):1198–203.

49. Apisarnthanarax S, Barry A, Cao M, et al. External Beam Radiation Therapy for Primary Liver Cancers: An ASTRO Clinical Practice Guideline. Pract Radiat Oncol 2022;12(1):28–51.

50. Shampain KL, Hackett CE, Towfighi S, et al. SBRT for HCC: Overview of technique and treatment response assessment. Abdom Radiol (NY) 2021;46(8): 3615–24.

51. Bush DA, Smith JC, Slater JD, et al. Randomized Clinical Trial Comparing Proton Beam Radiation Therapy with Transarterial Chemoembolization for Hepatocellular Carcinoma: Results of an Interim Analysis. Int J Radiat Oncol Biol Phys 2016; 95(1):477–82.

52. Sapisochin G, Barry A, Doherty M, et al. Stereotactic body radiotherapy vs. TACE or RFA as a bridge to transplant in patients with hepatocellular carcinoma. An intention-to-treat analysis. J Hepatol 2017;67(1):92–9.
53. Mohamed M, Katz AW, Tejani MA, et al. Comparison of outcomes between SBRT, yttrium-90 radioembolization, transarterial chemoembolization, and radiofrequency ablation as bridge to transplant for hepatocellular carcinoma. Adv Radiat Oncol 2016;1(1):35–42.
54. Wong TC, Lee VH, Law AL, et al. Prospective Study of Stereotactic Body Radiation Therapy for Hepatocellular Carcinoma on Waitlist for Liver Transplant. Hepatology 2021;74(5):2580–94.
55. Rim CH, Kim CY, Yang DS, et al. The role of external beam radiotherapy for hepatocellular carcinoma patients with lymph node metastasis: a meta-analysis of observational studies. Cancer Manag Res 2018;10:3305–15.
56. Wigg A, Hon K, Mosel L, et al. Down-staging of hepatocellular carcinoma via external-beam radiotherapy with subsequent liver transplantation: a case report. Liver Transplant 2013;19(10):1119–24.
57. Huo YR, Eslick GD. Transcatheter Arterial Chemoembolization Plus Radiotherapy Compared With Chemoembolization Alone for Hepatocellular Carcinoma: A Systematic Review and Meta-analysis. JAMA Oncol 2015;1(6):756–65.
58. Bai H, Gao P, Gao H, et al. Improvement of Survival Rate for Patients with Hepatocellular Carcinoma Using Transarterial Chemoembolization in Combination with Three-Dimensional Conformal Radiation Therapy: A Meta-Analysis. Med Sci Mon Int Med J Exp Clin Res 2016;22:1773–81.
59. Marrero JA, Kulik LM, Sirlin CB, et al. Diagnosis, Staging, and Management of Hepatocellular Carcinoma: 2018 Practice Guidance by the American Association for the Study of Liver Diseases. Hepatology 2018;68(2):723–50.
60. Sala M, Fuster J, Llovet JM, et al. High pathological risk of recurrence after surgical resection for hepatocellular carcinoma: an indication for salvage liver transplantation. Liver Transplant 2004;10(10):1294–300.
61. de Haas RJ, Lim C, Bhangui P, et al. Curative salvage liver transplantation in patients with cirrhosis and hepatocellular carcinoma: An intention-to-treat analysis. Hepatology 2018;67(1):204–15.
62. Liu F, Wei Y, Wang W, et al. Salvage liver transplantation for recurrent hepatocellular carcinoma within UCSF criteria after liver resection. PLoS One 2012;7(11): e48932.
63. Belghiti J, Cortes A, Abdalla EK, et al. Resection prior to liver transplantation for hepatocellular carcinoma. Ann Surg 2003;238(6):885–92 [discussion: 892-3].
64. Bertacco A, Vitale A, Mescoli C, et al. Sorafenib treatment has the potential to downstage advanced hepatocellular carcinoma before liver resection. Per Med 2020;17(2):83–7.
65. Vagefi PA, Hirose R. Downstaging of hepatocellular carcinoma prior to liver transplant: is there a role for adjuvant sorafenib in locoregional therapy? J Gastrointest Cancer 2010;41(4):217–20.
66. Vagefi PA, Hirose R. Sorafenib combined with locoregional therapy prior to liver transplantation for hepatocellular carcinoma: an update on a previous case report. J Gastrointest Cancer 2013;44(2):246–7.
67. Llovet JM, Ricci S, Mazzaferro V, et al. Sorafenib in advanced hepatocellular carcinoma. N Engl J Med 2008;359(4):378–90.
68. Cheng AL, Kang YK, Chen Z, et al. Efficacy and safety of sorafenib in patients in the Asia-Pacific region with advanced hepatocellular carcinoma: a phase III randomised, double-blind, placebo-controlled trial. Lancet Oncol 2009;10(1):25–34.

69. Kudo M, Finn RS, Qin S, et al. Lenvatinib versus sorafenib in first-line treatment of patients with unresectable hepatocellular carcinoma: a randomised phase 3 non-inferiority trial. Lancet 2018;391(10126):1163–73.

70. Tomonari T, Sato Y, Tanaka H, et al. Conversion therapy for unresectable hepato-cellular carcinoma after lenvatinib: Three case reports. Medicine (Baltim) 2020; 99(42):e22782.

71. Tran NH, Munoz S, Thompson S, et al. Hepatocellular carcinoma downstaging for liver transplantation in the era of systemic combined therapy with anti-VEGF/TKI and immunotherapy. Hepatology 2022;76(4):1203–18.

72. Bruix J, Chan SL, Galle PR, et al. Systemic treatment of hepatocellular carcinoma: An EASL position paper. J Hepatol 2021;75(4):960–74.

73. Psilopatis I, Damaskos C, Garmpi A, et al. FDA-Approved Monoclonal Antibodies for Unresectable Hepatocellular Carcinoma: What Do We Know So Far? Int J Mol Sci 2023;24(3).

74. Finn RS, Qin S, Ikeda M, et al. Atezolizumab plus Bevacizumab in Unresectable Hepatocellular Carcinoma. N Engl J Med 2020;382(20):1894–905.

75. Ahmed F, Onwumeh-Okwundu J, Yukselen Z, et al. Atezolizumab plus bevacizu-mab versus sorafenib or atezolizumab alone for unresectable hepatocellular car-cinoma: A systematic review. World J Gastrointest Oncol 2021;13(11):1813–32.

76. Yau T, Kang YK, Kim TY, et al. Efficacy and Safety of Nivolumab Plus Ipilimumab in Patients With Advanced Hepatocellular Carcinoma Previously Treated With Sor-afenib: The CheckMate 040 Randomized Clinical Trial. JAMA Oncol 2020;6(11): e204564.

77. Katariya NN, Lizaola-Mayo BC, Chascsa DM, et al. Immune Checkpoint Inhibitors as Therapy to Down-Stage Hepatocellular Carcinoma Prior to Liver Transplanta-tion. Cancers 2022;14(9).

78. Yin C, Baba T, He AR, et al. Immune checkpoint inhibitors in liver transplant re-cipients - a review of current literature. Hepatoma Research 2021;7(52).

79. Tabrizian P, Florman SS, Schwartz ME. PD-1 inhibitor as bridge therapy to liver transplantation? Am J Transplant 2021;21(5):1979–80.

80. Schnickel GT, Fabbri K, Hosseini M, et al. Liver transplantation for hepatocellular carcinoma following checkpoint inhibitor therapy with nivolumab. Am J Transplant 2022;22(6):1699–704.

81. Schmiderer A., Zoller H., Niederreiter M., et al., Liver transplantation after suc-cessful downstaging of a locally advanced hepatocellular carcinoma with sys-temic therapy, *Dig Dis*, 41(4),2023, 641-644.

82. Llovet JM, Castet F, Heikenwalder M, et al. Immunotherapies for hepatocellular carcinoma. Nat Rev Clin Oncol 2022;19(3):151–72.

83. Mazzaferro V, Citterio D, Bhoori S, et al. Liver transplantation in hepatocellular carcinoma after tumour downstaging (XXL): a randomised, controlled, phase 2b/3 trial. Lancet Oncol 2020;21(7):947–56.

84. Tabrizian P, Holzner ML, Mehta N, et al. Ten-Year Outcomes of Liver Transplant and Downstaging for Hepatocellular Carcinoma. JAMA Surg 2022;157(9):779–88.

85. Mehta N, Dodge JL, Grab JD, et al. National Experience on Down-Staging of He-patocellular Carcinoma Before Liver Transplant: Influence of Tumor Burden, Alpha-Fetoprotein, and Wait Time. Hepatology 2020;71(3):943–54.

Immunotherapy and Liver Transplantation

The Future or the Failure?

Parissa Tabrizian, MD, MSc[a,*], Allen Yu, MD, PhD[a],
Neha Debnath, MD[a], Bryan Myers, MD[a], Thomas Marron, MD, PhD[a]

KEYWORDS

- Liver transplantation • Hepatocellular carcinoma • Immunotherapy • Rejection
- Outcomes

KEY POINTS

- The increasing demand for liver transplantation (LT) for hepatocellular carcinoma (HCC) has led to the continued efforts to expand LT indications.
- Immunotherapy has revolutionized the treatment of advanced HCC over the past few years.
- HCC and other solid tumors exploit evolutionary conserved inhibitory immune checkpoints to evade antitumor immune response by upregulating cognate ligands or receptors capable of inhibiting antitumor immunity.

INTRODUCTION

A quarter century has passed since the milestone study by Mazzaferro and colleagues on liver transplantation (LT) for hepatocellular carcinoma (HCC).[1] The increasing demand for LT for HCC has led to the continued efforts to expand LT indications.[2] Downstaging (DS) to within Milan criteria has been incorporated into the organ allocation policy for HCC in the United States in 2017 and provides acceptable long-term survival.[3] The first randomized controlled trial has shown 5 year survival of 77%.[4] The United Network for Organ Sharing DS was recently incorporated in the updated Barcelona clinic liver cancer guidelines.[5] In addition, immunotherapy has revolutionized the treatment of advanced HCC over the past few years (**Fig. 1**).[6,7] There has been reluctance to use immunotherapy in transplant candidates due to scattered reports of severe rejection and graft loss.[8] The present review focuses on the rationale of neoadjuvant immune checkpoint inhibitor (ICI) in HCC, the experience of ICI in the pre- and posttransplant setting.

[a] Liver Transplant and Hepatobiliary Surgery, Recanati/Miller Transplantation Institute, Icahn School of Medicine at Mount Sinai, One Gustave L. Levy, New York, NY 10029, USA
* Corresponding author.
E-mail address: parissa.tabrizian@mountsinai.org

Surg Clin N Am 104 (2024) 163–182
https://doi.org/10.1016/j.suc.2023.07.009
0039-6109/24/© 2023 Elsevier Inc. All rights reserved.

surgical.theclinics.com

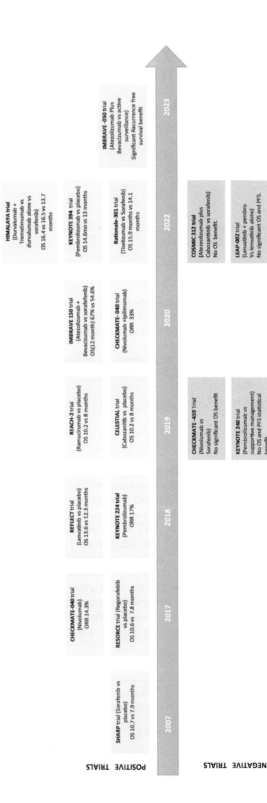

Fig. 1. Timeline of landmark positive and negative trials in HCC.

NEOADJUVANT IMMUNOTHERAPY RATIONALE

HCC and other solid tumors exploit evolutionary conserved inhibitory immune checkpoints to evade antitumor immune response by upregulating cognate ligands or receptors capable of inhibiting antitumor immunity. FDA-approved antibodies blocking PD-L1, CTLA-4, and LAG3 have demonstrated the ability to enhance antitumor immunity in clinically meaningful ways, and there are dozens of additional checkpoints and immunosuppressive pathways that are being therapeutically targeted in the tumor microenvironment. Recent landmark studies including the IMbrave150 and HIMALAYA trials have established the role of immunotherapy as the new standard of care for advanced HCC, whereas the role in earlier stage is still being explored.[6,7]

In early-stage HCC, surgical treatment or ablation is the mainstay of curative treatment. However, even among patients with tumors as small as 2 cm there is a nearly a 70% risk of recurrence.[9] Given that recurrence is typically not in the tumor bed, the primary reason for this high risk of recurrence is believed to be early dissemination of micrometastatic disease not evaluable at the time of surgical resection, and no perioperative approach has significantly decreased the risk of recurrence until recently when IMbrave050 study announced that adjuvant atezolizumab with bevacizumab treatment for early-stage HCC showed improvement in recurrence-free survival.[10,11] This is the first time any systemic therapy has shown conclusive benefit among patients with resectable HCC in a phase 3 clinical trial.[10,11] Tumors with significant immune infiltration at the time of resection—specifically high density of CD8+ T cells in the tumor and resected margin—are associated with a significantly low rate of recurrence following surgical resection for HCC, lending to the hypothesis that immune surveillance may play a role in risk of recurrence. This observation supports the theory that perioperative immunotherapy may aid in controlling the primary tumor as well as the all-too-common micrometastatic disease that is the nidus for recurrence.[12] Neoadjuvant or perioperative (neoadjuvant and adjuvant) immunotherapy is postulated to be superior to adjuvant immunotherapy because preoperative immunotherapy enhances the antitumor immunity, likely by means of priming new T-cell responses against the tumor neoantigens, whereas the tumor is still remains in vivo.[13] In the adjuvant setting, there is comparatively less immune priming and activation because the only neoantigens that linger in the body are from micrometastatic disease.[14] This hypothesis is supported by significant preclinical data,[13] and although it is unlikely that this clinical question will successfully be queried in HCC, the recent SWOG S1801 trial in melanoma showed that pre- and postoperative pembrolizumab led to better event-free survival (EFS) compared with adjuvant pembrolizumab alone, with a hazard ratio of 0.58.[15] Furthermore, tumors that are smaller in size might be associated with lower levels of clonal heterogeneity with lesser loss of heterozygosity, leading to more durable responses than those seen in the advanced/metastatic setting. This can potentially increase the chances of a stronger immune response against clonally conserved neoantigens leading to long-lasting benefits.[16] Based on randomized phase 3 trials, neoadjuvant immunotherapy by itself or with combination of chemotherapy has become standard line of therapy for triple-negative breast cancer and non small cell lung cancer (NSCLC) with promising phase 2 and 3 clinical trial data in multiple other tumor types.[17–19]

ONGOING TRIALS IN NEOADJUVANT IMMUNOTHERAPY IN HEPATOCELLULAR CARCINOMA

One of the first published trials regarding immunotherapy in the neoadjuvant setting in HCC was among patients with locally advanced disease. All patients had high-risk tumor features for which upfront surgical resection was not feasible. Nivolumab with cabozantinib was used to assess the possibility of DS tumors to enable curative-intent resection.[20] The trial enrolled 15 patients out of which 12 underwent resection; 5 patients had a major pathologic response (defined as ≥90% necrosis), with 1 patient attaining complete pathologic response. None of the patients experienced any treatment-related adverse event that precluded them to get surgery. Immunohisto-chemistry showed that the responder samples had a noticeably increased density of CD138+ cells in the region of the tumor with IgA-negative B cells.

Another phase 2 study presented the results of neoadjuvant cemiplimab in patients who met the criteria for surgical resection in early-stage HCC.[21] Twenty-one patients were enrolled in the trial and 20 patients effectively underwent surgery. The trials primary end point was significant tumor necrosis (defined by 70% or more necrosis of the resected tumor) which was seen in 4 of 20 tumors. There were no grade 4 or 5 adverse events. Immunohistochemistry analysis showed the increased density of CD8$^+$ T-cell infiltration in patients with 50% or greater necrosis in comparison with the patients with little to no necrosis. Another phase 2 study assessed the tolerability and safety of perioperative immunotherapy in patients with resectable HCC.[22] The trial enrolled 30 patients out of which 27 were randomly assigned to either nivolumab (13 patients) versus nivolumab plus ipilimumab (14 patients). The studies' primary endpoint was to assess the tolerability and safety of nivolumab with or without ipilimumab. Grade 3 to 4 adverse events were noted to be higher among patients who received nivolumab plus ipilimumab (43%) versus nivolumab alone (23%). None of the patients in either group had delays in their surgery due to any grade 3 or worse adverse events. Three (33%) of nine patients with nivolumab had a major pathologic response (defined as ≥70% necrosis in the resected tumor area) compared with three (27%) out of eleven patients with nivolumab plus ipilimumab. In addition, immunohistochemistry showed a substantial increase in T cells (CD3$^+$, CD8$^+$, and CD45RO$^+$ cells), B cells (CD20$^+$ cells), and immune cells expressing granzyme B, PD-1, and PD-L1 in the posttreatment tissue samples of the patients who had major pathologic response. Several other early phase clinical trials of novel checkpoints and combinations are being conducted with promising results (**Table 1**).[20–30]

A recent phase III trial (IMBRAVE 050) evaluating the use of atezolizumab in combination with bevacizumab in the adjuvant setting in patients with high risk of recurrence showed a statistically significant improvement in the RFS compared with active surveillance alone.[23] This is the first positive trial in the adjuvant setting post-resection in HCC patients.

IMMUNOTHERAPY PRE-LIVER TRANSPLANTATION

The role of ICIs in the pretransplant setting is unclear, and as would be expected there have been reports of allograft rejection when ICIs have been used posttransplant in patients with recurrent HCC.[31] Although clinical trials in the pretransplant setting are difficult to run in a standardized fashion given the heterogeneity of clinical progression and time-to-transplant, many patients who have been listed for transplant have received immunotherapy for HCC, and case series have demonstrated that ICI use before LT can be safe.[32–34] Here, the authors review their experience with ICI and liver transplants at a single tertiary referral center and describe the available literature to date. ICI therapy has received much attention given its success in a variety of cancers. They are considered to be the final choice for patients with recurrent tumors after transplantation. Preoperative ICIs have not been well studied, but the previously

Table 1
Ongoing neoadjuvant immunotherapy trials for resectable hepatocellular carcinoma

NCT/Identifier	Country	Neoadjuvant Treatment Arm	Primary Endpoints	Secondary Endpoints	Status
NCT03299946	US	Cabozantinib + nivolumab + surgery	Safety	Percentage of participants with complete response/MPRs, objective response rate (ORR), median overall survival (OS), disease-free survival (DFS)	Results available (Ho, Zhu et al,[20] 2021)
NCT03916627	US	Cemiplimab	Significant tumor necrosis (STN) at the time of surgery	DFS, overall response rate (ORR), OS	Results available (Marron, Fiel et al,[21] 2022)
NCT03222076	US	Ipilimumab + nivolumab	Safety	Objective response rate, time to progression, progression-free survival (PFS), surgical conversion rate	Results available (Kaseb, Hasanov et al,[22] 2022)
NCT04123379	US	Nivolumab/nivolumab + BMS-813160/nivolumab + BMS-986253	Major pathologic response (MPR) + Significant tumor necrosis (STN)	Percent of individuals who experience radiographic response, PFS, OS	Recruiting (No interim results available)
NCT04857684	US	SBRT + atezolizumab + bevacizumab	Proportion of patients with grade 3–4 treatment-related adverse events	Objective response rate (ORR), complete response (CR), OS, recurrence-free survival (RFS) after resection	Recruiting (No interim results available)
NCT04658147	US	Nivolumab + relatlimab	Number of patients who proceed to surgery	Objective response rate (ORR), OS, DFS	Recruiting (No interim results available)
NCT05194293	US	Durvalumab + regorafenib	Objective response rate (ORR)	PFS, RFS, Pathologic CR	Not yet recruiting
NCT05701488	US	Durvalumab + tremelimumab/durvalumab + tremelimumab + SIRT	Safety	Best radiologic response, best pathologic response, median OS, median PFS, CD8+/CD4+T-cell level, dendritic cell level, cytokines level, number of participants with surgical complications	Not yet recruiting

(continued on next page)

Table 1
(continued)

NCT/Identifier	Country	Neoadjuvant Treatment Arm	Primary Endpoints	Secondary Endpoints	Status
NCT03630640	France	Nivolumab	Local RFS	Intra-segmental/extra-segmental distant recurrence, OS	Results available (Harris)[24]
NCT03510871	Taiwan	Nivolumab plus ipilimumab	Percentage of subjects with tumor shrinkage after study drug treatment	Not mentioned	Results available (Su, Lin et al,[25] 2021)
NCT04615143	China	Tislelizumab combined lenvatinib/tislelizumab alone	DFS	Objective response rate, MPR	Results available (Chen, Wang et al,[26] 2022)
NCT03867370	China	Toripalimab + lenvatinib	MPR, CPR	OS, objective response rate, PFS	Results available (Shi, Ji et al,[27] 2021)
NCT04930315	China	Camrelizumab + apatinib	1-y tumor recurrence-free rate	OS, RFS, MPR	Result available (Bai, Chen et al,[28] 2022)
NCT03682276	UK	Ipilimumab + nivolumab	Delay to surgery, safety	Objective response rate, pathologic response rate	Results available (Pinato, Cortellini et al,[29] 2021)
NCT04297202	China	Apatinib combined with SHR-1210 (an anti-PD-1 inhibitor)	Major pathologic response	Pathologic CR, objective response (ORR), RFS, OS	Results available (Xia, Tang et al,[30] 2022)
NCT04727307	Multicenter in Europe	Neoadjuvant atezolizumab and adjuvant atezolizumab + bevacizumab in combination with percutaneous radiofrequency ablation	RFS	Not mentioned	Recruiting (No interim results available)
NCT04224480	Singapore	Pembrolizumab	HCC recurrence	Not mentioned	Recruiting (No interim results available)
NCT04954339	Korea	Atezolizumab plus bevacizumab	Pathologic CR	PFS, radiological response, (RFS)	Recruiting No interim results available)

NCT ID	Location	Intervention	Primary outcome	Secondary outcome	Status
NCT04521153	China	Camrelizumab + apatinib mesylate	3-y event-free survival (EFS)	OS, DFS, EFS	Recruiting (No interim results available)
NCT05277675	China	Tislelizumab/sintilimab + lenvatinib/bevacizumab + RFA	1-y RFS, 1-y OS	Procedure-related complications	Recruiting (No interim results available)
NCT05185531	China	Tislelizumab + stereotactic body radiotherapy	Delay to surgery, pathologic response rate	DFS, OS	Recruiting (No interim results available)
NCT05137899	Canada	Atezolizumab/bevacizumab	Proportion of patients who proceed to surgery	Response rate, PFS	Recruiting (No interim results available)
NCT05225116	China	Sintilimab + lenvatinib + radiotherapy	Proportion of patients who proceed to surgery	MPR, objective response rate (ORR), median overall survival (mOS), RFS	Recruiting (No interim results available)
NCT04727307	Multicenter in Europe	Neoadjuvant atezolizumab and adjuvant atezolizumab + bevacizumab in combination with percutaneous radiofrequency ablation	RFS	Not mentioned	Recruiting (No interim results available)
NCT05185739	UK	Pembrolizumab and lenvatinib	Major pathologic response rate	Radiological response rate, relapse-free survival	Recruiting (No interim results available)
NCT05250843	China	TACE/HAIC + lenvatinib + sintilimab	RFS	Adverse events	Not yet recruiting
NCT05389527	China	Pembrolizumab + lenvatinib	MPR	Pathologic CR (pCR), objective response rate (ORR), DFS, OS	Not yet recruiting
NCT05440864	Canada, Spain, Italy	Tremelimumab + durvalumab	Grade 3 adverse events (AEs) or immune-related adverse events	Number of patients who experience a surgical delay, overall response rate (ORR), pathologic response rate	Not yet recruiting
NCT04850157	China	Tislelizumab + IMRT	Relapse-free survival	Objective response rate (ORR), OS,	Not yet recruiting
NCT04850040	China	Camrelizumab + apatinib mesylate + oxaliplatin	MPR	ORR, 1-y tumor recurrence-free rate RFS, DFS	Not yet recruiting
NCT05471674	Hong Kong	Nivolumab	Pathologic tumor response rate	Recurrence-free survival, OS, short-term surgery outcomes	Completed (awaiting results)

published reports have observed increased chances at receiving transplants and a cure, improved outcomes of high-risk patients, and have the potential to DS lesions before transplant.[32–34]

The authors listed and successfully transplanted nine patients with HCC between 2017 and 2020, who were receiving nivolumab for pretransplant tumor treatment, with the last dose being within 4 weeks of transplant.[34] At median follow-up of 16 months posttransplant, the authors did not find any instances of severe allograft rejections, tumor recurrences, or deaths. In their literature search, the authors found reports of an additional 52 patients who received pre-liver transplant immunotherapy, as summarized in **Table 2**.[8,32,33,35–46]

Of the available data on the aggregated patients, 69% were male, with a mean age of 54 years. All patients received immunotherapy to treat HCC as their primary malignancy, with hepatitis C virus (HCV) as the leading underlying disorder in 29% of patients, HBV in 22%, and alcoholic liver disease in 7%. Cirrhosis in this population achieved an incidence of 24%. Graft rejection was reported in 33% of patients, with the mean time to rejection being 9 days, with given data. This is within the previously published rate of rejection of 30% to 40%.[47] However, liver biopsies in patients who had rejections are not routinely confirmed. Thus, at times, it is unclear if the immunosuppression was reduced for other indications. Recurrence occurred in 11% of patients, and the mortality rate was 5%. It has been hypothesized that PD1/PD-L1 expression plays a role in donor graft failure. There have been cases that correlate upregulation of PD-L1 in the allograft, which may have a protective effect which prevents early rejection. Patients treated with nivolumab who received a liver transplant within one half-life of the drug experienced acute rejection 75% of the time. The graft PD-1 status in our analysis is largely unreported but is positive in those who were recorded and exhibited rejection.

Another important factor to elucidate is the timing between the last dose of immunotherapy and liver transplant. The literature suggests a waiting period of 4 to 8 weeks.[48] The serum half-life of nivolumab in patients with cancer is approximately 27 days, and other PD-1/PD-L1 inhibitors have similarly long half-lives, and this should be taken into consideration when planning for a liver transplant and planning posttransplant immunosuppression time course. Some reports have expressed concern that the effects of immunotherapy may linger due to the presence of delayed toxicity.[48] However, there have been reports where no rejection was seen even within 1 week of treatment, and in general, acute rejection can be adequately treated by immunosuppressants.[38,49] In their review, the authors have found that all rejections but one, occurred within a 3-month window of ICI cessation.[34] This suggests that approximately three half-lives, or 3 months, of observation would be necessary before LT to avoid rejection. In the case of durvalumab, successful DS of HCC before liver transplant has been shown to require at least a 3-month washout period.[45] A large meta-analysis performed with a focus on solid tumors demonstrated that PD-1 inhibitors had superior overall survival (HR 0.75), over PD-L1 inhibitors.[50] However, additional prospective trials are necessary to solidify this finding. The choice of PD-1 inhibitors (nivolumab, pembrolizumab) or PD-L1 inhibitors (atezolizumab) has also not been well studied. In other cancers such as NSCLC, there seems no difference in response rate between PD-1 and PD-L1 inhibitors, and both side effect profiles are favorable.[51] In theory, PD-1 inhibitors are able to block their interaction with both PD-L1 and PD-L2 receptors and may provide additional benefit over PD-L1 inhibitors.

Induction therapy is commonly used for kidney, heart, and lung transplantation, but controversial in liver transplant. In theory, induction immunosuppression can improve

Table 2
Cases of immunotherapy use in pretransplant patients

Patients	Age (Years)	Underlying Disease	Immunotherapy	Time from Last Dose	Rejection	Outcome	Citation
1	66	HCV	Atezolizumab, bevacizumab	2 mo	–	No recurrence	Abdelrahim et al,[35] 2021
1	64	HCV	Nivolumab	0.5 mo	Mod to severe	Resolved rejection	Aby et al,[36] 2022
1	39	HBV	Toripalimab, lenvatinib	3 mo	Acute	Death	Chen et al,[37] 2021
1	64	–	Nivolumab	7 d	–	Recurrence	Chen Z et al,[38] 2021
1	47	–	Nivolumab	4 mo	–	Recurrence	Chen Z et al,[38] 2021
1	50	–	Nivolumab	2 mo	–	No recurrence	Chen Z et al,[38] 2021
1	38	–	Nivolumab	2 mo	–	No recurrence	Chen Z et al,[38] 2021
1	67	–	Nivolumab	2 mo	–	No recurrence	Chen Z et al,[38] 2021
8	63 (average)	HCV/HBV/NASH	Nivolumab	3 mo (average)	2 rejections	2 graft losses	Dave et al,[39] 2022
1	60	HCV	Nivolumab	1.5 mo	Acute	Graft loss	Dehghan et al,[40] 2021
1	14	–	Pembrolizumab	4.5 mo	–	No recurrence	Kang et al,[41] 2022
1	63	NASH	Nivolumab, ipilimumab	2 mo	–	No recurrence	Lizaola-Mayo et al,[32] 2021
1	65	HCV	Nivolumab	8 d	Acute	Death	Nordness et al,[8] 2020
1	68	HCV	Nivolumab	10 mo	–	No recurrence	Peterson et al,[42] 2021
7	53 (average)	–	Pembrolizumab, lenvatinib	1.3 mo	Acute	Resolved rejection	Qiao et al,[43] 2021
1	61	HCV	Nivolumab	1.5 mo	Acute	Graft loss	Schnickel et al,[44] 2022
1	65	HCV	Nivolumab	10 d	Acute	Salvaged graft	Schnickel et al,[44] 2022
1	71	HBV	Nivolumab	83 mo	–	No recurrence	Schnickel et al,[44] 2022

(continued on next page)

Table 2
(continued)

Patients	Age (Years)	Underlying Disease	Immunotherapy	Time from Last Dose	Rejection	Outcome	Citation
1	65	HCV	Nivolumab	4 mo	-	No recurrence	Schnickel et al,[44] 2022
1	68	HCV	Nivolumab	6 mo	-	No recurrence	Schnickel et al,[44] 2022
1	62	Alcoholic	Nivolumab	5 mo	-	No recurrence	Schnickel et al,[44] 2022
1	61	HBV	Durvalumab	3 mo	-	No recurrence	Schwacha-Eipper et al,[33] 2020
9	57 (average)	HBV	Nivolumab	1 mo	Mild	Resolved rejection	Sogbe et al,[45] 2021
1	37	HBV	Atezolizumab, lenvatinib	-	Severe	Death	Tabrizian et al,[34] 2021
16	51 (average)	HBV/alcohol	Nivolumab (2), pembrolizumab (7), sintilimab (4), camrelizumab (2), all four (1)	1.5 mo (average)	Acute (9)	Recurrence (5)	Wang et al,[46] 2023
63	52			7.4 mo	33%		

posttransplant organ function, decrease the risk of acute rejection, and decrease steroid dependence. In a large retrospective cohort study, induction therapy was associated with lower risk of death (aHR 0.90) and graft failure (aHR 0.91). It was also associated with greater improvement of GFR posttransplant and reduced the risk of acute rejection in the first year (OR 0.87).[52]

Patient selection is another important factor that requires additional prospective studies. It is unknown whether ICI would be more efficacious in high-risk groups such as down-staged patients, high AFP, high-risk pathology, or prior locoregional therapy. Management of immunosuppression in patients who are treated with ICI pre-liver transplant is also another question of contention without a consensus. Immunosuppression is integral for graft protection, yet it may also negate the positive antitumor effects afforded by immunotherapy. Graft loss has occurred even on high dose of immunosuppression.[47] However, it was found that treatment with at least one drug other than corticosteroids for baseline immunosuppression has been associated with a lower risk of rejection.[53] Research investigating the impact of pre-liver transplant immunotherapy use is ongoing. The use of ICI and locoregional therapy has shown promise as bridge therapy before transplant (**Table 3**).[47,54–65] The PLENTY202001 trial examines the safety and efficacy of pembrolizumab with neoadjuvant lenvatinib in the treatment of HCC before liver transplant. Preliminary data were favorable and promising. Open-label Dulect2020-1 investigates the safety and efficacy of durvalumab with lenvatinib in patients with HCC before liver transplant. MEDI4736 investigates whether durvalumab and tremelimumab for HCC before liver transplant is effective. These trials are still ongoing and enrolling patients.

Although immunotherapy has been quickly developing into the future of therapy in oncology, it is not without its limitations. Many patients with cancer do not seem to respond to immunotherapy or their response remains short-lived. Recurrence may be due to poorly understood mechanisms, and although our perceived rate was 11%, it was as high as 30% in one series. Identification of predictors of treatment response still remains a challenge. PD-L1 expression does not seem to correlate with treatment response to ICIs; however, tumor mutational burden, microsatellite instability, and CD8+ presence in the tumor microenvironment have been loosely associated with positive response.[66] Immunotherapy-related adverse events are also common, with the highest being GI symptoms. Grade 3 or higher adverse events include neutropenia, hypertension, and lymphopenia.[67]

Last, although deceased donor liver transplants (DDLT) have been the primary source of organs, given the organ shortage, the patient may choose to pursue a living donor liver transplant (LDLT), especially if they are ineligible or unlikely to receive DDLT. With an overall donor mortality rate of 0.4%, LDLTs also have a high complication rate of 40% in donors.[67,68] There are additional ethical considerations such as being under internal or external pressure to donate to a loved one. Etiologies of liver failure that are excluded from DDLT may be considered for LDLT including alcoholic hepatitis and patients that fall outside of Milan criteria but are at high risk of relapse or recurrence. It is of utmost importance for all parties to have open communication, ensure complete informed consent, and both donors and recipients are aware of the risks and benefits to each respective party.

IMMUNOTHERAPY POST-LIVER TRANSPLANT AND ITS ASSOCIATED HEPATOTOXICITY

Transplant recipients are at an increased risk of malignancies which represent a major cause of mortality in the late (five or more years with preserved graft function)

Table 3
Ongoing neoadjuvant immunotherapy trials for hepatocellular carcinoma before liver transplant

NCT/Identifier	Country	Neoadjuvant Treatment Arm	Primary End Points	Secondary Endpoints	Status
NCT04425226	China	Pembrolizumab + lenvatinib in before liver transplant	Recurrence-free survival (RFS)	Disease control rate (DCR), percentage of participants who experience an adverse event (AE), objective response rate (ORR	Recruiting (No interim results available)
NCT04443322	China	Durvalumab + lenvatinib before liver transplant	Progression-free survival (PFS, RFS)	ORR, OS, percentage of participants who experience an AE	Recruiting (No interim results available)
NCT05339581	China	IMRT(intensity-modulated radiotherapy) combined with PD-1 blockade and lenvatinib before transplant	Portal vein tumor thrombus-related response and necrosis rate	PFS, ORR, time to progression (TTP), duration of response (DOR), alpha-fetoprotein response (AFP-R)	Not yet recruiting
NCT05185505	US	TACE + atezolizumab + bevacizumab before liver transplant	Theproportion of liver transplant with graft rejection	ORR, RFS, OS	Not yet recruiting

posttransplant period.[69] This excessive risk is thought to be primarily driven by the need for immunosuppression in transplant recipients, dysregulating the cancer-immunity cycle.[70] The therapeutic challenge arises when malignancies occur or recur as often seen in HCC and the need for balancing the prevention of graft rejection with cancer-directed therapies. HCC tumor recurrence is reported to occur in 15% to 20% of LT cases performed for HCC.[71] Tumor recurrence in this population has a poor prognosis with median survival ranging between 7 and 16 months.[71] In addition to HCC, transplant recipients are at a much higher risk of developing cutaneous malignancies, in particular squamous cell carcinomas, although the true incidence is not known as these are not frequently captured in cancer registries.[69]

There is an overall lack of adjuvant therapies post-LT. The STORM trial (Sorafenib as Adjuvant Treatment in the Prevention of Recurrence of Hepatocellular Carcinoma) was a randomized, double-blinded placebo-controlled study that evaluated sorafenib as adjuvant prevention of HCC after surgical resection or ablation.[72] In 2015, a prospective arm of the study evaluated 14 post-LT transplant patients with high-risk HCC, most of which had underlying HCV. These patients had poorly differentiated tumors or vascular invasion pre-LT and were started on differing doses of sorafenib.[72] The patients were followed with scheduled surveillance for HCC recurrence. Four patients in this group developed HCC recurrence within the study period with a median recurrence-free survival of 716 days.[72] With regard to the tolerability of sorafenib, one patient developed graft rejection and died while most had mild hematologic or non-hematologic adverse events managed with dose interruptions or adjustments. Despite the small sample size, the outcomes seen with adjuvant sorafenib therapy in this patient population may warrant further evaluation, but preliminary results do not seem promising at preventing recurrence.

In contrast to disease prevention, several studies and case reports have examined the utility of using immunotherapy as a treatment for disease recurrence (eg, HCC) or new malignancies (eg, melanoma, non-small cell lung carcinoma). Most recently, Di Marco and colleagues published perhaps the most promising data advocating for immunotherapy for HCC recurrence in LT population.[73] In their study, the five patients who received adjuvant nivolumab and bevacizumab had a statistically significant increase in overall survival compared with those receiving salvage therapy. In another such study conducted in 2018, a cohort of seven LT recipients were treated with PD-1 inhibitors for HCC ($n = 5$) or melanoma ($n = 2$). Graft rejection was seen in two out of the seven patients, complete treatment response was seen in only one patient, whereas the remainder either had disease progression or discontinued therapy.[55] A systematic review of several smaller studies conducted by Gassmann and colleagues found higher rates of graft rejection after administration of anti-PD-1 antibodies (9 of 16, 56%) but also demonstrated higher rates of treatment response (11 of 16, 68%).[47] The investigators concluded the devastating risk profile associated with immunomodulators as it pertains to graft loss must be weighed against the promising response being seen for treatment of these malignancies in non-LT patients. **Table 4** lists the case reports found in the literature with adjuvant immunotherapy in post-LT patients.

A common theme seen with immunotherapy for post-LT patients is the associated intrinsic hepatotoxicity of the medications along with the increased rates of graft rejection due to the increased immune response. ICIs such as anti PD-1 and anti CTLD-4 antibodies have a reported incidence of hepatotoxicity ranging from 11% to 29% with a hepatocellular pattern of liver damage being most common. Anti PD-1 inhibitors have also been shown to cause cholestatic pattern of liver injury.[74] Symptoms vary from asymptomatic elevations in liver function tests and jaundice to acute liver failure.

Table 4
Adjuvant immunotherapy in post-liver transplantation patients

Reference	Indication for LT	Years from Transplant	Indication for Immunotherapy	Immunotherapy Agent	Duration of Immunotherapy	Response to Immunotherapy	Rejection
DeLeon et al,[55] 2018	HCC	2.7	HCC	Nivolumab	1.2 mo	Disease progression	No
	HCC	7.8	HCC	Nivolumab	1.1 mo	Disease progression	No
	HCC	3.7	HCC	Nivolumab	1.3 mo	Disease progression	No
	HCC	1.2 y	HCC	Nivolumab	0.3 mo	Multiorgan failure	No
	HCC	1.1 y	HCC	Nivolumab	0.9 mo	N/A	Yes; mild
	HCC	5.5 y	Melanoma	Pembrolizumab	9.5 mo	Complete response	No
Al Jarroudi et al,[56] 2020	HCC	3 y	HCC	Nivolumab	2 mo	Disease progression	Yes; moderate
	HCC	2 y	HCC	Nivolumab	2.5 mo	Disease progression	No
	HCC	5 y	HCC	Nivolumab	3 mo	Disease progression	No
Gassmann et al,[47] 2018	HCC	2 y	HCC	Nivolumab	0.25 mo	N/A	Yes; fulminant liver failure
Kuo et al,[57] 2018	HCC	4.5 y	Melanoma	Ipilimumab followed by pembrolizumab	20 mo	Partial response	No
Varkaris et al,[58]	HCC	8 y	HCC	Pembrolizumab	3 mo	Disease progression	No
Kumar et al,[59] 2019	HCC	2 y	HCC	Nivolumab	0.25 wk	N/A	Yes; mild
Gomez et al,[60] 2018	HCC	2 y	HCC	Nivolumab	1 mo	N/A	Yes; moderate
Friend et al,[61] 2017	HCC	3 y	HCC	Nivolumab	0.75 mo	N/A	Yes; fulminant liver failure
	HCC	1 y	HCC	Nivolumab	0.25 mo	N/A	Yes; fulminant liver failure
Anugwom et al,[62] 2020	HCC	5 y	Non-small cell lung carcinoma	Nivolumab	2 mo	N/A	Yes; fulminant liver failure
Rammohan et al,[63] 2018	HCC	4 y	HCC	Pembrolizumab and Sorafenib	3 mo	Complete response	No
Amjad et al,[64] 2020	HCC	1 y	HCC	Nivolumab	6 mo	Complete response	Yes; mild
Pandey et al,[65] 2020	HCC	7.5 y	HCC	Ipilimumab	12 mo	Complete response	Yes; mild
Morales et al,[66] 2015	HCC	3 y	Melanoma	Ipilimumab	6 mo	Partial response	Yes; mild

Abbreviation: N/A, not available.

Often the hepatotoxic effects become evident after two to four cycles and can resolve with cessation of the offending agent and steroids.[75] However, fatal cases of acute liver failure have been reported. In post-LT patients, the rate of acute rejection leading to graft loss varies widely but one systemic review found the incidence to be nearly one-third of patients treated with ICIs experienced some degree of graft rejection.[31] Another study found an acute rejection of solid organ grafts occurring in 40% of patients after initiation of ICIs with over two-thirds of those patients progressing to end-stage organ failure.[74]

SUMMARY

Immunotherapy has revolutionized the treatment of advanced HCC over the past few years. Improved outcomes have been demonstrated in the use of neoadjuvant therapy from early phase trials in various solid tumor types. As more and more studies are performed and immunotherapy is more universally adopted, it shows immense promise not only for the multimodal treatment approach for HCC but also for bridging therapy to liver transplants. Although initial concerns for graft rejection were high due to the mechanism of these immune checkpoint therapies, the cases presented in the literature have shown a rejection incidence of 24%, these can readily be treated with immunosuppressants and reduced with a 3-month washout period. Additional research and studies need to be conducted to better ascertain risk assessment regarding usage of immunotherapies in the context of pre-liver transplants.

Treatment of disease recurrence in post-LT patients represents a challenging clinical scenario between balancing effective therapy with preservation of liver graft function. Much of the available research on immunotherapy post-LT to date demonstrates poor treatment response. Moreover, acute graft loss secondary to immunotherapy poses a real danger to starting these cancer-directed therapies. These complex patients require a multidisciplinary approach to their care with a thoughtful risk–benefit discussion before initiating adjuvant immunotherapy.

CLINICS CARE POINTS

- Downstaging to within Milan criteria has been incorporated into the organ allocation policy for hepatocellular carcinoma (HCC) in the United States in 2017 and provides acceptable long-term survival.
- Indications for liver transplantation (LT) in HCC continue to expand.
- Several early-phase clinical trials of novel checkpoints and combinations have shown promising results pre-resection in patients with HCC.
- There has been reluctance to use immunotherapy in transplant candidates due to scattered reports of severe rejection and graft loss.
- Data suggest that approximately three half-lives, or 3 months, of observation would be necessary before liver transplantation to avoid rejection.
- Research investigating the impact of pre-liver transplant immunotherapy use is ongoing.
- Results on immunotherapy post-LT to date demonstrate poor treatment response and need to be further investigated.

DISCLOSURE

No financial disclocures.

REFERENCES

1. Mazzaferro V, Regalia E, Doci R, et al. Liver transplantation for the treatment of small hepatocellular carcinomas in patients with cirrhosis. N Engl J Med 1996;334:693–9.
2. Yao FY, Fidelman N. Reassessing the boundaries of liver transplantation for hepatocellular carcinoma: Where do we stand with tumor down-staging? Hepatology 2016;63(3):1014–25.
3. Tabrizian P, Holzner M, Mehta N, et al. Ten-Year outcomes of Liver Transplant and Downstaging for Hepatocellular carcinoma. JAMA Surg 2022;157(9):779–88.
4. Mazzaferro V, Citterio D, Bhoori S, et al. Liver transplantation in hepatocellular carcinoma after tumour downstaging (XXL): a randomised, controlled, phase 2b/3 trial. Lancet Oncol 2020;21:947–56.
5. Reig M, Forner A, Rimola J, et al. BCLC strategy for prognosis prediction and treatment recommendation: The 2022 update. J Hepatol 2022;76(3):681–93.
6. Finn RS, Qin S, Ikeda M, et al. Atezolizumab plus Bevacizumab in Unresectable Hepatocellular Carcinoma. N Engl J Med 2020;382(20):1894–905.
7. Abou-Alfa GK, Lau G, Kudo M, et al. Tremelimumab plus Durvalumab in Unresectable Hepatocellular Carcinoma. NEJM Evidence 2022;1(8). EVIDoa2100070.
8. Nordness MF, Hamel S, Godfrey CM, et al. Fatal hepatic necrosis after nivolumab as a bridge to liver transplant for HCC: Are checkpoint inhibitors safe for the pretransplant patient? Am J Transplant 2020;20(3):879–83.
9. Marron TU, Schwartz M, Corbett V, et al. Neoadjuvant Immunotherapy for Hepatocellular Carcinoma. J Hepatocell Carcinoma 2022;9:571–81.
10. Hack SP, Spahn J, Chen M, et al. IMbrave 050: a Phase III trial of atezolizumab plus bevacizumab in high-risk hepatocellular carcinoma after curative resection or ablation. Future Oncol 2020;16(15):975–89.
11. Chow P, Chen M, Cheng A-L, et al. IMbrave050: phase 3 study of adjuvant atezolizumab + bevacizumab versus active surveillance in patients with hepatocellular carcinoma (HCC) at high risk of disease recurrence following resection or ablation. American Association for Cancer Research (AACR) Annual Conference; 2023.
12. Gabrielson A, Wu Y, Wang H, et al. Intratumoral CD3 and CD8 T-cell Densities Associated with Relapse-Free Survival in HCC. Cancer Immunol Res 2016;4(5): 419–30.
13. Liu J, Blake SJ, Yong MC, et al. Improved Efficacy of Neoadjuvant Compared to Adjuvant Immunotherapy to Eradicate Metastatic Disease. Cancer Discov 2016; 6(12):1382–99.
14. Blank CU, Rozeman EA, Fanchi LF, et al. Neoadjuvant versus adjuvant ipilimumab plus nivolumab in macroscopic stage III melanoma. Nature medicine 2018;24(11):1655–61.
15. Patel SP, Othus M, Chen Y, et al. Neoadjuvant–adjuvant or adjuvant-only pembrolizumab in advanced melanoma. N Engl J Med 2023;388(9):813–23.
16. Pinato DJ, Fessas P, Sapisochin G, et al. Perspectives on the Neoadjuvant Use of Immunotherapy in Hepatocellular Carcinoma. Hepatology 2021;74(1):483–90.
17. Schmid P, Cortes J, Dent R, et al. VP7-2021: KEYNOTE-522: Phase III study of neoadjuvant pembrolizumab + chemotherapy vs. placebo + chemotherapy, followed by adjuvant pembrolizumab vs. placebo for early-stage TNBC. Ann Oncol 2021;32(9):1198–200.
18. Forde PM, Spicer J, Lu S, et al. Neoadjuvant Nivolumab plus Chemotherapy in Resectable Lung Cancer. N Engl J Med 2022;386(21):1973–85.

19. Topalian SL, Bhatia S, Amin A, et al. Neoadjuvant Nivolumab for Patients With Resectable Merkel Cell Carcinoma in the CheckMate 358 Trial. J Clin Oncol 2020;38(22):2476–87.
20. Ho WJ, Zhu Q, Durham J, et al. Neoadjuvant Cabozantinib and Nivolumab Converts Locally Advanced HCC into Resectable Disease with Enhanced Antitumor Immunity. Nat Cancer 2021;2(9):891–903.
21. Marron TU, Fiel MI, Hamon P, et al. Neoadjuvant cemiplimab for resectable hepatocellular carcinoma: a single-arm, open-label, phase 2 trial. The Lancet Gastroenterology & Hepatology 2022;7(3):219–29.
22. Kaseb AO, Hasanov E, Cao HST, et al. Perioperative nivolumab monotherapy versus nivolumab plus ipilimumab in resectable hepatocellular carcinoma: a randomised, open-label, phase 2 trial. Lancet Gastroenterol Hepatol 2022;7(3):208–18.
23. https://www.gene.com/media/press-releases/14981/2023-01-18/genentechs-tecentriq-plus-avastin-is-the.
24. Harris J. Early Data Shows Neoadjuvant Nivolumab Potentializes Electroporation in HCC.
25. Su Y, Lin Y, Hsiao C, et al. P-124 Nivolumab plus ipilimumab as neoadjuvant therapy for potentially resectable hepatocellular carcinoma. Ann Oncol 2021;32:S141.
26. Chen S, Wang Y, Xie W, et al. 710P Neoadjuvant tislelizumab for resectable recurrent hepatocellular carcinoma: A non-randomized control, phase II trial (TALENT). Ann Oncol 2022;33:S867.
27. Shi Y-H, Ji Y, Liu W-R, et al. A phase Ib/II, open-label study evaluating the efficacy and safety of Toripalimab injection (JS001) or combination with Lenvatinib as a neoadjuvant therapy for patients with resectable hepatocellular carcinoma (HCC). Cancer Res 2021;81(13_Supplement):486.
28. Bai X, Chen Y, Zhang X, et al. 712P CAPT: A multicenter randomized controlled trial of perioperative versus postoperative camrelizumab plus apatinib for resectable hepatocellular carcinoma. Ann Oncol 2022;33:S868.
29. Pinato DJ, Cortellini A, Pai M, et al. PRIME-HCC: Phase Ib study of neoadjuvant ipilimumab and nivolumab prior to liver resection for hepatocellular carcinoma. J Clin Oncol 2021;39(15_suppl):e16131–.
30. Xia Y, Tang W, Qian X, et al. Efficacy and safety of camrelizumab plus apatinib during the perioperative period in resectable hepatocellular carcinoma: a single-arm, open label, phase II clinical trial. J ImmunoTherapy Cancer 2022;10(4):e004656.
31. Yin C, Baba T, He AR, et al. Immune checkpoint inhibitors in liver transplant recipients - a review of current literature. Hepatoma Research 2021;7:52.
32. Lizaola-Mayo BC, Mathur AK, Borad M-J, et al. Immunotherapy as a Downstaging Tool for Liver Transplantation in Hepatocellular Carcinoma. Official J Am Coll Gastroenterol | ACG 2021;116(12):2478–80.
33. Schwacha-Eipper B, Minciuna I, Banz V, et al. Immunotherapy as a Downstaging Therapy for Liver Transplantation. Hepatology 2020;72(4):1488–90.
34. Tabrizian P, Florman SS, Schwartz ME. PD-1 inhibitor as bridge therapy to liver transplantation? Am J Transplant 2021;21(5):1979–80.
35. Abdelrahim M, Esmail A, Umoru G, et al. Immunotherapy as a Neoadjuvant Therapy for a Patient with Hepatocellular Carcinoma in the Pretransplant Setting: A Case Report. Curr Oncol 2022;29(6):4267–73.
36. Aby ES, Lake JR. Immune Checkpoint Inhibitor Therapy Before Liver Transplantation-Case and Literature Review. Transplant Direct 2022;8(4):e1304.

37. Chen GH, Wang GB, Huang F, et al. Pretransplant use of toripalimab for hepato-cellular carcinoma resulting in fatal acute hepatic necrosis in the immediate post-operative period. Transpl Immunol 2021;66:101386.

38. Chen Z, Hong X, Wang T, et al. Prognosis after liver transplantation in patients treated with anti-PD-1 immunotherapy for advanced hepatocellular carcinoma: case series. Ann Palliat Med 2021;10(9):9354–61.

39. Dave S, Yang K, Schnickel GT, et al. The Impact of Treatment of Hepatocellular Carcinoma With Immune Checkpoint Inhibitors on Pre- and Post-liver Transplant Outcomes. Transplantation 2022;106(6):e308–9.

40. Dehghan Y, Schnickel GT, Hosseini M, et al. Rescue liver re-transplantation after graft loss due to severe rejection in the setting of pre-transplant nivolumab ther-apy. Clin J Gastroenterol 2021;14(6):1718–24.

41. Kang E, Martinez M, Moisander-Joyce H, et al. Stable liver graft post anti-PD1 therapy as a bridge to transplantation in an adolescent with hepatocellular carci-noma. Pediatr Transplant 2022;26(3):e14209.

42. Peterson J, Stanek S, Kalman R, et al. Nivolumab as a Bridge to Liver Transplan-tation in Advanced Hepatocellular Carcinoma. Am J Gastroenterol 2021;116:S1159.

43. Qiao ZY, Zhang ZJ, Lv ZC, et al. Neoadjuvant Programmed Cell Death 1 (PD-1) Inhibitor Treatment in Patients With Hepatocellular Carcinoma Before Liver Trans-plant: A Cohort Study and Literature Review. Front Immunol 2021;12:653437.

44. Schnickel GT, Fabbri K, Hosseini M, et al. Liver transplantation for hepatocellular carcinoma following checkpoint inhibitor therapy with nivolumab. Am J Transplant 2022;22(6):1699–704.

45. Sogbe M, Lopez-Guerra D, Blanco-Fernandez G, et al. Durvalumab as a Suc-cessful Downstaging Therapy for Liver Transplantation in Hepatocellular Carci-noma: The Importance of a Washout Period. Transplantation 2021;105(12):e398–400.

46. Wang T, Chen Z, Liu Y, et al. Neoadjuvant programmed cell death 1 inhibitor before liver transplantation for HCC is not associated with increased graft loss. Liver Transplant 2023. https://doi.org/10.1097/LVT.0000000000000083.

47. Gassmann D, Weiler S, Mertens JC, et al. Liver Allograft Failure After Nivolumab Treatment-A Case Report With Systematic Literature Research. Transplant Direct 2018;4(8):e376.

48. Tran NH, Munoz S, Thompson S, et al. Hepatocellular carcinoma downstaging for liver transplantation in the era of systemic combined therapy with anti-VEGF/TKI and immunotherapy. Hepatology 2022;76(4):1203–18.

49. Haanen J, Carbonnel F, Robert C, et al. Management of toxicities from immuno-therapy: ESMO Clinical Practice Guidelines for diagnosis, treatment and follow-up. Ann Oncol 2017;28(suppl_4):iv119–42.

50. Duan J, Cui L, Zhao X, et al. Use of Immunotherapy With Programmed Cell Death 1 vs Programmed Cell Death Ligand 1 Inhibitors in Patients With Cancer: A Sys-tematic Review and Meta-analysis. JAMA Oncol 2020;6(3):375–84.

51. Pillai RN, Behera M, Owonikoko TK, et al. Comparison of the toxicity profile of PD-1 versus PD-L1 inhibitors in non-small cell lung cancer: A systematic analysis of the literature. Cancer 2018;124(2):271–7.

52. Bittermann T, Hubbard RA, Lewis JD, et al. The use of induction therapy in liver transplantation is highly variable and is associated with posttransplant outcomes. Am J Transplant 2019;19(12):3319–27.

53. Rizzo A, Brandi G. Biochemical predictors of response to immune checkpoint inhibitors in unresectable hepatocellular carcinoma. Cancer Treat Res Commun 2021;27:100328.

54. Wang Y. Managing immunotherapy related organ toxicities: a practical guide. Springer International Publishing AG; 2022.

55. DeLeon TT, Salomao MA, Aqel BA, et al. Pilot evaluation of PD-1 inhibition in metastatic cancer patients with a history of liver transplantation: the Mayo Clinic experience. J Gastrointest Oncol 2018;9(6):1054–62.

56. Al Jarroudi O, Ulusakarya A, Almohamad W, et al. Anti-Programmed Cell Death Protein 1 (PD-1) Immunotherapy for Metastatic Hepatocellular Carcinoma After Liver Transplantation: A Report of Three Cases. Cureus 2020;12(10):e11150.

57. Kuo JC, Lilly LB, Hogg D. Immune checkpoint inhibitor therapy in a liver transplant recipient with a rare subtype of melanoma: a case report and literature review. Melanoma Res 2018;28(1):61–4.

58. Varkaris A, Lewis DW, Nugent FW. Preserved Liver Transplant After PD-1 Pathway Inhibitor for Hepatocellular Carcinoma. Am J Gastroenterol 2017;112(12):1895–6.

59. Kumar Shiva MD, MHA1. 2235 Nivolumab-Induced Severe Allograft Rejection in Recurrent Post-Transplant Hepatocellular Carcinoma. Am J Gastroenterol 2019; 114:S1251.

60. Gomez Paul MD1, Naim Alan MD1, Zucker, et al. A Case of Hepatocellular Carcinoma (HCC) Immunotherapy Inducing Liver Transplant Rejection: 2416. Am J Gastroenterol 2018;113:S1347.

61. Friend BD, Venick RS, McDiarmid SV, et al. Fatal orthotopic liver transplant organ rejection induced by a checkpoint inhibitor in two patients with refractory, metastatic hepatocellular carcinoma. Pediatr Blood Cancer 2017;64(12).

62. Anugwom C, Leventhal T. Nivolumab-Induced Autoimmune-Like Cholestatic Hepatitis in a Liver Transplant Recipient. ACG Case Rep J 2020;7(7):e00416.

63. Rammohan A, Reddy MS, Farouk M, et al. Pembrolizumab for metastatic hepatocellular carcinoma following live donor liver transplantation: The silver bullet? Hepatology 2018;67(3):1166–8.

64. Amjad W, Kotiah S, Gupta A, et al. Successful Treatment of Disseminated Hepatocellular Carcinoma After Liver Transplantation With Nivolumab. J Clin Exp Hepatol 2020;10(2):185–7.

65. Pandey A, Cohen DJ. Ipilumumab for hepatocellular cancer in a liver transplant recipient, with durable response, tolerance and without allograft rejection. Immunotherapy 2020;12(5):287–92.

66. Morales RE, Shoushtari AN, Walsh MM, et al. Safety and efficacy of ipilimumab to treat advanced melanoma in the setting of liver transplantation. J Immunother Cancer 2015;3:22.

67. Dobosz P, Stepien M, Golke A, et al. Challenges of the Immunotherapy: Perspectives and Limitations of the Immune Checkpoint Inhibitor Treatment. Int J Mol Sci 2022;23(5). https://doi.org/10.3390/ijms23052847.

68. Abecassis MM, Fisher RA, Olthoff KM, et al. Complications of living donor hepatic lobectomy–a comprehensive report. Am J Transplant 2012;12(5):1208–17.

69. Engels EA, Pfeiffer RM, Fraumeni JF, et al. Spectrum of Cancer Risk Among US Solid Organ Transplant Recipients. JAMA 2011;306(17):1891–901.

70. Vulasala SSR, Onteddu NK, Kumar SP, et al. Advances and effectiveness of the immunotherapy after liver transplantation. World J Gastrointest Surg 2022;14(6): 629–31.

71. Filgueira NA. Hepatocellular carcinoma recurrence after liver transplantation: Risk factors, screening and clinical presentation. World J Hepatol 2019;11(3): 261–72.

72. Siegel AB, El-Khoueiry AB, Finn RS, et al. Phase I trial of sorafenib following liver transplantation in patients with high-risk hepatocellular carcinoma. Liver Cancer 2015;4(2):115–25.

73. Di Marco L, Pivetti A, Foschi FG, et al. Feasibility, safety, and outcome of second-line nivolumab/bevacizumab in liver transplant patients with recurrent hepatocellular carcinoma. Liver Transplant 2023;29(5):559–63.

74. d'Izarny-Gargas T, Durrbach A, Zaidan M. Efficacy and tolerance of immune checkpoint inhibitors in transplant patients with cancer: A systematic review. Am J Transplant 2020;20(9):2457–65.

75. LiverTox. Clinical and research information on drug-induced liver injury [internet]. Bethesda (MD): National Institute of Diabetes and Digestive and Kidney Diseases; 2012. Nivolumab. [Updated 2020 Apr 29].

Liver Transplantation for Hilar Cholangiocarcinoma

Christopher J. Sonnenday, MD, MHS*

KEYWORDS

- Hilar cholangiocarcinoma • Liver transplantation • Neoadjuvant therapy
- Transplant oncology

KEY POINTS

- Liver transplantation may be appropriate for patients with unresectable hilar cholangiocarcinoma, with tumors less than 3 cm, and no evidence of extrahepatic disease including no regional nodal metastases.
- Neoadjuvant chemoradiation followed by liver transplantation is associated with a 60% 5-year survival among appropriately selected patients.
- Hilar cholangiocarcinoma that occurs in the setting of primary sclerosing cholangitis, without evidence of extrahepatic disease, may be treated with neoadjuvant chemoradiation followed by liver transplantation.

The application of liver transplantation to the treatment of hepatobiliary malignancy has a circuitous and sometimes stumbling history. Like hepatocellular carcinoma (HCC), the history of hilar cholangiocarcinoma (hCCA) dates to the first transplants performed.[1] Specifically, the third transplant reported by Thomas Starzl in his initial series in 1963: "was a 67-year-old male with progressive jaundice.... Exploratory operation was performed on 3 June 1963, and an intrahepatic duct cell carcinoma was found which had obstructed both the right and left main hepatic ducts." The recipient received a liver from a donor after circulatory death, suffered complications of infection and bile peritonitis, and died on day 7. Other early recipients with biliary cancer as their indication for transplant suffered similarly poor short-term outcomes, including early post-transplant recurrence of their malignancy.[2]

For the indications for liver transplantation to expand responsibly for oncologic indications, established principles of surgical oncology must be observed. First and foremost, *tumor biology* needs to be understood and accommodated. Applying total hepatectomy and organ replacement to hepatobiliary malignancy is not a replacement for biologic selection, and in fact, the post-transplant immunosuppression may

Department of Surgery, University of Michigan Health, F6686 UH-South, 1500 East Medical Center Drive, Ann Arbor, MI 48109-5296, USA
* Corresponding author.
E-mail address: csonnend@umich.edu

Surg Clin N Am 104 (2024) 183–196
https://doi.org/10.1016/j.suc.2023.09.004
0039-6109/24/© 2023 Elsevier Inc. All rights reserved.

augment the impact of occult metastatic disease and even accelerate the patient's recurrence and death. Like HCC, understanding the *biology of any underlying liver disease* and its impact of the patient's candidacy for resection of other therapies is important as well, especially in the case of hCCA occurring in the setting of underlying primary sclerosing cholangitis (PSC) as discussed below. In addition to biology, the *technical adequacy* of hepatectomy and transplant must be considered, especially in the case of extrahepatic cancer such as hCCA. Failure to achieve a negative margin (R0 resection) with transplantation would be predicted to have equally high recurrence risk to hepatic resection with positive margins (R1 or R2 resection). Finally, the *logistics of obtaining a liver for transplant*, utilization of resources, availability of organs, allocation priority, and the role of living donor liver transplantation (LDLT), must all be considered.

EPIDEMIOLOGY AND RISK FACTORS

Cholangiocarcinoma (CCA), an infiltrative tumor of the biliary epithelial cells known for its associated dense desmoplastic reaction and associated hepatic dysfunction caused by biliary obstruction and sepsis, may often present in advanced stages or in central locations that preclude definitive resection.[3] Total hepatectomy and liver transplantation seems to offer definitive therapy to patients with unresectable CCA, but it has taken decades to identify which patients are most appropriate for this therapy. In addition, it is recognized that CCA tumors may vary significantly in their clinical behavior and prognosis based on location (intrahepatic, hilar/perihilar, extrahepatic) and the presence or absence of background liver disease (PSC, cirrhosis). The application of resection and transplant to intrahepatic CCA is dealt with in other chapters of this issue.

CCA is a cancer of increasing incidence in the United States, which may be explained by an approximate tripling of the age-adjusted incidence of *intrahepatic* CCA over the last 30 years.[4] Interestingly, recent data suggest that the incidence of *extrahepatic* CCA may be decreasing.[5] These trends in incidence may be explained in part by relevant risk factors associated with the development of CCA, with the increase in intrahepatic CCA associated with the increased prevalence of viral hepatitis, cirrhosis, and metabolic-associated fatty liver disease.[6] Both intrahepatic and extrahepatic CCA are strongly associated with biliary tract disease, specifically PSC. Patients with PSC seem to have a lifetime risk of CCA of at least 10%, and patients with PSC and associated inflammatory bowel disease may have a lifetime incidence of 30% or higher.[7,8] Although no prospectively validated screening methods exist for the early diagnosis of CCA, PSC patients seem to benefit from annual surveillance for biliary malignancies. Current American Association for the Study of Liver Diseases (AASLD) practice guidelines suggest annual contrast-enhanced MRI with magnetic resonance cholangiopancreatography (MRCP), with or without carbohydrate antigen 19-9 (CA 19-9) serum testing. Patients under the age of 18 years, or with small duct disease, do not seem to benefit from screening due to a markedly lower incidence of malignancy.[9]

DIAGNOSIS AND STAGING

A significant portion of the poor prognosis associated with CCA may be attributed to the challenges that this tumor presents in terms of diagnosis, leading to frequent delays in initiation of therapy and progressive decline in patient performance status and hepatic function. Hilar and extrahepatic CCA most often present with obstructive jaundice. Cholangitis at initial presentation is rare among patients without PSC and patients who have not had previous biliary instrumentation. Weight loss and malnutrition are common among jaundiced patients with CCA and may progress relatively rapidly with delays in biliary decompression and diagnosis. Laboratory evaluation will be consistent with the degree of biliary obstruction, with marked cholestasis and hypoalbuminemia common in patients with complete biliary obstruction. Ultrasound is the most common initial imaging test, which can be helpful in determining the level of obstruction (hilar, with associated intrahepatic ductal dilatation or distal, with associated intrahepatic and extrahepatic ductal dilatation). Many patients will often then be referred for endoscopic retrograde cholangiopancreatography (ERCP) but it is preferred when possible to obtain cross-sectional imaging first, as local extent of disease may be easier to interpret before biliary instrumentation. Contrast-enhanced MRI with MRCP is the preferred study for CCA diagnosis and treatment planning but may be augmented by the addition of liver CT which can provide higher fidelity images of the vasculature for determination of resectability and surgical planning.

Obtaining a tissue diagnosis in cases of hilar or extrahepatic CCA may be challenging, and in some cases, clinical decision-making may occur without a definitive diagnosis. ERCP with brushings of a concerning biliary stricture evaluated by cytology has a relatively low sensitivity for diagnosing extrahepatic CCA, which may be augmented using fluorescence in situ hybridization (FISH).[10] Percutaneous or transperitoneal (via endoscopic ultrasound [EUS] or surgical biopsy) tissue sampling of hCCA should be avoided, as it risks tumor seeding and excludes patients from consideration for transplantation.[11] Serum values of CA 19-9 may help support a diagnosis of CCA, and markedly high values (>1000 U/mL) raise concern for occult metastatic disease, often within the peritoneum.[12] Limitations of using CA 19-9 as a diagnostic tool include the fact that values will be markedly elevated in jaundiced patients, including patients with biliary obstruction of nonmalignant causes, and individuals who do not express the Lewis antigen (approximately 7%–10% of the population) will not express CA 19-9 regardless of diagnosis.[13] A more sensitive and specific biomarker for CCA is definitely needed.

Staging of hCCA includes establishing the presence or absence of extrahepatic disease, assessment of regional nodes, and determination of resectability. Metastatic disease to extrahepatic sites other than regional lymph nodes is an absolute contraindication to surgical therapy including transplantation, as there are essentially no long-term survivors among patients with distant disease. Regional nodal disease is a contraindication to liver transplantation, and a significant risk factor for recurrence and diminished survival (at best 20% at 5 years) following resection.[14,15] For patients with hCCA, determination of resectability is complex and involves determination of the likelihood of achieving a negative margin (R0) resection, the options for biliary and vascular reconstruction, and the size and health of the future liver remnant.[16] Resectability may be predicted by the modified T stage system proposed by Blumgart based on the determination of the involvement of second-order biliary radicles, hepatic artery and/or portal vein involvement, and associated lobar atrophy from chronic biliary obstruction.[17] Extended hepatic resections for hCCA are complex procedures with high potential morbidity and mortality, risks that may be further increased by advanced patient age, smaller future liver remnant, presence of associated cholangitis, and persistent jaundice at the time of resection.[18]

SELECTION FOR LIVER TRANSPLANTATION FOR HILAR CHOLANGIOCARCINOMA

Unresectable patients with hCCA who are proven not to have regional nodal disease (by fine needle aspiration via EUS and confirmed by lymphadenectomy at staging laparotomy) may be candidates for liver transplantation following neoadjuvant chemo-radiotherapy. Radial tumor diameter should not exceed 3 cm (**Fig. 1**). Patients with PSC who have hCCA (including resectable disease), particularly those with advanced liver disease and also proven to not have nodal disease, are also best served by liver transplantation as their hepatic dysfunction and cholestasis makes them poor resection candidates.

Central to achieving acceptable outcomes in liver transplantation for hCCA is developing a robust multidisciplinary approach to patient selection. Common pitfalls for transplant programs early in their experience with this disease is to presume that their liver transplant program, who may have significant experience in patient selection for HCC, have the expertise to determine resectability in this complex patient population. Hepatobiliary surgery (non-transplant) input is central to determining resectability and endorsing transplant evaluation in appropriate patients. Transplant programs have created this resource in varied manners, but having review by a hepatobiliary surgeon experienced in resection of hCCA evaluate patients in a setting independent of the transplant evaluation is essential. Multidisciplinary tumor board review including partners in surgical oncology, medical oncology, radiation oncology, and hepatology should review patients before initiating a transplant evaluation, in a process that is independent of the liver transplant selection committee. The selection process should be expected to be stringent, as less than 10% of patients presenting with hCCA seem to be appropriate for liver transplantation from medical and oncologic criteria.[19]

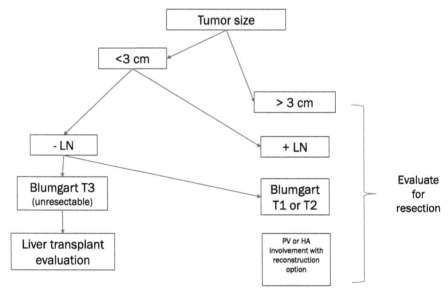

Fig. 1. Selection algorithm for hilar cholangiocarcinoma. Blumgart staging is as follows: T1: tumor involving biliary confluence with unilateral extension to second-order biliary radicles; T2: tumor involving biliary confluence with unilateral extension to second-order biliary radicles with: ipsilateral portal vein involvement, or ipsilateral hepatic atrophy; T3: tumor involving biliary confluence with bilateral extension to second-order biliary radicles; or unilateral extension to second-order biliary radicles with contralateral portal vein involvement; or unilateral extension to second-order biliary radicles with contralateral hepatic lobar atrophy; or main or bilateral portal venous involvement. *Adapted from* Matsuo, K. et al. The Blumgart preoperative staging system for hilar cholangiocarcinoma: analysis of resectability and outcomes in 380 patients. Journal of the American College of Surgeons 215, 343–355 (2012).

Defining resectability in hCCA is not simple itself, as it relies on surgeon experience and interpretation of imaging, and the nuances of imaging (as discussed in a previous chapter of this edition). Surgical experience suggests that radiographic review of these tumors tends to overestimate vascular involvement (particularly the involvement of the right hepatic artery, which most often abuts the posterior aspect of hilar biliary tumors) and underestimate the biliary involvement (as even direct cholangiography is unable to determine the degree of linear ductal and periductal involvement of these tumors). The relative risk and logistics of liver transplantation compared with a vascular reconstruction (eg, segmental hepatic artery or portal vein resection and reconstruction) or complex biliary reconstruction to multiple intrahepatic ducts is based on available expertise and experience, as direct comparisons of these therapies are not available. Once nodal status is evaluated, patients with positive portal nodes with locally advanced disease might even be reconsidered for resection by some surgeons, because they do not have a transplant option in that circumstance. In that specific instance, neoadjuvant protocols before an attempt at resection should be considered and prospectively studied.[20,21] Again, these decisions should be thoroughly discussed and vetted in a multidisciplinary tumor board where both the tumor and patient factors are fully considered.

Beyond the technical decision-making, patient fitness and functional status are primary factors in consideration of these advanced therapies for hCCA. Robust data exist about the morbidity and mortality risk for surgical resection for hCCA, with age functioning as a profound risk magnifier, especially among patients with prior cholangitis and small liver remnants.[18] Similarly, transplant protocols for hCCA are long and intense with risk of cholangitis, progressive malnutrition, and progressive debilitation. Reports even from experienced centers suggest a notable incidence (up to 30%) of patient dropout due to progressive frailty or other complications, not just for tumor progression.[22] Given hCCA often occurs in older patients, having a standardized approach to evaluating and tracking patient fitness/frailty is highly recommended for this population. Progressive fatigue following radiation and intermittent cholangitis related to stent malfunction are both primary drivers of ongoing functional decline, and these patients should be reevaluated frequently while undergoing neoadjuvant therapy and awaiting transplant (ideally every 2–4 weeks, with regular laboratory studies to assess for progressive cholestasis, treatment side effects, or signs of infection). Finally, severity of underlying liver disease may also compromise the ability of patients to complete the neoadjuvant protocol, as model for end-stage liver disease (MELD) greater than 20 was associated with a threefold increased risk of dropout in the Mayo Clinic experience.[22]

NEOADJUVANT PROTOCOLS

The principles of neoadjuvant therapy for hCCA in the pre-transplant setting are like neoadjuvant strategies from other diseases, with the added nuance (or "benefit") of preparing for a complete explant of the therapeutic target. Neoadjuvant therapy provides a biologic test period, as more aggressive behaving tumors that progress through treatment would not likely benefit from transplant. Furthermore, patients are more likely to complete intended therapy as opposed to relying on post-transplant therapy which is challenging in the context of immunosuppression and could be deferred due to surgical complications or other factors that complicate recovery. Finally, reduction in intraductal or radial extent of viable tumor due to neoadjuvant chemoradiation may increase the likelihood of achieving an R0 resection at the time of total hepatectomy with excision of the extrahepatic biliary tree. In addition to these advantages of neoadjuvant therapy, the neoadjuvant radiation therapy given to hCCA candidates for transplant aims at delivering extremely high localized doses given that there is not a need for surgical reconstruction of the treated tissues. Although concern exists about the collateral vascular complications that may occur because of this high-dose radiation delivered to the hilum, total hepatectomy eliminates the need to dissect or reconstruct bile ducts that have been radiated, which is a challenge in the setting of neoadjuvant radiation therapy given before attempt at surgical resection.

Although protocols vary from center to center, all must contain critical elements as detailed below. Furthermore, Organ Procurement and Transplantation Network (OPTN) policy require that programs have an approved protocol containing the elements described in **Box 1** for patients to receive a CCA MELD exception score at the time of listing.[23] Neoadjuvant protocols for hCCA include the following essential elements.

- *Establishment of CCA diagnosis* by documenting a malignant-appearing stricture with either diagnostic cytology or biopsy, CA 19-9 greater than 100 U/mL, or aneuploidy by FISH.
- *Unresectable hilar mass* not exceeding radial diameter greater than 3 cm.

Box 1
Organ Procurement and Transplantation Network Policy 9.5.A: Requirements for cholangiocarcinoma MELD score exceptions

A candidate will receive an MELD or pediatric end-stage liver disease (PELD) score exception for CCA, if the candidate's transplant program meets all the following qualifications:

1. Submits a written protocol for patient care to the Liver and Intestinal Organ Transplantation Committee that must include all of the following:
   i. Candidate selection criteria
   ii. Administration of neoadjuvant therapy before transplantation
   iii. Operative staging to exclude any patient with regional hepatic lymph node metastases, intrahepatic metastases, or extrahepatic disease
   iv. Any data requested by the Liver and Intestinal Organ Transplantation Committee

2. Documents that the candidate meets the diagnostic criteria for hilar CCA with a malignant appearing stricture on cholangiography and at least one of the following:
   - Biopsy or cytology results demonstrating malignancy
   - Carbohydrate antigen 19-9 greater than 100 U/mL in the absence of cholangitis
   - Aneuploidy
   - Hilar mass, which is less than 3 cm in radial diameter.

The tumor must be considered unresectable because of technical considerations or underlying liver disease.

3. Submits cross-sectional imaging studies. If cross-sectional imaging studies demonstrate a mass, the mass must be single and less than 3 cm in radial (perpendicular to the duct) diameter. The longitudinal extension of the stricture along the bile duct is not considered in the measurement of a mass.

4. Documents the exclusion of intrahepatic and extrahepatic metastases by cross-sectional imaging studies of the chest and abdomen within 90 days before submission of the initial exception request.

5. Assesses regional hepatic lymph node involvement and peritoneal metastases by operative staging after completion of neoadjuvant therapy and before liver transplantation. Endoscopic ultrasound-guided aspiration of regional hepatic lymph nodes may be advisable to exclude patients with obvious metastases before neoadjuvant therapy is initiated.

6. Transperitoneal aspiration or biopsy of the primary tumor (either by endoscopic ultrasound, operative, or percutaneous approaches) must be avoided because of the high risk of tumor seeding associated with these procedures.

- *Staging operation to exclude occult peritoneal and nodal metastatic disease* performed after completion of neoadjuvant therapy and before liver transplantation. EUS with fine needle aspiration (FNA) sampling of portal nodes should be considered before transplant evaluation and initiation of neoadjuvant chemoradiation.
- *Staging cross-sectional imaging of the chest and abdomen* documenting the lack of metastatic disease within 90 days of listing for transplant and every 90 days while listed for transplant.
- *Exclusion criteria* include transperitoneal biopsies of the primary tumor by percutaneous, endoscopic, or operative approaches and documentation of metastatic disease by imaging or staging examinations.

Because the primary neoadjuvant modality given before transplant for hCCA has been radiation therapy, the systemic chemotherapy regimens typically given have been primarily aimed at radiosensitization, with a maintenance regimen given while awaiting transplantation. The initial University of Nebraska and Mayo clinic regimens included daily bolus fluorouracil (5-FU) but migrated to continuous infusion 5-FU.[24,25] Maintenance capecitabine is then typically given for maintenance chemotherapy while awaiting transplant. Other programs have preferred to use gemcitabine as a single agent (most commonly) or in combination with cisplatin. In published studies, capecitabine seems to be the most common maintenance regimen. There is much interest in targeted therapies for CCA as oncogenic mutations are identified for which selective inhibitors are available. However, currently identified mutations for the hilar variant of CCA are less common than seen in intrahepatic CCA, and no neoadjuvant protocols using targeted agents have yet been developed.[26]

Variation in the technique and dosage of radiotherapy also exists, and there are no comparative trials to identify an optimal technique in this unique population. Conventional external beam radiotherapy is a mainstay of most published regimens (1.5–2 Gy per fraction to a total dose of ~50 Gy), though centers have reported the use of stereotactic body radiotherapy (SBRT: higher dose fractions of 6–10 Gy over 5–6 fractions). Variability exists in the inclusion of boost doses to nodal basins in the porta and celiac axis, with no cohort data to allow meaningful comparisons in outcome in this patient population. A recent survey of US centers performing liver transplantation for hCCA suggests significant variation in total dose, suggesting that there is opportunity for further standardization of neoadjuvant treatment regimens.[27]

TREATMENT DROPOUT

Published series suggest that 20% to 30% of patients will drop out after neoadjuvant chemoradiation, before transplantation.[22,28] More than half of all dropouts occur at the time of the staging operation (laparoscopy or laparotomy with portal node dissection), which in some protocols occurs before listing while other centers do the staging operation immediately before or at the time of transplantation. Another third of patients will develop evidence of progression of disease (typically appearance of intrahepatic metastases or extrahepatic disease) on surveillance imaging. The remainder of dropouts are due to non-cancer-related causes (frailty, infection, comorbid disease), attesting to the rigorous nature of the neoadjuvant protocols and the inherent risks of the disease.

TECHNICAL DETAILS

Although the outcome among patients with hCCA undergoing liver transplantation is driven primarily by selection, the management of these patients is technically demanding and requires meticulous attention to detail throughout the listing period and at the time of transplant.

The staging operation includes evaluation of the peritoneal cavity for occult metastatic disease, typically done by laparoscopy, and portal lymph node sampling, which may be done through minimally invasive or open techniques. There are advantages and disadvantages of placing the timing of the staging operation closer to the time of completion of neoadjuvant therapy versus closer to the time of transplantation. Advantages of performing the staging operation soon after the completion of neoadjuvant radiation include making a decision about listing for transplant with more complete information (and therefore lowering the risk of dropout after listing, which has programmatic impact), allowing one to complete the portal dissection sooner after the radiation when the porta is less fibrotic with cleaner planes, and decreasing the likelihood of the patient's disappointment of a long waiting time for transplant only to dropout later. In contrast, moving the staging operation closer to the time of transplant potentially allows diagnosis of occult metastatic disease that progressed while waiting for transplant, removes the low risk of a delay in listing due to a complication of the staging operation, and may prevent scarring and adhesion from the staging operation that complicates portal dissection at the time of transplant. Importantly, in published multicenter data, the timing of the staging operation did not seem to have an impact on post-transplant survival.

The portal lymph node sampling should aim to excise nodes in the hepatoduodenal ligament (station 12) and along the common hepatic artery (station 8). Ideally, one should avoid dissection beyond the proximal aspect of the anterior hepatic artery lymph node, preserving the more proximal common hepatic artery as undissected should it be needed as an inflow target for transplant given that the more distal artery is in the radiation field. Approaching the staging portal node dissection from a minimally invasive technique is a nice option in experienced hands, as it clearly yields less scarring to encounter later at the time of transplant and avoids an upper abdominal incision within the radiation field that must be approached again later.

The relative value of living donor liver transplant (LDLT) versus deceased donor liver transplant (DDLT) for hCCA has been debated. Before OPTN policy allowing a pathway to an MELD exception for CCA, LDLT had the obvious advantage of a clear pathway to transplant when available and avoids the uncertainty of prolonged waiting time. In the setting of LDLT, the staging operation can either be done in the days leading up to the transplant or on the day of transplant before beginning the donor operation. The disadvantages of LDLT are primarily related to the necessity to use the radiated recipient portal vein and hepatic artery for inflow or to obtain additional vascular conduit to allow creation of a portal venous extension graft for the donor segmental portal vein, and/or to create an aortic conduit or interposition graft to provide arterial inflow from a source that has not been previously radiated. Although vascular complications are increased in LDLT at baseline relative to DDLT, more recent studies do not suggest that these risks are excessively high in hCCA patients following neoadjuvant radiation.[22]

In the setting of DDLT, allograft selection should be made in anticipation of a more complex hepatectomy and the need for potential vascular reconstruction. Good quality grafts that can require longer cold ischemia time, or use of machine perfusion to mitigate the impact of a longer recipient hepatectomy, should be considered. Good quality donor venous and arterial conduit should be procured to provide options for vascular reconstruction. A backup recipient should be identified and ideally called in for preoperative evaluation, such that the donor allograft could be rapidly reallocated to the backup recipient if metastatic disease is found at the time of recipient hepatectomy.

The recipient hepatectomy following neoadjuvant radiation, long-term indwelling biliary stents, and an infiltrative cancer can be somewhat unpredictable. These patients do not typically have portal hypertension or coagulopathy but the planes in the porta can be obliterated. The first priority should be a thorough exploration looking for occult peritoneal metastases and sampling any remaining suspicious nodal material in the porta. Depending on how long after radiation transplant is occurring, there may be no distinct nodal tissue, only dense fibrosis that can be hard to dissect and sample. Accessing the hepatic artery outside the porta can be the most prudent move, isolating the common hepatic artery and proceeding distally cautiously, as a first move. The common bile duct is then dissected distally and divided at the level of the pancreatic head. Stents are removed from their transampullary position and a distal biliary margin sent for frozen section. The distal duct is oversewn at the pancreatic head with fine absorbable suture. Unfortunately, with long-term stent placement and chronic inflammation the distal margin can be hard to interpret even by skilled pathologists. Proceeding with a pancreaticoduodenectomy at the time of transplant may be done for a definitively positive distal margin, but it clearly adds substantial perioperative risk in a situation where the oncologic benefit is questionable. Most experienced centers are very reticent to consider patients with more bulky hilar tumors that appear to have significant distal extension, as these patients anecdotally seem to do worse both in terms of perioperative risk and face poor oncologic outcomes.

The portal vein is then dissected cautiously, as it can be friable following radiation. It may be prudent to complete the final exposure of the portal vein after mobilization of the rest of the liver to avoid risk of injury before the liver is ready to be excised. The normally wide-open plane at the foramen of Winslow between the posterior aspect of the portal vein and the anterior aspect of the inferior vena cava can be obliterated following portal radiation and inflammation and should be dissected carefully as it would be in a redo transplant setting. There has been some debate about whether caval preservation is appropriate in the setting of CCA, but all the usual advantages of avoiding a bicaval clamp exist and certainly there do not seem to be inferior oncologic outcomes for hCCA in LDLT, in which the cava is preserved.

Once the liver is mobilized, consideration should be given to the need for vascular conduit. Some centers have routinely done supraceliac or infrarenal aortic conduit using donor iliac artery in hCCA cases. If that is the case, it may be prudent to systemically heparinize, place the aortic occlusion clamp and sew the proximal anastomosis of the vascular conduit before completing the hepatectomy. This allows it to be completed in a controlled manner without the pressure of time, and the transplant arterial inflow can be reestablished before or immediately after reperfusion. Once the proximal anastomosis of the conduit is completed, the aortic clamp is removed, and a gentle clamp placed on the proximal conduit until arterial reperfusion. The recipient hepatectomy is then completed and graft implantation is performed through standard means according to surgeon preference. In the case of DDLT, adequate donor vessel length should facilitate arterial and portal venous anastomoses without additional extension grafts. In the case of LDLT, additional conduit may be needed both to extend the portal vein (as it is quite difficult to preserve the hilum of the portal vein in these cases) and to provide an interposition graft or aortic conduit for the arterial reconstruction. Again, appropriate conduit should be considered and acquired before the transplant to allow options for reconstruction.

Biliary reconstruction is typically completed with a Roux-en-Y choledochojejunostomy (DDLT) or hepaticojejunostomy (LDLT) using standard techniques. Although many centers routinely use choledochoduodenostomy for biliary reconstruction in PSC and other situations that approach may not be prudent in hCCA patients in whom the duodenum has been radiated and the risk of technical complications may already be higher than other transplant recipients.

POSTOPERATIVE CARE AND COMPLICATIONS

Post-transplant care proceeds according to usual protocols, with vigilant attention for technical complications. Given the vascular reconstruction(s) often needed in these cases, regular daily surveillance Doppler ultrasound should be considered for the first 3 to 7 days post-transplant. Therapeutic anticoagulation is typically not indicated but prophylactic postoperative anticoagulation and aspirin for arterial reconstructions should be strongly considered. If drains were placed, monitoring for biliary leak, and occult pancreatic injury from a difficult portal dissection, should be considered before drain removal. Although alternative immunosuppressive regimens containing mammalian target of rapamycin (mTOR) inhibitors (eg, everolimus) have been considered in the setting of transplant for malignancy, there are no definitive trials suggesting a benefit in the setting of hCCA and most centers use standard three-drug immunosuppression (tacrolimus, mycophenolate mofetil, and prednisone taper).

Surveillance post-transplant should proceed in a manner similar to standard practice following resection for hCCA, with contrast-enhanced cross-sectional imaging (MRI or CT) of the abdomen and serum CA 19-9 measured every 3 to 4 months for 3 years and then every 6 months for a total of 5 years. Chest CT should be performed annually. PET-CT does not have a value in standard surveillance but could be added if suspicious areas are identified on cross-sectional imaging or in the setting of a rising CA 19-9. Median time to recurrence in published series is just under 2 years, with recurrences occurring out to 4 to 5 years.

The role of adjuvant chemotherapy following liver transplantation has been considered, but no studies have documented a benefit. A recent European trial was closed due to poor accrual, with the majority of the small number of patients enrolled unable to tolerate adjuvant gemcitabine due to side effects.[29] At the present time, post-transplant chemotherapy should be reserved for patients with recurrence or perhaps rare patients with unexpectedly concerning explant pathology.

In addition to the usual post-transplant technical and immunosuppression-related complications, hCCA patients seem to face a significantly increased risk of vascular complications, typically related to the arterial reconstruction. Early reports from the Mayo Clinic described a vascular complication rate as high as 40%, with some graft losses reported due to delayed hepatic artery thrombosis.[30] More recent reports suggest a major vascular complication rate closer to 20%, with fewer complications leading to graft loss, suggesting that standardized radiation protocols and more careful patient selection may allow mitigation of vascular catastrophes. A recent multicenter international study of high-volume liver transplant centers with protocols for hCCA suggested a 90-day mortality rate of less than 5% in "benchmark" cases, which is consistent or better than outcomes in patients with other indications for liver transplantation.[31]

ONCOLOGIC OUTCOMES

The Mayo Clinic experience with neoadjuvant brachytherapy and systemic chemotherapy, coupled with strict patient selection, documented approximately 70% 5-year survival among hCCA patients following liver transplantation.[28] Unique features of the Mayo Clinic cohort include a substantial number of CCA patients with underlying PSC, who appear to have potential earlier diagnosis, more favorable tumor biology, and better long-term prognosis.[32] Protocols from other centers have modified the

Mayo protocol slightly, including other radiation therapy modalities such as SBRT,[25] and achieved 60% 5-year survival in a patient cohort largely made up of de novo CCA patients without PSC.[22]

Multicenter published experience with transplant for hCCA consistently report 5-year recurrence-free survival rates of approximately 60%. Intention to treat survival, including all patients who enter hCCA protocols with intent to transplant, is approximately 40% to 45% reflecting the substantial dropout from progression or occult metastatic disease at staging in this population. Much has been made of comparisons to similar node-negative patients who undergo resection, with arguments made that liver transplantation offers better outcomes in this "head-to-head" comparison.[25] Although true that liver transplantation may offer some survival benefit driven primarily by an increased ability to achieve an R0 resection, this may reflect the challenge of patient selection with currently available imaging. A comparison of patients with similar oncologic characteristics who undergo planned resection versus planned transplant reveal very similar overall outcomes, arguing against extending liver transplantation to patients considered resectable.[33] Clearly ongoing study is needed to continue to refine patient selection for this complex patient population.

The predictors of cancer recurrence in available trials include higher tumor grade, presence of perineural or vascular invasion, and identification of node-positive disease on explant pathology.[10] Patients with positive distal biliary margins, and patients who undergo pancreaticoduodenectomy to achieve a negative margin, appear to have double the risk of post-transplant recurrence. In the early Mayo Clinic experience, tumor radial size greater than 3 cm was associated with a significant increased risk of recurrence, which is why that remains an exclusion criterion in most current protocols.[34] Factors associated with improved prognosis after transplant include CCA that occurs in the setting of PSC (approximately half the risk of recurrence when compared with de novo CCA patients) and the presence of complete pathologic response on explant pathology.[10,35]

Survival after recurrence is poor, with median survival regardless of therapeutic interventions reported as approximately 6 months. Site of recurrence is typically the abdomen (peritoneum, nodal, and intrahepatic metastases), although distant sites of recurrence (lung, bone) have been reported.

In summary, liver transplantation has been established as an effective therapy for unresectable hCCA in highly selected node-negative patients. Protocol dropout occurs in up to 30% of patients before transplant, but post-transplant morbidity and mortality is quite low in this complex population. Multidisciplinary patient selection and meticulous perioperative care facilitate excellent outcomes in experienced centers. Further study is needed to consider expansion of selection criteria in this population and to evolve neoadjuvant regimens to include more standardized radiation protocols and expansion of systemic therapies.

CLINICS CARE POINTS

- Multidisciplinary evaluation of eligible patients with hilar cholangiocarcinoma (hCCA), including evaluation for resection by an experienced hepatobiliary surgeon, is critical to appropriate selection of candidates for liver transplantation.

- Appropriate staging evaluation to rule out extrahepatic disease, including endoscopic ultrasound with fine needle aspiration of portal nodes, is necessary before initiating neoadjuvant chemoradiation for hCCA in a liver transplant protocol.

- A staging operation, including exploration of the peritoneum for occult metastatic disease and portal lymphadenectomy to document a lack of nodal metastases, is required following the completion of neoadjuvant radiation therapy and before liver transplantation. There are advantages and disadvantages of performing this operation either before listing or closer to the time of transplantation.

- Both deceased donor and living donor liver transplantation may achieve acceptable outcomes when applied to hCCA patients following neoadjuvant chemoradiation. Vascular conduit may be needed for arterial or venous reconstruction, especially at the time of living donor liver transplantation.

- Risk factors for recurrent disease following liver transplantation include higher tumor grade, presence of perineural or vascular invasion, identification of node-positive disease on explant pathology, and patients with a positive distal margin and/or those requiring pancreaticoduodenectomy at the time of transplant.

DISCLOSURE

The author has nothing to disclose.

REFERENCES

1. STARZL TE, Marchioro TL, Von Kaulla KN, et al. Homotransplantation of the liver in humans. Surg Gynecol Obstet 1963;117:659.
2. Neuberger JM, Adams DH. Liver transplantation. Baillière's Clin Gastroenterology 2004;3:231–52.
3. KLATSKIN G. Adenocarcinoma of the hepatic duct at its bifurcation within the porta hepatis. an unusual tumor with distinctive clinical and pathological features. Am J Med 1965;38:241–56.
4. Saha SK, Zhu AX, Fuchs CS, et al. Forty-Year Trends in Cholangiocarcinoma Incidence in the U.S.: Intrahepatic Disease on the Rise. Oncol 2016;21:594–9.
5. Sharma P, Yadav S. Demographics, tumor characteristics, treatment, and survival of patients with Klatskin tumors. Ann Gastroenterol 2018;31:231–6.
6. Gupta A, Dixon E. Epidemiology and risk factors: intrahepatic cholangiocarcinoma. Hepatobiliary Surg Nutr 2017;6:101–4.
7. Claessen MMH, Vleggaar FP, Tytgat KMAJ, et al. High lifetime risk of cancer in primary sclerosing cholangitis. JOURNAL OF HEPATOLOGY 2009;50:158–64.
8. Trivedi PJ, Crothers H, Mytton J, et al. Effects of Primary Sclerosing Cholangitis on Risks of Cancer and Death in People With Inflammatory Bowel Disease, Based on Sex, Race, and Age. Gastroenterology 2020;159(3):915–28.
9. Bowlus CL, Arrivé L, Bergquist A, et al. AASLD practice guidance on primary sclerosing cholangitis and cholangiocarcinoma. Hepatology 2023;77(2): 659–702.
10. Moreno Luna LE, Kipp B, Halling KC, et al. Advanced cytologic techniques for the detection of malignant pancreatobiliary strictures. Gastroenterology 2006;131(4): 1064–72.
11. Heimbach JK, Sanchez W, Rosen CB, et al. Trans-peritoneal fine needle aspiration biopsy of hilar cholangiocarcinoma is associated with disease dissemination. HPB : the official journal of the International Hepato Pancreato Biliary Association 2011;13:356–60.
12. Patel AH, Harnois DM, Klee GG, et al. The utility of CA 19-9 in the diagnoses of cholangiocarcinoma in patients without primary sclerosing cholangitis. Am J Gastroenterol 2000;95:204–7.
13. Tempero MA, Uchida E, Takasaki H, et al. Relationship of carbohydrate antigen 19-9 and Lewis antigens in pancreatic cancer. Cancer Res 1987;47(20):5501–3.

14. Hemming AW, Reed AI, Fujita S, et al. Surgical management of hilar cholangio-carcinoma. Ann Surg 2005;241:693–9, discussion: 699–702].
15. Rocha FG, Matsuo K, Blumgart LH, et al. Hilar cholangiocarcinoma: the Memorial Sloan-Kettering Cancer Center experience. J Hepato-Biliary-Pancreatic Sci 2010; 17:490–6.
16. Mansour JC, Aloia TA, Crane CH, et al. Hilar cholangiocarcinoma: expert consensus statement. HPB (Oxford) 2015;17(8):691–9.
17. Matsuo K, Rocha FG, Ito K, et al. The Blumgart preoperative staging system for hilar cholangiocarcinoma: analysis of resectability and outcomes in 380 patients. J Am Coll Surg 2012;215(3):343–55.
18. Olthof PB, Wiggers JK, Groot Koerkamp B, et al. Postoperative Liver Failure Risk Score: Identifying Patients with Resectable Perihilar Cholangiocarcinoma Who Can Benefit from Portal Vein Embolization. J Am Coll Surg 2017;225(3):387–94.
19. Vugts JJA, Gaspersz MP, Roos E, et al. Eligibility for Liver Transplantation in Patients with Perihilar Cholangiocarcinoma. Ann Surg Oncol 2021;28(3):1483–92.
20. Grendar J, Grendarova P, Sinha R, et al. Neoadjuvant therapy for downstaging of locally advanced hilar cholangiocarcinoma: a systematic review. HPB 2014;16: 297–303.
21. Silver CM, Joung RH, Logan CD, et al. Neoadjuvant therapy use and association with postoperative outcomes and overall survival in patients with extrahepatic cholangiocarcinoma. J Surg Oncol 2023;127(1):90–8.
22. Darwish Murad S, Kim WR, Harnois DM, et al. Efficacy of neoadjuvant chemora-diation, followed by liver transplantation, for perihilar cholangiocarcinoma at 12 US centers. Gastroenterology 2012;143(1):88–98.e3.
23. "Organ Procurement and Transplant Network (OPTN) Policies". 2023. Available at: https://optn.transplant.hrsa.gov/media/eavh5bf3/optn_policies.pdf. Accessed September 4, 2023.
24. Sudan D, DeRoover A, Chinnakotla S, et al. Radiochemotherapy and transplan-tation allow long-term survival for nonresectable hilar cholangiocarcinoma. Am J Transplant 2002;2(8). 774–749.
25. Rea DJ, Heimbach JK, Rosen CB, et al. Liver transplantation with neoadjuvant chemoradiation is more effective than resection for hilar cholangiocarcinoma. Ann Surg 2005;242(3):451–8.
26. Rizzo A, Ricci AD, Cusmai A, et al. Systemic Treatment for Metastatic Biliary Tract Cancer: State of the Art and a Glimpse to the Future. Curr Oncol 2022;29(2): 551–64.
27. Keltner SJ, Hallemeier C, Wang K, et al. Neoadjuvant Therapy Regimens for Hilar Cholangiocarcinoma Before Liver Transplant. Am J Clin Oncol 2023;46(6):276–8.
28. Darwish Murad S, Kim WR, Therneau T, et al. Predictors of pretransplant dropout and posttransplant recurrence in patients with perihilar cholangiocarcinoma. Hepatology 2012;56(3):972–81.
29. Schmelzle M, Benzing C, Fischer L, et al. Feasibility and Efficacy of Adjuvant Chemotherapy With Gemcitabine After Liver Transplantation for Perihilar Cholan-giocarcinoma - A Multi-Center, Randomized, Controlled Trial (pro-duct001). Front Oncol 2022;12:910871.
30. Mantel HT, Rosen CB, Heimbach JK, et al. Vascular complications after ortho-topic liver transplantation after neoadjuvant therapy for hilar cholangiocarcinoma. Liver Transpl 2007;13(10):1372–81.
31. Breuer E, Mueller M, Doyle MB, et al. Liver Transplantation as a New Standard of Care in Patients With Perihilar Cholangiocarcinoma? Results From an Interna-tional Benchmark Study. Ann Surg 2022;276(5):846–53.

32. Heimbach JK, Gores GJ, Haddock MG, et al. Predictors of disease recurrence following neoadjuvant chemoradiotherapy and liver transplantation for unresectable perihilar cholangiocarcinoma. Transplantation 2006;82(12):1703–7.

33. Croome KP, Rosen CB, Heimbach JK, et al. Is Liver Transplantation Appropriate for Patients with Potentially Resectable De Novo Hilar Cholangiocarcinoma? J Am Coll Surg 2015;221:130–9.

34. Rosen CB, Heimbach JK, Gores GJ. Surgery for cholangiocarcinoma: the role of liver transplantation. HPB 2008;10:186–9.

35. Welling TH, Feng M, Wan S, et al. Neoadjuvant stereotactic body radiation therapy, capecitabine, and liver transplantation for unresectable hilar cholangiocarcinoma. Liver Transpl 2014;20(1):81–8.

How to Determine Unresectability in Hilar Cholangiocarcinoma

Catherine G. Pratt, MD[a], Jenna N. Whitrock, MD[a],
Shimul A. Shah, MD, MHCM[a,b], Zhi Ven Fong, MD, MPH, DrPH[c],*

KEYWORDS

- Hilar cholangiocarcinoma • Klatskin tumor • Vascular invasion • Transplant
- Unresectability • Resectability

KEY POINTS

- Overall incidence and disease-specific mortality is on the rise for hilar cholangiocarcinoma.
- Margin negative (R0) resection is the strongest predictor for survival.
- Preoperative evaluation for resectability is challenging given the tumors proximity and possible invasion into to the *porta hepatis*.
- No clinical staging system readily predicts resectability.
- A multidisciplinary, holistic, and individualized approach gives the best evaluation.

BACKGROUND

Cholangiocarcinoma (CCA) is a cancer arising from the biliary epithelium and represents the second most common primary liver tumor following hepatocellular carcinoma. CCAs are typically classified anatomically into three distinct entities: intrahepatic, hilar/perihilar, and distal.[1] Its overall incidence and disease-specific mortality has been on the rise likely secondary to improved diagnostic modalities for detection of these tumors as well as the increasing burden of liver disease such as viral hepatitis and fatty liver disease.[2,3]

---

[a] Cincinnati Research in Outcomes and Safety in Surgery (CROSS) Research Group, Department of Surgery, University of Cincinnati College of Medicine, 231 Albert Sabin Way, ML 0558, Cincinnati, OH 45267-0558, USA; [b] Division of Transplantation, Department of Surgery, University of Cincinnati College of Medicine, 231 Albert Sabin Way, MSB 2006C, ML 0519, Cincinnati, OH 45267-0558, USA; [c] Division of Surgical Oncology and Endocrine Surgery, Department of Surgery, Mayo Clinic Arizona, Mayo Clinic College of Medicine, 5777 East Mayo Boulevard, Phoenix, AZ 85054, USA
* Corresponding author.
E-mail address: Fong.Zhi@mayo.edu
Twitter: @CPrattMD (C.G.P.); @JennaWhitrockMD (J.N.W.); @shimulshah73 (S.A.S.); @ZhiVen-FongMD (Z.V.F.)

Surg Clin N Am 104 (2024) 197–214
https://doi.org/10.1016/j.suc.2023.09.001
0039-6109/24/© 2023 Elsevier Inc. All rights reserved.
surgical.theclinics.com

Hilar CCAs (hCCAs) were first described by Dr Altemeier in 1957 and again by Dr Klatskin in 1965 and comprise 40% to 60% of all diagnosed CCAs.[1,4] There are an estimated 3000 cases of hilar and distal (extrahepatic) CCAs diagnosed annually in the United States, but over one-half to two-thirds of hCCAs are determined to be surgically unresectable at the time of presentation.[5,6] Indolent symptoms lead to delays in diagnosis, and patients often present with late-stage disease with tumor invasion into critical adjacent structures. Unfortunately, most of the patients with unresectable hCCA will succumb to their disease within 12 months of initial presentation, with approximately 50% of untreated patients not surviving beyond 3 to 4 months.[1]

Owing to the aggressive nature of these tumors, surgical resection with negative margins (R0) is the only curative treatment and the strongest predictor of favorable survival.[4] However, the proximity of hCCAs to the *porta hepatis* makes determining resectability, particularly the locoregional assessment, challenging. Yet, this assessment is critical in the decision for and to prevent delays in the next best steps of treatment. This article aims to review the determination of unresectability in hilar CCA in three parts: the preoperative assessment, the intraoperative assessment, and key steps of surgical resection, as well as treatment options for unresectable tumors.

STAGING AND CONSIDERATIONS FOR RESECTION

To determine suitability for resection, a holistic view of patient and tumor characteristics must be considered. Following diagnosis, the preoperative workup includes evaluating the patient's performance status, locoregional factors and surrounding structure involvement, the future liver remnant (FLR), and the biology of the tumor. This is followed by the intraoperative assessment, which confirms that locoregional factors continue to support the possibility of an R0 resection.

Several staging systems have been developed to classify hilar disease. The Bismuth–Corlette system delineates four overarching types: Type I—tumor involving the distal bile duct to the hepatic duct confluence, Type II—tumor extending to and involving the hepatic duct confluence, Type IIIa/b—tumor involving the hepatic duct confluence and extending to the proximal right/left hepatic duct (RHD/LHD), and Type IV—tumor extending from the hepatic duct confluence bilaterally to the proximal hepatic ducts and secondary biliary radicals or multicentric tumors (**Fig. 1**).[4,7] The American Joint Committee on Cancer (AJCC) combines tumor size and/or vascular invasion with evaluation of nodal and/or metastatic disease into the traditional TNM staging.[4] The Jarnagin–Blumgart system describes three types of biliary tree tumor involvement with or without portal vein (PV) invasion and/or hepatic lobar atrophy: T1—tumor involving the hepatic duct confluence with unilateral extension to right or left biliary radicals; T2—tumor involving the hepatic duct confluence with unilateral extension and ipsilateral PV invasion or ipsilateral hepatic lobar atrophy; and T3—tumor involving the hepatic duct confluence with bilateral extension to biliary radicals, or unilateral extension to biliary radicals with contralateral PV invasion, or unilateral extension with contralateral hepatic lobar atrophy, or main or bilateral PV invasion (**Fig. 2**).[8] Of these, no current staging system stratifies patients based on preoperative resectability. The Bismuth system describes the extent of tumor involvement of the biliary tree, the AJCC system focuses on pathologic criteria, and the Blumgart system adds consideration for involvement of the PV and the presence of lobar atrophy, but does not account for arterial involvement.[1,6] Thus, a combination of established staging and preoperative resection planning should be used.

The most definitive locoregional criteria for unresectability are bilateral involvement of secondary biliary radicals, bilateral involvement of the hepatic artery (HA)

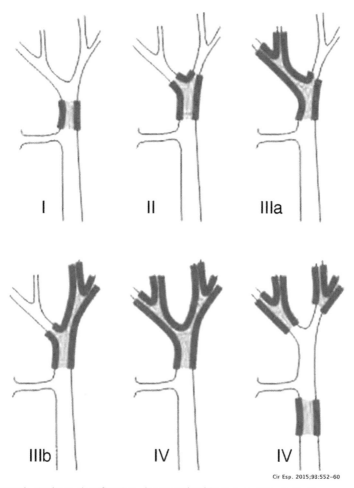

Cir Esp. 2015;93:552–60

Fig. 1. Bismuth–Corlette classification. (*From* "Klatskin Tumor: Diagnosis, Preoperative Evaluation and Surgical Considerations",[7] with permission.)

or portal venous branches, involvement of the PV main trunk proximal to the bifurcation, or unilateral HA or portal venous encasement with involvement of the contralateral secondary biliary radicals. Beyond locoregional factors, patient's medical fitness and ability to tolerate an operation as well as the presence of distant metastases are additional key considerations when determining the resectability of CCAs (**Fig. 3**).

PREOPERATIVE ASSESSMENT
Patient Factors

Although they do not represent the resectability of hCCA in its strictest sense, patient factors and ability to tolerate major surgery are critical components of the initial evaluation. This is especially true when considering surgical resection of hCCA is associated with postoperative morbidity and mortality rates ranging from 40% to 70% and 5% to 15%, respectively, even at high-volume referral centers.[5,9] This is compared with 20% to 50% morbidity and 1% to 5% mortality for liver resections in general.[10–13]

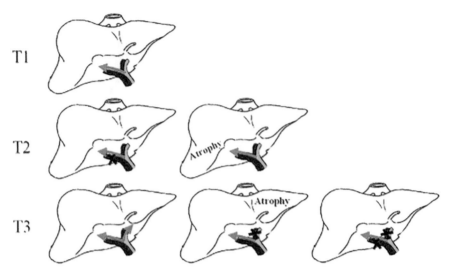

Fig. 2. Jarnagin–Blumgart classification. (*From* "The Blumgart Preoperative Staging System for Hilar Cholangiocarcinoma: Analysis of Resectability and Outcomes in 380 Patients",[8] with permission.)

To assess a patient's medical fitness and ability to tolerate surgery, several strategies can be used.

The use of preoperative surgical risk calculators such as the Revised Cardiac Risk Index or the Charlson Comorbidity Index (CCI) can be helpful to assess the likelihood of major morbidity or mortality in the perioperative period.[14,15] Frailty is another factor that can be assessed preoperatively via scoring systems such as the modified frailty index. Several studies have shown that those with increased levels of preoperative frailty are at increased risk for postoperative complications, including mortality after

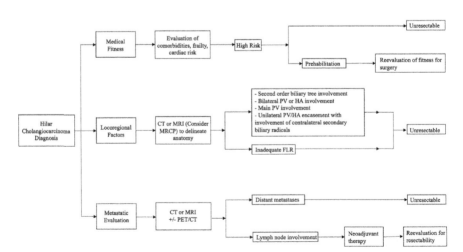

Fig. 3. Diagram demonstrating preoperative workup and evaluation for unresectability. CT, computed tomography; FLR, future liver remnant; MRCP, magnetic resonance cholangiopancreatography.

major surgery.[16] Functional status should also be assessed in patients being evaluated for major surgery and is a reliable predictor of perioperative cardiac events. Informal questioning regarding activities of daily living can be performed, though more formal assessment scales exist, such as the Duke Activity Status Index and Eastern Cooperative Oncology Group performance assessment.[17] Patients with good preoperative fitness and functional status are unlikely to require further testing; however, those who are found to have poor preoperative functional status, a high comorbidity burden, or increased frailty may benefit from more rigorous preoperative testing.[14]

All patients with established coronary artery disease should undergo preoperative electrocardiogram (ECG). For those without a known cardiac history, obtaining an ECG preoperatively may serve as a useful baseline given the high-risk nature of the operation. In patients who are found to be at increased cardiac risk and have poor functional status preoperatively, further cardiac testing should be performed as delineated in the algorithm in **Fig. 4**. Typically, these patients require pharmacologic stress testing followed by coronary revascularization if indicated before surgery.[14]

In patients who are medically high-risk, participation in a prehabilitation program before surgery may help optimize their preoperative fitness.[15] Prehabilitation programs may include a variety of activities known to improve physiologic reserve such as physical exercise, dietary interventions and nutrition counseling, smoking and alcohol cessation counseling, and psychological support.[18] Prehabilitation should typically begin 1 month before surgery, though its timing can depend on the urgency of surgery and no definite guidelines regarding adequate duration of prehabilitation programs have been established. Participation in a prehabilitation program is particularly appealing and convenient if neoadjuvant treatment is pursued.

Locoregional Factors

Given the complexity of the portal anatomy, a comprehensive preoperative assessment of locoregional structures relies on high-quality, accurate imaging. Despite

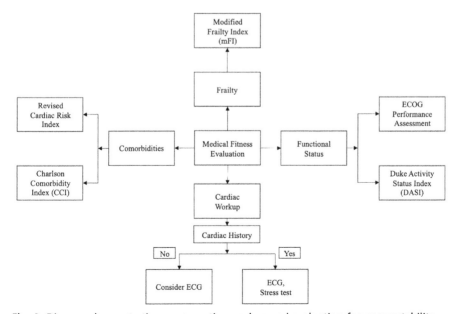

Fig. 4. Diagram demonstrating preoperative workup and evaluation for unresectability.

extensive preoperative workup, 40% to 50% of preoperatively resectable patients are still determined to be unresectable at the time of surgical exploration.[5] Currently, computed tomography (CT) and MRI are considered the standard imaging modalities for hCCA with comparable sensitivity (90% to 97%) and specificity (60% to 81%) for determining resectability.[19] High-resolution CT can accurately depict a thickened bile duct and show evidence of tumor invasion into liver parenchyma or hilar vessels (**Fig. 5**). MRI with magnetic resonance cholangiopancreatography can provide unique insight into biliary anatomy, and although its ability to provide comprehensive vascular evaluation is considered suboptimal compared with CT (**Fig. 6**), it serves as an acceptable alternative or adjunct modality.[19] At our institution, patients typically undergo CT scan with intravenous contrast with arterial, portal venous, and delayed phases for preoperative workup, given its more granular discrimination of *porta* structure involvement as compared with MRI. Regardless of modalities used, cross-sectional imaging should include a minimum of three phases. Specifically, early and late portal venous phases allow optimal delineation of tumor involvement of hepatic arteries and delayed phases of more than 6 minutes (typically 10 minutes) can improve the sensitivity of determining the full extent of tumor invasion.[20]

Many patients will also undergo endoscopic retrograde cholangiopancreatography (ERCP) with cholangiogram as an additional diagnostic modality. This is typically obtained before and after drain placement for biliary decompression with stenting to relieve CCA-related obstructive jaundice or cholangitis. A pre-decompression cholangiogram displays upstream dilated ducts secondary to stricturing from the cancer and provides significant insight into the extent of biliary tree involvement by the tumor.[4,21] This said, an ERCP is typically not pursued solely for diagnostic purposes if biliary obstruction is not present due to its associated risks.[21] If biliary decompression is necessary, biopsy via brushings or spyglass can be obtained simultaneously, though this is not routinely required for resectable cases with reasonable clinical suspicion.[4]

Following the completion of imaging, evaluation of locoregional factors when determining resectability predicates strongly on bilateral structure involvement (**Fig. 7**). All second-order biliary tree involvement (Bismuth Type IV) is considered unresectable disease (see **Figs. 1** and **6**). Likewise, bilateral involvement of either the PV or HA is classically regarded as unresectable (see **Figs. 5** and **6**; **Fig. 8**). Invasion or occlusion of the main PV proximal to the bifurcation also precludes surgical resection.[1]

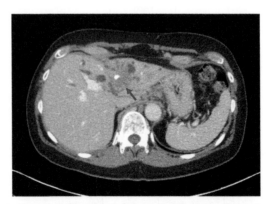

Fig. 5. CT demonstrating an infiltrative left hepatic lobe mass (*arrow*) resulting in central biliary obstruction. The mass results in occlusion of the left portal vein and branches with irregular attenuation of the left hepatic arteries.

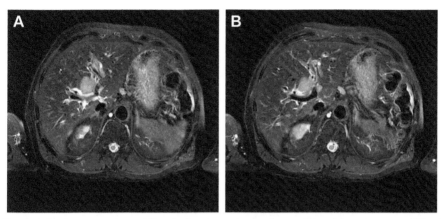

Fig. 6. MRI demonstrating a hilar cholangiocarcinoma (*arrows*) involving the central/distal right hepatic duct and left hepatic duct to its second-order branches with tumor encasement of the right hepatic artery and abutment of the proximal left hepatic artery.

Consideration for resection with unilateral structure involvement is more nuanced and is more often of concern when anticipating the necessity of a right hepatectomy for R0 resection. Contralateral lobe atrophy from the involved biliary segment may result in inadequate FLR following resection and thus exclude surgical intervention (see **Fig. 8**). An FLR of at least 25% to 30% of the preoperative, non-atrophied volume with preserved vascular inflow and outflow and adequate biliary drainage is considered sufficient to decrease the risk of postoperative hepatic insufficiency.[22,23] It is critical to note that this assumes a healthy FLR, with more remnant required (30%–40%) should the patient have varying degrees of nonalcoholic fatty liver disease or has received hepatotoxic chemotherapy.[19,22]

To minimize the risk of hepatic insufficiency after major hepatectomy, especially when a right or extended hepatectomy is required, the anticipated FLR must be analyzed through volumetric or functional assessment. A three-dimensional assessment of liver parenchyma, vasculature, and tumor allows for a volumetric calculation of the anticipated remaining liver following resection as a percentage of the total preoperative volume.[22] Alternatively, dynamic functional tests such as indocyanine green (ICG) clearance or hepatobiliary scintigraphy (HBS) with technetium-99m (Tc-99) are available to evaluate the preoperative global liver function and FLR. Volumetric assessment alone can overestimate liver function, and utilization of functional

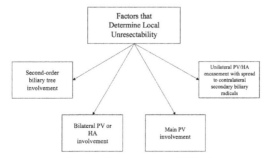

Fig. 7. Diagram demonstrating locoregional unresectability factors.

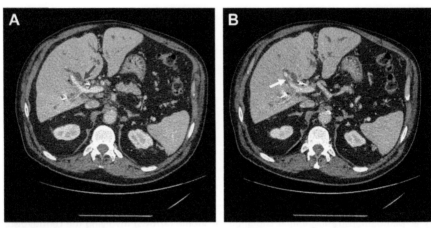

Fig. 8. CT demonstrating biliary hilar stricture consistent with cholangiocarcinoma with atrophic right hepatic lobe. There is mild right and moderate left intrahepatic biliary dilation (*A, red arrow*) and apparent encasement and narrowing of the proximal left portal vein at the hepatic hilum (*B, white arrow*).

assessment has been shown to better estimate the FLR and avoid postresection hepatic insufficiency.[24] The recent inaugural European "Consensus Guidelines for Preoperative Liver Function Assessment Before Hepatectomy" strongly recommends volumetric assessment and functional assessment with ICG clearance with a conditional recommendation for HBS.[25] Notable limitations exist within current functional assessment modalities in that both ICG and Tc-99 clearance are affected by hyperbilirubinemia and cholestatic states.[24,25] No analogous guidelines have been published in the United States to date.

In addition, preoperative biliary drainage should be considered as it allows for a less congested, non-cholestatic FLR. Although no benefit has been shown for an FLR of greater than 30%, lower incidences of hepatic insufficiency and mortality postoperatively have been demonstrated in patients with an FLR of less than 30% who underwent preoperative biliary drainage.[26] Furthermore, studies conducted in Europe have demonstrated a mortality benefit in patients who received preoperative biliary drainage before right hepatectomy.[27,28] No benefit for preoperative biliary drainage before left hepatectomy was shown, which corresponds to the benefit demonstrated in patients with an FLR of greater than 30%.[27,28]

For patients with an inadequate predicted FLR, there are several treatment options available, which should be individualized to the patient's specific circumstance. PV embolization (PVE) has long been the gold standard modality to induce hypertrophy in the contralateral lobe for patients with inadequate FLR. PVE redirects blood flow to the contralateral lobe and thereby induces hypertrophy by approximately 30% in 6 to 8 weeks.[29] An alternate technique that capitalizes on the same concept is radiological simultaneous portohepatic vein embolization (RASPE, sometimes also termed total hepatic venous deprivation), whereby the ipsilateral portal and hepatic veins are both embolized. RASPE has been demonstrated to achieve higher rates of hypertrophy, with studies reporting hypertrophy rates of more than 60%.[30] The DRAGON trial is a collaborative group of international centers that performed a head-to-head comparison of the two modalities and reported that RASPE-induced greater contralateral hypertrophy (59% vs 48%, $P = .02$), was associated with higher resection rates

(90% vs 68%, $P = .002$), and had comparable morbidity as well as mortality rates when compared with PVE.[31]

A final consideration in operative planning is management of the caudate lobe. Given its location and biliary drainage patterns, caudate lobe bile ducts have been implicated with microscopic invasion in 24% to 98% of patients on retrospective review.[32] A recent review of the literature suggests that routine caudate lobe resection may increase the rate of an R0 resection with a reported fivefold increase in overall survival (OS) and without a significant increase in perioperative morbidity.[32,33] However, substantial limitations are present with regard to selection bias, power, and generalizability beyond high-volume centers. Conversely, as the caudate lobe represents 5% to 10% of the liver mass,[33] preservation of the lobe increases the FLR in patients requiring an extended right hepatectomy with a resultant borderline FLR. Although caudate lobe resection is indicated in cases of obvious tumor involvement, its resection in cases without obvious involvement is not without additional risk. Owing to its location with respect to the inferior vena cava, portal venous inflow, middle and left hepatic veins, and unique biliary drainage, caudate resection requires additional intraoperative planning and may add risk of postoperative complications.[32,33] As such, while generally recommended, an individualized approach should be made regarding caudate lobe resection in hCCA cases with questionable tumor involvement of the caudate lobe.

Biological Factors

When evaluating resectability for hilar CCA, the biology of the cancer must be considered. This is determined preoperatively through any evidence for locoregional lymph node involvement and the tumor response to neoadjuvant systemic therapy. Locoregional lymph node involvement is a critical prognostic factor and is associated with more than 50% reduction in survival for patients with node-positive tumors.[6] However, patients with N1 disease (regional nodes within the *porta hepatis*) should still be considered for surgical resection (**Fig. 9**). N2 nodal disease that involves disease spread to periaortic, pericaval, superior mesenteric, or celiac nodes and, on the other hand, indicates more advanced disease that may preclude resection.[34] There is an estimated 7-month increase in OS between N1 positive patients who undergo resection compared with N1 positive patients who do not complete surgical resection.[35] However, recurrence-free survival (RFS) is limited to less than 7 years for all node-positive

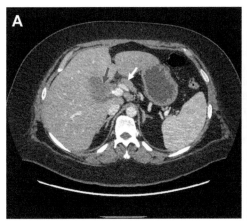
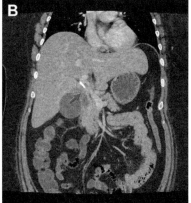

Fig. 9. CT demonstrating an ill-defined hypodense hilar mass (*A, B red arrows*) with enlarging periportal lymph nodes (*A, white arrow*).

disease.[36] Although patients with N1 and limited N2 disease had 5-year OS rates of 19.2% and 11.5%, respectively,[37] most patients N2 disease has limited data to suggest increased survival following resection and has an estimated OS closer to that of metastatic disease, arguing against the rationale for surgical resection.[37]

Distant metastatic disease represents tumor spread beyond that of direct extension or nodal involvement of the hCCA. Evidence of distant metastatic disease on preoperative imaging or when encountered early on in surgical resection precludes surgical resection, and patients should be referred for palliative therapy.[23] Although preoperative cross-sectional imaging with CT or MRI can detect suspicious lymph nodes or metastatic disease, its sensitivity is limited, and radiographically occult metastases still occur 10% to 30% of the time.[4] PET/CT has the highest sensitivity and specificity to detect both lymph node and distant metastatic disease[19] and is an important component of the preoperative staging workup that can drastically alter the treatment approach and strategy.

Owing to the concern for radiographically occult metastatic disease, staging laparoscopy could be considered for patients with more advanced disease on preoperative imaging. For large tumors with vascular involvement or for those with equivocal lymph nodes or distant lesions of concern, staging laparoscopy could spare patients the morbidity of a nontherapeutic laparotomy. Staging laparoscopy has been shown to identify occult peritoneal metastatic disease in between 10% and 20% of Blumgart T2 and T3 lesions with negative preoperative imaging.[4,23] Although the continued improvement of radiographic modalities and increasing utilization of PET/CT has increased the preoperative detection of metastatic disease, staging laparoscopy still detects advanced disease, which precludes resection for one in seven patients in contemporary series and remains a clinically beneficial tool for select patients.[4,22] The utility of peritoneal washings obtained during staging laparoscopy is still questionable, with smaller series demonstrating minimal yield[38] and others demonstrating an association between positive cytology and portal venous invasion.[39] Further validation is required before it can be routinely recommended.

For patients with large infiltrating hCCAs or significant locoregional lymphadenopathy with no apparent distant disease, another approach is to test the disease's biology with neoadjuvant systemic therapy. By using a neoadjuvant approach, patients who go on to develop progressive or metastatic disease on treatment are spared a morbid operation. The SWOG 1815 single-arm phase II trial using gemcitabine, cisplatin, and nab-paclitaxel in patients with advanced biliary tract cancers demonstrated encouraging OS and PFS of 19.2 and 11.8 months, respectively.[40] However, enthusiasm around the regimen dampened when its phase III, two-arm trial demonstrated no difference in survival outcomes when compared with gemcitabine and cisplatin.[41] The TOPAZ-1 trial evaluating gemcitabine, cisplatin, and durvalumab demonstrated a statistically significant difference in survival outcomes when compared with patients receiving gemcitabine and cisplatin, although its clinical impact of survival difference (12.8 months in the Durvalumab group vs 11.5 months in the control arm, $P = .02$) is debated.[42] Efforts are being focused on determining the ideal regimen for patients with advanced disease, and these patients should be treated in the context of a clinical trial whenever possible.

INTRAOPERATIVE ASSESSMENT
Technical Considerations

The operative approach should proceed with selective staging laparoscopy when appropriate, and in the absence of radiographically occult metastases, followed by partial hepatectomy with en bloc bile duct resection and portal lymphadenectomy, and concluding with Roux-en-Y hepaticojejunostomy reconstruction. Although the initial approach and exposure may proceed in a routine manner, notable differences exist between right and left portal anatomy, which dictate the procedure progression.[22] Safe dissection of the *porta hepatis* is paramount, as injury to the uninvolved, contralateral structures could preclude surgical resection in its entirety. In this section, the authors cover basic anatomic principles and operative steps when approaching right-sided and left-sided hCCAs.

Porta Anatomy

Although variations in hepatic ductal, arterial, and portovenous anatomy are common, some anatomic principles are consistent and important to understand to facilitate a safe *porta hepatis* dissection. First, the hepatic arterial bifurcation typically lies fairly inferior to the hepatic ductal and portovenous bifurcations and away from major structures (**Fig. 10**). Once the hilar plate is lowered, dissection can be safely initiated in the space above the hepatic arterial bifurcation given its ease of access and distance from major structures. Second, the right HA (RHA) frequently "knuckles out" posterior and lateral to the common bile duct (CBD), coursing up the hilum into the right liver (see **Fig. 10**). It can be easily identified if the CBD is retracted medially, and care should be taken not to injure it. Third, the lateral edge of the transition from the main PV to right PV (RPV) is typically a smooth contour because of its linear alignment (see **Fig. 10**). This is opposed to the left PV (LPV) that bifurcates almost at a tangential angle

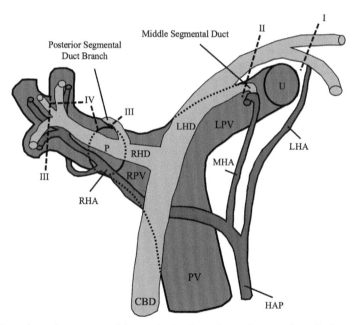

Fig. 10. *Porta hepatis* anatomy with standard orientation, relative order of bifurcation, and angles. CBD, common bile duct; HAP, hepatic artery proper; LHA, left hepatic artery; LHD, left hepatic duct; LPV, left portal vein; MHA, middle hepatic artery; P, right posterior section; PV, portal vein; RHA, right hepatic artery; RHD, right hepatic duct; RPV, right portal vein; U, umbilical portion of LPV. Numerals corresponding to Couinaud's liver segments. I: extended right hepatectomy, II: right hepatectomy, III: left hepatectomy, IV: extended left hepatectomy. (*Adapted from* "Assessing resectability in cholangiocarcinoma",[43] with permission.)

from the main PV. As such, the RPV can only be safely distinguished from the main PV once dissection reveals the LPV branching off medially from the main trunk. In addition, there is frequently a posterior sector branch posterior to the RPV where dissection is frequently initiated, and care should be taken to avoid injury to it. Finally, the LHD typically courses superior and parallel to the LPV (see **Fig. 10**), and as such, the LPV can be used as a landmark to identify or avoid injury to the LHD.

Right-sided hilar cholangiocarcinoma

The surgical approach for resectable right-sided hCCA is as follows: First, the left HA (LHA) is isolated and encircled with a vessel loop. Next, the RHA is identified as it exits posteriorly and lateral to the CBD and encircled with a vessel loop. The RHA and CBD are then retracted medially to expose the portal venous bifurcation. The LPV is then identified and isolated. At this time, the hCCA is then palpated to confirm there is no involvement of the LHA and LPV. If those structures remain free from invasion, the RHA can then be divided. This facilitates the RPV exposure. Care must be taken to avoid injuring a posterior segment V venous branch as the RPV is circumferentially dissected and then divided with a vascular staple load. The LHD typically courses superior and parallel to the LPV and can be identified accordingly. Here, a segment of the LHD that is uninvolved by tumor can be selected for transection and margins sent for frozen section if indicated. The LHD classically has additional extrahepatic length than the RHD, which allows for easier establishment of appropriate margin and setup for the Roux-en-Y hepaticojejunostomy. After transection, the LHD is marked with suture for easier identification for the eventual anastomosis.

Left-sided hilar cholangiocarcinoma

The surgical approach for resectable left-sided hCCA is as follows: First, the RHA is isolated and encircled with a vessel loop as it exists posterior and lateral to the CBD. Next, the RPV is exposed and identified by retracting the RHA anteromedially. Additional exposure may be necessary and is readily accomplished through anteromedial retraction of the CBD using a vein retractor. Care must be taken to identify the presence of a posterior segment V venous branch as the posterior surface of the RPV is dissected. At this time, the hCCA is then palpated to confirm there is no involvement of the RHA and RPV. If those structures remain free from invasion, the LHA and LPV can then be divided. This facilitates complete isolation of the RHD. Here, a segment of the RHD that is uninvolved by tumor can be selected for transection, marked with suture, and margins sent for frozen section if indicated.

Additional intraoperative considerations

The utility of intraoperative frozen section analysis of the proximal bile duct to ensure an R0 resection is debated. Although an R0 resection remains a significant prognostic factor, it has also been shown that successful re-resection of the proximal bile duct margin when an initial margin was positive for tumor does not improve long-term outcomes.[43] A retrospective cohort study of additional bile duct margin cases in Japan found an RFS and OS of 47 and 63 months in patients with an initial R0 resection compared with an RFS and OS of 16 and 25 months in those with an initial positive margin.[44] Of note, they found no significant difference in RFS or OS between cases in which an additional bile duct margin provided an R0 resection and cases with a final positive margin,[44] suggesting that an initially positive resection margin reflects tumor biology as opposed to technical inadequacies. In some cases, an additional proximal margin is obtained only with significant difficulty with increased operative morbidity. It can also necessitate a more complex bilioenteric reconstruction and contribute to additional postoperative complications. Given the potentially high risk and apparent minimal benefit to additional margin attainment, it is not unreasonable to forgo this practice, though a case-by-case approach should be used.

Furthermore, the impact of an R1 resection (margins positive for microscopic disease) on OS is controversial. A cohort study of 79 patients who underwent R1 resection followed by adjuvant chemoradiation and 51 patients with nonmetastatic, locally advanced hCCA who did not undergo surgical resection demonstrated that OS was more favorable in patients who had an R1 resection (18.9 months vs 5.0 months, $P < .001$).[45] However, the retrospective study should be interpreted in the context of its study design. The resected patients likely had more localized disease because they were explored with curative intent, and the patients deemed unresectable and who were not explored likely had more advanced disease. In addition, a separate cohort study demonstrated that R1 resection was associated with similar OS when compared with R0 resection only in the absence of lymphovascular and perineural invasion.[46] This further reinforces that cancer biology ultimately dictates overall prognosis and that the added morbidity of more radical resection is likely not justified when adjuvant therapies such as chemoradiation can be used.

Vascular resection and reconstruction can be considered when PV or HA invasion does not preclude resection. When evaluating vascular involvement and need for resection, short-term risks must be weighed against the potential for improved long-term outcomes. LPV resection can generally be achieved without additional difficulty, and reconstruction can proceed with end-to-end anastomosis with or without the use of an interposition graft.[34] Grafting can often be avoided due to the long extrahepatic course of the LPV and its ease of access at the umbilical fissure[47] (see **Fig. 10**). The RPV is typically shorter and bifurcates earlier. Its involvement frequently requires grafting during reconstruction and can implicate multiple RPV branches depending on the location of the RPV bifurcation.[47] If possible, PV resection and reconstruction planning should be performed preoperatively to decrease intraoperative morbidity. However, it is not uncommon to encounter more significant tumor involvement than appreciated on preoperative imaging.

Although PV resection is considered relatively straight-forward, HA resection and reconstruction carry higher rates of morbidity and mortality.[47] Tumor infrequently invades the LHA given its anatomic separation from the biliary confluence. As it runs along the left edge of the hepatoduodenal ligament, tumor invasion of the LHA would only occur with near complete encasement of the hepatoduodenal ligament, in which case it renders the hCCA unresectable. RHA involvement of a left-predominant hCCA is more common given its proximity to the anterior and posterior surface of the biliary confluence.[47] However, its preservation or reconstruction following removal for an R0 resection is critical for the FLR following a left or extended left hepatectomy. Overall, high-volume referral centers and those with living donor liver transplantation programs have improved outcomes for resections involving either PV or HA reconstruction.[22,47]

TREATMENT OPTIONS IN THE EVENT OF UNRESECTABILITY

When a patient with hCCA is not a candidate for resection, other treatment modalities can be considered in the context of a multidisciplinary team approach. The most common first-line treatment of patients with unresectable hCCA is systemic chemotherapy, typically with gemcitabine and cisplatin. This combination was first demonstrated to increase survival in the Advanced Biliary Cancer (ABC)-01 trial followed by the ABC-02 trial.[48] As mentioned previously, the SWOG S1815 trial evaluated the effect of adding nab-paclitaxel to the regimen with promising results; however, the phase III study was not able to replicate the success found in the initial phase II study.[41,48,49]

The addition of immunotherapeutic agents such as durvalumab has been evaluated in the phase III TOPAZ-1 trial, which showed improved OS in advanced biliary tract cancers compared with chemotherapy alone, though the benefit was marginal and it is important to note that extrahepatic CCA only made up a small subset of the population of this study.[44,50]

Radiation therapy is another treatment modality that can be used in the management of unresectable hCCA in addition to chemotherapy. The addition of radiation therapy to systemic chemotherapy was shown to improve quality of life and local control in the phase II SWOG S0809 trial in 2015.[42] Studies have suggested that stereotactic body radiation therapy (SBRT) may have advantages and lead to increased OS over conventional radiotherapy in patients with unresectable but localized hCCA when combined with systemic therapy. However, those with extensive regional lymph node metastases may still benefit more from conventional radiation therapy combined with systemic therapy to avoid SBRT to high-risk areas.[51]

Liver transplantation is another emerging treatment modality for unresectable hCCA in highly selected patients (tumors <3 cm in radial diameter without lymph node involvement) in conjunction with neoadjuvant chemoradiotherapy.[52–54] Over the last decade, with the improvement of immunosuppression therapy and perioperative care, liver transplant has been trialed as a viable treatment option for patients with unresectable hCCA. Studies including the Mayo Clinic Group's experience and a large retrospective review of 12 US centers by Darwish Murad and colleagues have shown promising results with 60% to 65% 5-year survival rates in highly selected patients following neoadjuvant chemotherapy.[5,55] Patients with primary sclerosing cholangitis (PSC) are one of the select groups, which may benefit from liver transplant. Those with PSC are typically younger, female, and are diagnosed at an earlier stage, all representing factors associated with favorable post-transplant survival.[53,56,57] PSC-associated hCCA is also more frequently associated with multifocal disease, and these patients more frequently have underlying liver disease, which are additional reasons that transplant is favored in this group.[53,56,57] Of note, 5-year survival of as high as 70% can be achieved in this population after liver transplant when combined with neoadjuvant chemotherapy.[5,57,58]

SUMMARY

hCCA is a biologically aggressive disease for which the only curative treatment remains surgical resection. The intersection of the patient's physical reserve, locoregional tumor involvement of *porta hepatis* structures, predicted resection requirements with resultant FLR, and accurate assessment of metastatic disease heavily influence patient selection and their ultimate ability to undergo surgical resection. A multidisciplinary, holistic, and individualized approach to patient selection is critical to accurately determine resectability and optimize clinical outcomes for patients with hCCA.

CLINICS CARE POINTS

- The overall incidence and disease-specific mortality of hilar cholangiocarcinoma is increasing, likely secondary to improved diagnostic modalities for detection and the increasing burden of liver disease.
- Over one-half to two-thirds of cases are deemed surgically unresectable at presentation.
- Surgical resection with negative margins (R0) is the only curative treatment and the strongest predictor of favorable survival.

- The preoperative workup should include evaluating the patient's performance status, locoregional factors and surrounding structure involvement, the future liver remnant (FLR), and the biology of the tumor.
- No current staging system stratifies hCCA patients based on preoperative resectability.
- The most definitive locoregional criteria for unresectability are bilateral involvement of secondary biliary radicals, bilateral involvement of the hepatic artery or portal venous branches, involvement of the portal vein main trunk proximal to the bifurcation, or unilateral hepatic artery or portal venous encasement with involvement of the contralateral secondary biliary radicals.
- Surgical resection of hCCA is associated with high postoperative morbidity and mortality rates compared with liver resections in general.
- CT and MRI are the standard imaging modalities for hCCA (with or without PET/CT).
- Assuming a healthy liver, an FLR of at least 25% to 30% is considered sufficient to decrease the risk of postoperative hepatic insufficiency.
- The inaugural European "Consensus Guidelines" strongly recommend both volumetric assessment and functional assessment with indocyanine green clearance for preoperative assessment of liver function before hepatectomy.
- Preoperative biliary drainage should be considered for obstructive symptoms and hilar cholangiocarcinoma (hCCA) patients with an FLR of less than 30%.
- An individualized approach to caudate lobe resection in hCCA is critical to optimize postoperative outcomes.
- Patients with N1 disease should still be considered for surgical resection; however, N2 involvement and distant metastasis preclude surgical resection.
- Staging laparoscopy should be considered for patients with more advanced disease on preoperative imaging.
- Safe dissection of the *porta hepatis* is paramount.
- Successful re-resection of an initially positive margin of the proximal bile duct does not improve long-term outcomes.
- Benefits of a positive margin for microscopic disease (R1) resection are debated and current evidence suggests that the potential for benefit does not outweigh the added morbidity.
- Studies are ongoing to optimize systemic therapy for unresectable hCCA.
- Liver transplantation is an emerging treatment modality for unresectable hCCA in highly selected patients in conjunction with neoadjuvant chemoradiotherapy.

DISCLOSURE

The authors have nothing to disclose.

REFERENCES

1. Jarnagin W, Winston C. Hilar cholangiocarcinoma: diagnosis and staging. HPB (Oxford) 2005;7(4):244–51.
2. Khan SA, Toledano MB, Taylor-Robinson SD. Epidemiology, risk factors, and pathogenesis of cholangiocarcinoma. HPB 2008;10(2):77–82.
3. Palmer WC, Patel T. Are common factors involved in the pathogenesis of primary liver cancers? A meta-analysis of risk factors for intrahepatic cholangiocarci-noma. J Hepatol 2012;57(1):69–76.

4. Fong ZV, Brownlee SA, Qadan M, et al. The clinical management of cholangiocarcinoma in the united states and Europe: a comprehensive and evidence-based comparison of guidelines. Ann Surg Oncol 2021;28(5):2660–74.

5. Soares KC, Kamel I, Cosgrove DP, et al. Hilar cholangiocarcinoma: diagnosis, treatment options, and management. Hepatobiliary Surg Nutr 2014;3(1):18–34.

6. Rocha FG, Matsuo K, Blumgart LH, et al. Hilar cholangiocarcinoma: the Memorial Sloan-Kettering Cancer Center experience. J Hepatobiliary Pancreat Sci 2010; 17(4):490–6.

7. Molina V, Sampson J, Ferrer J, et al. Klatskin tumor: diagnosis, preoperative evaluation and surgical considerations. Cir Esp 2015;93(9):552–60.

8. Matsuo K, Rocha FG, Ito K, et al. The Blumgart preoperative staging system for hilar cholangiocarcinoma: analysis of resectability and outcomes in 380 patients. J Am Coll Surg 2012;215(3):343–55.

9. Dewulf M, Verrips M, Coolsen MME, et al. The effect of prehabilitation on postoperative complications and postoperative hospital stay in hepatopancreatobiliary surgery a systematic review. HPB 2021;23(9):1299–310.

10. Lancaster RT, Tanabe KK, Schifftner TL, et al. Liver resection in veterans affairs and selected university medical centers: results of the patient safety in surgery study. J Am Coll Surg 2007;204(6):1242.

11. Vauthey JN, Pawlik TM, Abdalla EK, et al. Is Extended Hepatectomy for Hepatobiliary Malignancy Justified? Ann Surg 2004;239(5):722–32.

12. Andres A, Toso C, Moldovan B, et al. Complications of Elective Liver Resections in a Center With Low Mortality: A Simple Score to Predict Morbidity. Arch Surg 2011;146(11):1246–52.

13. Vasavada B, Patel H. Postoperative mortality after liver resection for hepatocellular carcinoma—a systematic review. Metanalysis and metaregression of studies published in the last 5 years. Surg Pract 2022;26(2):123–30.

14. Fleisher LA, Fleischmann KE, Auerbach AD, et al. 2014 ACC/AHA Guideline on Perioperative Cardiovascular Evaluation and Management of Patients Undergoing Noncardiac Surgery. Circulation 2014;130(24):e278–333.

15. Laor A, Tal S, Guller V, et al. The Charlson Comorbidity Index (CCI) as a Mortality Predictor after Surgery in Elderly Patients. Am Surg 2016;82(1):22–7.

16. Nidadavolu LS, Ehrlich AL, Sieber FE, et al. Preoperative Evaluation of the Frail Patient. Anesth Analg 2020;130(6):1493–503.

17. Azam F, Latif MF, Farooq A, et al. Performance Status Assessment by Using ECOG (Eastern Cooperative Oncology Group) Score for Cancer Patients by Oncology Healthcare Professionals. Case Rep Oncol 2019;12(3):728–36.

18. Joliat GR, Kobayashi K, Hasegawa K, et al. Guidelines for Perioperative Care for Liver Surgery: Enhanced Recovery After Surgery (ERAS) Society Recommendations 2022. World J Surg 2023;47(1):11–34.

19. Zhang H, Zhu J, Ke F, et al. Radiological imaging for assessing the respectability of hilar cholangiocarcinoma: a systematic review and meta-analysis. BioMed Res Int 2015;2015:e497942.

20. Engelbrecht MR, Katz SS, van Gulik TM, et al. Imaging of Perihilar Cholangiocarcinoma. Am J Roentgenol 2015;204(4):782–91.

21. Rassam F, Roos E, van Lienden KP, et al. Modern work-up and extended resection in perihilar cholangiocarcinoma: the AMC experience. Langenbeck's Arch Surg 2018;403(3):289–307.

22. Lidsky ME, Jarnagin WR. Surgical management of hilar cholangiocarcinoma at Memorial Sloan Kettering Cancer Center. Ann Gastroenterol Surg 2018;2(4): 304–12.

23. Schulick RD. Criteria of unresectability and the decision-making process. HPB (Oxford) 2008;10(2):122–5.
24. Tomassini F, Giglio MC, De Simone G, et al. Hepatic function assessment to predict post-hepatectomy liver failure: what can we trust? A systematic review. Updates Surg 2020;72(4):925–38.
25. Primavesi F, Maglione M, Cipriani F, et al. E-AHPBA–ESSO–ESSR Innsbruck consensus guidelines for preoperative liver function assessment before hepatectomy. Br J Surg 2023;znad233. https://doi.org/10.1093/bjs/znad233.
26. Kennedy TJ, Yopp A, Qin Y, et al. Role of preoperative biliary drainage of liver remnant prior to extended liver resection for hilar cholangiocarcinoma. HPB 2009;11(5):445–51.
27. Farges O, Regimbeau JM, Fuks D, et al. Multicentre European study of preoperative biliary drainage for hilar cholangiocarcinoma. Br J Surg 2013;100(2):274–83.
28. Nuzzo G, Giuliante F, Ardito F, et al. Improvement in perioperative and long-term outcome after surgical treatment of hilar cholangiocarcinoma: results of an Italian multicenter analysis of 440 patients. Arch Surg 2012;147(1):26–34.
29. van Lienden KP, van den Esschert JW, de Graaf W, et al. Portal Vein Embolization Before Liver Resection: A Systematic Review. Cardiovasc Intervent Radiol 2013;36(1):25–34.
30. Laurent C, Fernandez B, Marichez A, et al. Radiological Simultaneous Portohepatic Vein Embolization (RASPE) Before Major Hepatectomy: A Better Way to Optimize Liver Hypertrophy Compared to Portal Vein Embolization. Ann Surg 2020;272(2):199.
31. Heil J, Korenblik R, Heid F, et al. Preoperative portal vein or portal and hepatic vein embolization: DRAGON collaborative group analysis. Br J Surg 2021;108(7):834–42.
32. Gilbert RWD, Lenet T, Cleary SP, et al. Does Caudate Resection Improve Outcomes of Patients Undergoing Curative Resection for Perihilar Cholangiocarcinoma? A Systematic Review and Meta-Analysis. Ann Surg Oncol 2022;29(11):6759–71.
33. Dinant S, Gerhards MF, Busch ORC, et al. The importance of complete excision of the caudate lobe in resection of hilar cholangiocarcinoma. HPB 2005;7(4):263–7.
34. Otto G, Romaneehsen B, Hoppe-Lotichius M, et al. Hilar cholangiocarcinoma: resectability and radicality after routine diagnostic imaging. J Hepatobiliary Pancreat Surg 2004;11(5):310–8.
35. Buettner S, van Vugt JLA, Gaspersz MP, et al. Survival after resection of perihilar cholangiocarcinoma in patients with lymph node metastases. HPB 2017;19(8):735–40.
36. Groot Koerkamp B, Wiggers JK, Allen PJ, et al. Recurrence Rate and Pattern of Perihilar Cholangiocarcinoma after Curative Intent Resection. J Am Coll Surg 2015;221(6):1041–9.
37. Aoba T, Ebata T, Yokoyama Y, et al. Assessment of Nodal Status for Perihilar Cholangiocarcinoma: Location, Number, or Ratio of Involved Nodes. Ann Surg 2013;257(4):718.
38. Martin RCGI, Fong Y, DeMatteo RP, et al. Peritoneal Washings Are Not Predictive of Occult Peritoneal Disease in Patients with Hilar Cholangiocarcinoma. J Am Coll Surg 2001;193(6):620.
39. Matsukuma S, Nagano H, Kobayashi S, et al. The impact of peritoneal lavage cytology in biliary tract cancer (KHBO1701): Kansai Hepato-Biliary Oncology Group. Cancer Reports 2021;4(2):e1323.

40. Shroff RT, Javle MM, Xiao L, et al. Gemcitabine, Cisplatin, and nab-Paclitaxel for the Treatment of Advanced Biliary Tract Cancers: A Phase 2 Clinical Trial. JAMA Oncol 2019;5(6):824–30.

41. Shroff RT, Guthrie KA, Scott AJ, et al. SWOG 1815: A phase III randomized trial of gemcitabine, cisplatin, and nab-paclitaxel versus gemcitabine and cisplatin in newly diagnosed, advanced biliary tract cancers. J Clin Orthod 2023;41(4_suppl):LBA490.

42. Oh DY, Ruth He A, Qin S, et al. Durvalumab plus Gemcitabine and Cisplatin in Advanced Biliary Tract Cancer. NEJM Evid 2022;1(8). https://doi.org/10.1056/EVIDoa2200015. EVIDoa2200015.

43. Neuhaus P, Thelen A. Radical surgery for right-sided Klatskin tumor. HPB 2008; 10(3):171–3.

44. Kawano F, Ito H, Oba A, et al. Role of Intraoperative Assessment of Proximal Bile Duct Margin Status and Additional Resection of Perihilar Cholangiocarcinoma: Can Local Clearance Trump Tumor Biology? A Retrospective Cohort Study. Ann Surg Oncol 2023;30(6):3348–59.

45. Schiffman SC, Reuter NP, McMasters KM, et al. Overall survival peri-hilar cholangiocarcinoma: R1 resection with curative intent compared to primary endoscopic therapy. J Surg Oncol 2012;105(1):91–6.

46. Kovalenko YA, Zharikov YO, Konchina NA, et al. Perihilar cholangiocarcinoma: A different concept for radical resection. Surgical Oncology 2020;33:270–5.

47. Serrablo A, Serrablo L, Alikhanov R, et al. Vascular Resection in Perihilar Cholangiocarcinoma. Cancers 2021;13(21):5278.

48. Halder R, Amaraneni A, Shroff RT. Cholangiocarcinoma: a review of the literature and future directions in therapy. Hepatobiliary Surg Nutr 2022;11(4):55566.

49. Nab-Paclitaxel and Biliary Tract Cancer OS | SWOG. https://www.swog.org/news-events/news/2023/01/20/nab-paclitaxel-and-biliary-tract-cancer-os. Accessed August 20, 2023.

50. National Comprehensive Cancer Network. Treatment by cancer type - biliary tract cancers. NCCN; 2023. https://www.nccn.org/guidelines/category_1.

51. Wang N, Huang A, Kuang B, et al. Progress in Radiotherapy for Cholangiocarcinoma. Front Oncol 2022;12:868034.

52. Keltner SJ, Hallemeier C, Wang K, et al. Neoadjuvant Therapy Regimens for Hilar Cholangiocarcinoma Before Liver Transplant. Am J Clin Oncol 2023;46(6):276.

53. Mansour JC, Aloia TA, Crane CH, et al. Hilar Cholangiocarcinoma: expert consensus statement. HPB (Oxford) 2015;17(8):691–9.

54. Ethun CG, Lopez-Aguiar AG, Anderson DJ, et al. Transplantation Versus Resection for Hilar Cholangiocarcinoma: An Argument for Shifting Treatment Paradigms for Resectable Disease. Ann Surg 2018;267(5):797.

55. Darwish Murad S, Kim WR, Harnois DM, et al. Efficacy of neoadjuvant chemoradiation, followed by liver transplantation, for perihilar cholangiocarcinoma at 12 US centers. Gastroenterology 2012;143(1):88–98, e3; quiz e14.

56. Bowlus CL, Arrivé L, Bergquist A, et al. AASLD practice guidance on primary sclerosing cholangitis and cholangiocarcinoma. Hepatology 2023;77(2):659.

57. Rea DJ, Heimbach JK, Rosen CB, et al. Liver Transplantation with Neoadjuvant Chemoradiation is More Effective than Resection for Hilar Cholangiocarcinoma. Ann Surg 2005;242(3):451–61.

58. Chapman R, Fevery J, Kalloo A, et al. Diagnosis and management of primary sclerosing cholangitis. Hepatology 2010;51(2):660–78.

Liver Transplant for Intrahepatic Cholangiocarcinoma

Olanrewaju A. Eletta, MBBS[a], Guergana G. Panayotova, MD[b],
Keri E. Lunsford, MD, PhD[b,*]

KEYWORDS

- Intrahepatic cholangiocarcinoma • Liver resection • Liver transplant
- Transplant oncology

KEY POINTS

- Cholangiocarcinoma is the second most common primary hepatic malignancy following hepatocellular carcinoma.
- There has been a marked global increase in the incidence of intrahepatic cholangiocarcinoma (iCCA). This aggressive cancer tends to be asymptomatic until late stages, leading most of the patients to present at advanced stages of the disease.
- Poor outcomes resulted in liver transplantation being formally contraindicated for patients with iCCA; however, recent advances in patient selection and neoadjuvant therapy have resulted in a paradigm shift in liver transplant oncology.

INTRODUCTION

Cholangiocarcinoma (CCA) is the second most common primary hepatic malignancy following hepatocellular carcinoma (HCC). It is an aggressive malignancy with an extremely poor prognosis arising from cholangiocytes in the biliary tract epithelium.[1,2]

Based on its anatomic location, it is classified into intrahepatic CCA (iCCA) and extrahepatic CCA, which includes perihilar CCA (pCCA) and distal CCA (dCCA).[3] Lesions above the hilar junction are classified as iCCA, constituting 5% to 10% of CCA. CCA occurring between the biliary hilum and the cystic duct are classified as pCCA. These are the most common, constituting 50% to 60% of CCA. CCA occurring distal to the cystic duct and proximal to the Ampulla of Vater are classified as dCCA, making up about 20% to 30% of CCA (**Fig. 1**).[3–5]

a Department of Surgery, Rutgers Robert Wood Johnson Medical School, 125 Paterson Street, MEB 596, New Brunswick, NJ 08901, USA; b Division of Transplant and HPB Surgery, Department of Surgery Rutgers, New Jersey Medical School, 185 South Orange Avenue, Newark, NJ 07103, USA
* Corresponding author.
E-mail address: keri.lunsford@rutgers.edu

Surg Clin N Am 104 (2024) 215–225
https://doi.org/10.1016/j.suc.2023.07.006
0039-6109/24/© 2023 Elsevier Inc. All rights reserved.

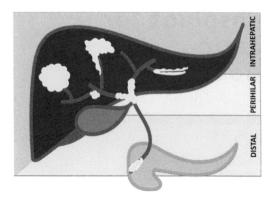

Fig. 1. Anatomic classification of cholangiocarcinoma.

There has been a marked global increase in the incidence of iCCA.[6–11] Over the past 4 decades, the incidence of iCCA has increased by approximately 2.3% annually (0.44–1.18 cases per 100,000; 128% increase from 1973 to 2012). It is unclear whether this represents an increase in the overall incidence of this complex disease or if it reflects improved detection and classification of previously undiagnosed or misdiagnosed disease.[2,12] Within the United States, the incidence of iCCA has also increased significantly.[2,6] Although iCCA may occur in a background of cirrhosis, it may also occur in the absence of known preexisting liver disease, and screening of such patients is limited. Despite advances in imaging and other diagnostic modalities, iCCA tends to be asymptomatic until late stages, leading most of the patients to present at advanced stages of disease; this limits the available management options, resulting in a less than 10% overall survival at 5 years following diagnosis.[1]

DIAGNOSIS
Imaging

CCAs are mostly asymptomatic, particularly in early stages of the disease. When symptomatic, pCCA and dCCA most frequently present with obstructive jaundice. Given its more peripheral location, obstructive jaundice is less frequent in patients with iCCA and occurs only in association with advanced disease or with more central location adjacent to larger biliary structures. The disease tends to be extremely aggressive, with a poor prognosis in advanced stages. In the absence of underlying liver disease, early detection is relegated to incidental findings on cross-sectional imaging done for other purposes, which accounts for about 20% to 25% of iCCA.[13] Patients with underlying cirrhosis are at higher risk for development of iCCA, but HCC is much more frequent. Misdiagnosis of iCCA based on imaging is common in this setting, especially in the absence of biopsy, and this results in a proportion of patients with iCCA receiving liver transplant for HCC being identified only on pathologic explant evaluation.

Ultrasonography, contrast-enhanced ultrasonography, computed tomography (CT), and MRI are indispensable in the diagnosis, staging, follow-up, and assessment of treatment response of CCA. Patterns of growth and tumor locations affect their diagnostic accuracy and utility as staging modalities. Multiphase contrast CT is considered the standard imaging method for preoperative assessment of iCCA, including noncontrast, arterial, portal venous, and delayed-phase contrasted imaging. It comprehensively evaluates the primary tumor, its relationship with adjacent structures, and identifies metastatic disease.[14] CT and MRI most commonly show arterial peripheral rim enhancement with progressive homogeneous contrast agent uptake until the delayed or stable uptake during late dynamic phases.[15] These imaging techniques notwithstanding, there is no specific radiologic pattern for iCCA. As such, histopathological or cytologic analysis is mandatory to confirm diagnosis.[16]

Imaging is also essential for diagnosis of metastatic disease during preoperative or pretransplant evaluation. Lymph node, peritoneal, lung, and bone metastases can commonly occur. During evaluation for liver transplant or resection, presence of extrahepatic disease can significantly affect candidate selection and postoperative recurrence risk. At our center, we prefer to initially evaluate patients with a multiphase contrasted CT of both the abdomen and pelvis, as drop metastases to the pelvis may occur. Contrasted MRI may be substituted when CT is contraindicated. We also routinely perform PET CT scans during the preoperative or pretransplant workup, and this is preferentially done before initiation of neoadjuvant therapy. Although magnetic resonance cholangiopancreatography, endoscopic retrograde cholangiopancreatography, and endoscopic ultrasound are not usually necessary for diagnosis, they can be useful adjuncts during preoperative and pretransplant assessment of extrahepatic disease (ie, in cases of suspicious lymphadenopathy) or assessment of biliary obstruction in more centrally located tumors. Furthermore, biliary imaging may be necessary to differentiate pCCA from iCCA.

Histopathology

Before the seventh edition of the American Joint Committee on Cancer (AJCC) Staging, iCCA was staged similarly to HCC. Intrahepatic CCA has a distinct molecular profile, several pathologic subtypes, and variable growth patterns.[13] Subtypes of iCCA are classified based on the growth pattern. These subtypes include mass-forming (MF-iCCA, most common), periductal infiltrating (PI-iCCA), and intraductal growing (**Fig. 2**).[3,13] Although MF-iCCA is associated with an intraparenchymal mass with distinct borders, PI-iCCA is characterized by tumor infiltration along the bile duct, often causing peripheral bile duct dilatation.[17]

Intrahepatic CCA also has variable histologic characteristics, including conventional, CCA, and rare variants.[18] Conventional iCCA is further subtyped based on the size or level of the affected duct as small bile duct iCCA and large bile duct iCCA. Small bile duct iCCA comprises small-sized tubular or acinar adenocarcinomas with nodular growth invading the liver parenchyma and no or minimal mucin production. It has been associated with chronic liver disease. On the other hand, large bile duct iCCA arises in large intrahepatic bile ducts and comprises mucin-producing columnar tumor cells arranged in a large duct or papillary architecture.[13,17–19] The heterogeneity of CCA at presentation presents challenges in diagnosing, staging, and managing this cancer.[5]

Given the importance of tumor biology in response to therapy as well as in potential application of emerging medical therapies for disease control, it is critical to supplement histopathologic data with genetic characterization of the tumors. Intrahepatic CCA is known to have a high mutational burden. We advocate for next-generation sequencing (NGS) analysis of all biopsy specimens. Profiling is again performed following tumor explant, as tumor mutation may change as a result of neoadjuvant therapy. Circulating tumor DNA from blood (ie, liquid biopsy) is sent to identify mutational variants and potential therapeutic targets in patients who lack sufficient biopsy tissue for NGS analysis. Although few chemotherapeutic agents targeting specific mutations are approved for first-line therapy, knowledge gained through NGS may identify targetable mutations for second-line or investigational treatments.

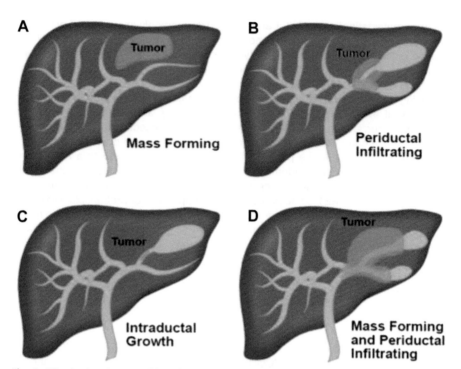

Fig. 2. Histologic subtypes of intrahepatic cholangiocarcinoma. (*A*) Mass forming. (*B*) Periductal infiltrating (*C*) Intraductal growth. (*D*) Mass forming and periductal infiltrating. (*From* Brown KM, Parmar AD, Geller DA. Intrahepatic cholangiocarcinoma. Surgical Oncology Clinics of North America. 2014;23(2):231–246. Doi:10.1016/j.soc.2013.10.004.)

SURGICAL MANAGEMENT OF INTRAHEPATIC CHOLANGIOCARCINOMA

A combination of medical and surgical therapy and an in-depth understanding of tumor biology is crucial for managing patients with iCCA.[3] Advances in molecular profiling and understanding of the genetic basis for these tumors are expanding, and the possibilities for targeted therapy against tumor mutations are rapidly evolving. Despite the advances in medical and locoregional interventional therapies, removal of the tumor remains the only widely accepted curative treatment.[5]

LIVER RESECTION

Liver resection with at least a portal lymphadenectomy is currently the standard of care and the only curative treatment option for iCCA.[1] The extent of lymphadenectomy for iCCA is a matter of debate and may vary based on surgeon preference, disease extent, and tumor location. Retrieval of at least 6 nodes is necessary for optimal pathologic staging following resection. Achievement of an R0 resection is the oncologic goal, with both gross and microscopically negative margin. Resectability depends on tumor location, its relation to vascular and biliary structures, the size of the future liver remnant (FLR), and the presence of extrahepatic disease. Extrahepatic disease, including positive lymph nodes beyond the hilum, is considered a relative contraindication to resection, given that surgery does not improve survival. At presentation, most patients are not candidates for resection due to factors such as tumor location, cirrhosis, portal hypertension, and multifocal disease.[20,21]

Resections may include both nonanatomic, as is the case for relatively small and peripheral lesions, or anatomic hepatectomies, as is the case with large tumors involving multiple segments. Most patients (50%–70%) with iCCA require major hepatectomies (resection of ≥ 3 segments) to achieve tumor-free margins due to the advanced stages at presentation. [22,23] Long-term retrospective database analysis suggests equivalent oncologic outcomes for minor versus major resections, with exception of close margins (1–4 mm) where minor resections show inferior recurrence-free survival.[3,24–26] Even with R0 resection, long-term outcomes are poor, with only 30% to 40% overall survival at 5 years, a cure rate of 9.7% (95% confidence interval, 6.1–13.4), and 60% to 70% recurrence.[1] Resection is contraindicated in patients with prohibitive comorbidities, bilateral multifocal or multicentric disease, macrovascular invasion, distant metastasis, and underlying liver disease. An FLR of less than 20% to 30% also prohibits resectability, particularly when the response to portal vein embolization techniques to grow the FLR has been inadequate.[3,27]

There has been a decrease in the morbidity and mortality associated with iCCA resection, 43% and 5%, respectively, in high-volume specialized centers.[3] Predictors of death and recurrence include age, tumor size, multiple lesions, lymphovascular invasion, and poor tumor differentiation.[4] The probability of cure ranges from 25.8% in patients with single, less than or equal to 5 cm disease, which is well differentiated without lymphovascular disease or periductal invasion to less than 0.1% in patients with all these risk factors.[28]

LIVER TRANSPLANTATION

Until recently, historically poor outcomes resulted in liver transplantation (LT) being formally contraindicated in patient with iCCA. Early studies demonstrated dismal overall survival (OS) with recurrence-free survival of 18% to 25% at 5 years[5,29]; however, patient selection was often suboptimal in early studies. Large tumor size and extension outside of the liver were common, and the utilization of neoadjuvant therapies was limited.[30] Because patients with known iCCA were excluded from transplant, many studies base transplant outcomes on patients with incidental or misdiagnosed tumors, and few prospective clinical trials have been performed.[1,5]

Despite this, replacement of the entire liver has theoretic benefit in iCCA. Advances in medical and interventional therapy as well as reevaluation of oncologic outcomes from other cancer types, such as HCC and pCCA, have reinstated consideration of LT as a viable treatment modality for iCCA.[1] Based on preliminary evidence of acceptable overall and recurrence-free survival outcomes for liver transplant in iCCA in more recent studies, the AASLD recently suggested that consideration of liver transplant for iCCA may be reasonable under research protocols.[31]

Several studies have retrospectively assessed the risk of recurrence of iCCA in patients with underlying cirrhosis who were misdiagnosed or incidentally found to have iCCA on explant pathology.

A multicenter retrospective analysis by Sapisochin and colleagues compared OS and recurrence-free survival following liver transplant in patients with iCCA (n = 27) or mixed hepatocholangiocarcinoma (HCC/CCA, n = 15) with that of HCC (n = 84). Outcomes were evaluated by tumor type, allowing a direct comparison between patients with iCCA and HCC. Patients with iCCA who had a solitary nodule less than or equal to 2 cm in diameter demonstrated a 5-year OS of 62% compared with 80% for matched HCC control. There was no significant difference in recurrence.[32,33]

A follow-up study, which included 17 major international transplant centers, was subsequently performed. This study retrospectively evaluated liver transplant outcomes from 2000 to 2013. Included patients again were identified based on explant, rather than pretransplant, diagnosis, and patients receiving pretransplant chemotherapy were excluded. Patients were subdivided into 2 groups: "very early" iCCA (≤2 cm) and "advanced" disease (solitary lesion >2 cm or multifocal disease). Cumulative risks of recurrence at 1, 3, and 5 years were 7%, 18%, and 18% in the very early iCCA group compared with 30%, 47%, and 61% in the advanced iCCA group (P = .01). The 1-year, 3-year, and 5-year actuarial survival rates were 93%, 84%, and 65%, respectively, in the very early iCCA group compared with 79%, 50%, and 45% in the advanced iCCA group (P = .02).[5,34] These 5-year recurrence rate and survival rates are within the range of currently accepted oncologic outcomes for HCC.

Subsequently, single-center analysis of patients undergoing liver transplant for HCC demonstrated that 7.1% of patients with HCC were found to have iCCA or mixed HCC/CCA on explant. Of these, OS for patients with early iCCA of mixed HCC/CCA was equivalent to that of patients undergoing liver transplant for HCC within Milan criteria, and recurrence-free survival was slightly inferior for iCCA.[5,35] Together, these studies suggest that select patients with liver-limited, small iCCA in a background of cirrhosis may be candidates for LT[5]; this is currently being further assessed through a multi-center prospective clinical trial.

Most patients with iCCA present at advanced stages, which makes it challenging to identify patients with "very early" iCCA. To evaluate the possibility of removing the 2 cm restriction in the aforementioned studies, a multicenter retrospective review comparing outcomes for liver resection and transplant in patients with iCCA was con-ducted by a group of French hepatobiliary centers. Their analysis included 45 patients with incidental iCCA or mixed HCC/CCA tumors with diameters between 2 and 5 cm. recurrence-free survival was 74% at 5 years, and transplant outcomes were similar to patients receiving liver transplant with tumor diameter less than or equal to 2 cm.[5,36] These data suggest that cirrhotic patients with tumors up to 5 cm might have accept-able outcomes following liver transplant in the absence of neoadjuvant therapy or with only locoregional therapy.

Although these outcomes are promising, most of the patients presenting with iCCA do not have underlying liver disease and present with more advanced disease burden. This raised the question of whether pretransplant medical therapy might augment recurrence risk for iCCA, as had been demonstrated for pCCA. The group from Univer-sity of California, Los Angeles was the first to demonstrate that adjuvant or neoadju-vant therapy in combination with liver transplant may improve survival for iCCA; however, results were difficult to interpret, given the combination of both hCCA and pCCA data in results.[5]

In collaboration with MD Anderson, Houston Methodist Hospital prospectively eval-uated the utility of pretransplant neoadjuvant chemotherapy in management of pa-tients with iCCA. In a paradigm shift from prior studies, the Methodist-MD Anderson protocol used tumor biology rather than tumor size to determine eligibility for liver transplant. Their protocol primarily used chemotherapeutic response as a proxy for favorable tumor biology. Selected patients had stable disease or disease response to chemotherapy for at least 6 months before transplant listing. Disease must be limited to the liver without evidence of lymph node metastases, but there is no limita-tion with regard to tumor size or multiplicity.

In 2018, they published the first prospective case series evaluating outcomes of liver transplant following neoadjuvant therapy. Serial cross-sectional imaging was used to ascertain disease stability, and all tumors were biopsy confirmed as iCCA. In the initial series, 6 patients with more than 6 months of radiographic stability or response to gemcitabine–cisplatin–based neoadjuvant chemotherapy were transplanted. The median tumor diameter was 10.5 cm, and the median number of lesions was 4. No tumor was less than 5 cm. Patients who had active disease on explant pathology received additional adjuvant chemotherapy. They found an OS and recurrence-free survival of 83% and 50% at 5 years, respectively.[4,32,37] Since then, 12 patients have undergone liver transplant on this strict protocol, with similar favorable outcomes[4]; this suggests that neoadjuvant chemotherapy may improve outcomes following liver transplant for patients with locally advanced unresectable iCCA. **Table 1** details the recent studies evaluating liver transplant in iCCA as well as the outcomes noted in those studies.

CLINICAL TRIALS IN LIVER TRANSPLANT FOR INTRAHEPATIC CHOLANGIOCARCINOMA: FUTURE TRENDS

Given candidacy for liver transplant depends on center policy rather than centrally regulated, there are multiple centers that have opened clinical protocols to consider patients with iCCA for transplant; these occur outside of a formal clinical trial setting. In addition, there are currently 4 formal clinical trials evaluating liver transplant as a treatment of iCCA.

- The Liver Transplantation for Non-Resectable Intrahepatic Cholangiocarcinoma: a Prospective Exploratory Trial (TESLA Trial. NCT04556214) is run out of Oslo University, Norway. It is an open-label study comprising a single group. It plans to enroll 15 participants. Inclusion criteria include ineligibility for liver resection (LR) based on the tumor's location or liver dysfunction. There must be no metastasis, and the participant must have good performance status. Participants must also have received at least 6 months of chemotherapy or locoregional therapy. They are evaluating OS as a primary outcome. Secondary outcomes include disease-free survival up to 10 years following transplant, adverse outcomes of surgery, and quality of life.
- Liver Transplantation for the Treatment of Early Stages of Intrahepatic Cholangiocarcinoma in Cirrhotic (NCT02878473) is a study run in University Health Network, Toronto and Hospital Clinic Spain. They are recruiting patients to meet an enrollment goal of 30 participants. This study has 5-year patient survival as the primary outcome and 5-year cumulative risk of recurrence after LT as the secondary outcome. To meet inclusion criteria, participants should have a biopsy-proven iCCA less than or equal to 2 cm, which is not amenable to liver resection, underlying liver cirrhosis, no metastasis, no lymphovascular invasion, and a cancer antigen 19-9 of less than or equal to 100 ng/mL.
- Liver Transplant for Stable, Advanced Intrahepatic Cholangiocarcinoma (NCT04195503) is a single-center, open-label clinical trial also recruiting out of University Health Network, Toronto. Patients with stable or regressing disease following a standard course of chemotherapy are included, and design is based off of the Houston Methodist/MD Anderson protocol. Selected patients must have unresectable iCCA with disease stability at least 6 months on neoadjuvant therapy. Appropriate candidates are considered for living donor liver transplant. They have an estimated enrollment of 10 participants. Primary and secondary outcomes are 5-year patient survival and disease-free survival, respectively. Inclusion criteria include good performance status, ineligibility for LR, absence of metastasis or lymphovascular invasion, and availability of a potentially appropriate living donor.
- Liver Transplantation in Patients With Incidental Hepatocellular-Cholangiocarcinoma and Intrahepatic Cholangiocarcinoma: A Single-center Experience (NCT04848805)

Table 1
Literature reported 5-year outcomes of liver transplants in patients with intrahepatic cholangiocarcinoma

Author	Groups	Number of Participants	Tumor Size	5-Year Overall Survival	5-y Recurrence (%)
Sapisochin et al[33] 2014	Total	29	—	45	29
	"Very early group"	8	≤2 cm	73	0
Sapisochin et al[33] 2014	"Very early iCCA only"	15	≤2 cm	65	18
	"Advanced" iCCA only	33	>2 cm	45	61
Facciuto et al[35] 2015	Total	32	—	57	66
	"Within Milan" group	10	0.8–4.8 cm. Median 2.5 cm	78	22
De Martin et al[36] 2020	Total	49	—	67	25
	< 2 cm tumor group	25	<2 cm	69	Not reported
	2–5 cm tumor group	24	2-5 cm	65	26
Lunsford et al[37] 2018	Total	6	≥ 5 cm. Median 10.5 cm	83	50

is a retrospective cohort study that evaluated 279 participants at Istanbul Demiroglu Bilim University in Turkey. The inclusion criteria are explant pathology of either HCC/CCA or iCCA and age greater than 18 years. Patients with explant pathology indicative of HCC are excluded. They assess the correlation between tumor diameter and multiplicity with recurrence.

CHALLENGES OF LIVER TRANSPLANT FOR INTRAHEPATIC CHOLANGIOCARCINOMA

In consideration of liver transplant for iCCA, patient selection is a challenge. More data are needed to identify patients at risk of recurrence with a higher degree of accuracy. Another significant challenge limiting the widespread acceptance of LT for iCCA is the limited access to donor liver allografts. Given the absence of underlying liver disease, patients with iCCA neither have high model for end-stage liver disease (MELD) scores nor qualify for exception points by current United Network for Organ Sharing (UNOS) Standards; this limits access to livers for patients with iCCA. As a result, deceased donor transplant for iCCA necessitates utilization of orphan livers that have been discarded by all other centers, and it is unclear as to whether use of these marginal grafts affects long-term outcomes. Current UNOS policy and transplant center evaluation metrics further limit the center's consideration of "experimental" protocols, especially in lower volume center. Living donor LT may also be a viable option for patients with appropriate tumor biology and response to neoadjuvant therapy; however, some opponents argue that living donor livers should not be used for an indication not currently recognized by UNOS.

Houston Methodist predominantly used extended criteria, orphan grafts for transplant recipients. Although most of the patients did well with these, one patient did experience early graft loss due to hepatic artery thrombosis, which was related to extensive arterial disease in the donor artery. Reproducible positive outcomes from multiple centers may set the groundwork for UNOS policies that will recognize iCCA as an indication for liver transplant and award MELD exception to these patients. Large-scale, prospective multicenter clinical trials are limited due to challenges with funding and donor organ availability. Adjuvant chemotherapy and local therapy may also be beneficial in long-term survival, especially in the absence of cirrhosis. A better understanding of tumor biology using next-generation sequencing technology may detect genetic abnormalities predicting biologically favorable disease, provide insight into the iCCA subgroups, and identify targeted therapeutic options.[38] Expression of programmed death ligand 1 and B7 homolog 1 has also been noted in iCCA, hence the question of the role of immunotherapy needs further exploration. The understanding of tumor biology provided by these will help direct LT in iCCA.[4,39]

CLINICS CARE POINTS

- Global incidence of intrahepatic CCA is on the increase.
- Most patients present at an advanced stage of the disease, which limits management options. Hence the disease has a very poor prognosis.
- Surgical resection is the current gold standard for iCCA management. However, contrary to prior findings, recent studies have shown liver transplant is potentially a viable treatment option in select patients.

DISCLOSURE

Dr Lunsford receives research funding from the NIH, United States NIDDK, United States K09DK118187, NIH NCI, United States R21CA267368, the New Jersey Health Foundation, United States (PC 106–21), and the American Society of Transplant Surgeons, United States. Other authors have no commercial or financial conflicts to disclose.

REFERENCES

1. Sapisochin G, Ivanics T, Heimbach J. Liver transplantation for intrahepatic cholangiocarcinoma: Ready for prime time? Hepatology 2022;75(2):455–72.
2. Saha SK, Zhu AX, Fuchs CS, et al. Forty-year trends in cholangiocarcinoma incidence in the U.S.: Intrahepatic disease on the rise. Oncol 2016;21(5):594–9.
3. Panayotova G, Guerra J, Guarrera JV, et al. The role of surgical resection and liver transplantation for the treatment of intrahepatic cholangiocarcinoma. J Clin Med 2021;10(11):2428.
4. McMillan RR, Saharia A, Abdelrahim M, et al. New breakthroughs for liver transplantation of cholangiocarcinoma. Current Transplantation Reports 2021; 8(1):21–7.
5. Panayotova GG, Paterno F, Guarrera JV, et al. Liver transplantation for cholangiocarcinoma: Insights into the prognosis and the evolving indications. Curr Oncol Rep 2020;22(5). https://doi.org/10.1007/s11912-020-00910-1.
6. Wu L, Tsilimigras DI, Paredes AZ, et al. Trends in the incidence, treatment and outcomes of patients with intrahepatic cholangiocarcinoma in the USA: Facility type is associated with margin status, use of lymphadenectomy and overall survival. World J Surg 2019;43(7):1777–87.
7. Altekruse SF, Petrick JL, Rolin AI, et al. Geographic variation of intrahepatic cholangiocarcinoma, extrahepatic cholangiocarcinoma, and hepatocellular carcinoma in

the United States. PLoS One 2015;10(4). https://doi.org/10.1371/journal.pone. 0120574.

8. Van Dyke AL, Shiels MS, Jones GS, et al. Biliary tract cancer incidence and trends in the United States by Demographic Group, 1999-2013. Cancer 2019; 125(9):1489–98.

9. Witjes CDM, Karim-Kos HE, Visser O, et al. Intrahepatic cholangiocarcinoma in a low endemic area: Rising incidence and improved survival. HPB 2012;14(11): 777–81.

10. von Hahn T, Ciesek S, Wegener G, et al. Epidemiological trends in incidence and mortality of hepatobiliary cancers in Germany. Scand J Gastroenterol 2011;46(9): 1092–8.

11. Khan SA, Emadossadaty S, Ladep NG, et al. Rising trends in Cholangiocarcinoma: Is the ICD classification system misleading us? J Hepatol 2012;56(4): 848–54.

12. Zamora-Valdes D, Heimbach JK. Liver transplant for Cholangiocarcinoma. Gastroenterol Clin N Am 2018;47(2):267–80.

13. Banales JM, Marin JJ, Lamarca A, et al. Cholangiocarcinoma 2020: The next horizon in mechanisms and management. Nat Rev Gastroenterol Hepatol 2020; 17(9):557–88.

14. Joo I, Lee JM, Yoon JH. Imaging diagnosis of intrahepatic and perihilar cholangiocarcinoma: Recent advances and challenges. Radiology 2018;288(1):7–13.

15. Rimola J, Forner A, Reig M, et al. Cholangiocarcinoma in cirrhosis: Absence of contrast washout in delayed phases by magnetic resonance imaging avoids misdiagnosis of hepatocellular carcinoma. Hepatology 2009;50(3):791–8.

16. Bridgewater J, Galle PR, Khan SA, et al. Guidelines for the diagnosis and management of intrahepatic cholangiocarcinoma. J Hepatol 2014;60(6):1268–89.

17. Lee AJ, Chun YS. Intrahepatic cholangiocarcinoma: The AJCC/UICC 8th edition updates. Chin Clin Oncol 2018;7(5):52.

18. Kendall T, Verheij J, Gaudio E, et al. Anatomical, histomorphological and molecular classification of Cholangiocarcinoma. Liver Int 2019;39(S1):7–18.

19. Aishima S, Oda Y. Pathogenesis and classification of intrahepatic cholangiocarcinoma: Different characters of perihilar large duct type versus peripheral small duct type. J Hepato-Biliary-Pancreatic Sci 2014;22(2):94–100.

20. Mazzaferro V, Gorgen A, Roayaie S, et al. Liver resection and transplantation for intrahepatic cholangiocarcinoma. J Hepatol 2020;72(2):364–77.

21. Paik KY, Jung JC, Heo JS, et al. What prognostic factors are important for resected intrahepatic cholangiocarcinoma? J Gastroenterol Hepatol 2008;23(5): 766–70.

22. Sotiropoulos GC, Bockhorn M, Sgourakis G, et al. R0 liver resections for primary malignant liver tumors in the noncirrhotic liver: A diagnosis-related analysis. Dig Dis Sci 2008;54(4):887–94.

23. de Jong MC, Nathan H, Sotiropoulos GC, et al. Intrahepatic Cholangiocarcinoma: An international multi-institutional analysis of prognostic factors and lymph node assessment. J Clin Oncol 2011;29(23):3140–5.

24. Si A, Li J, Yang Z, et al. Impact of anatomical versus non-anatomical liver resection on short- and long-term outcomes for patients with intrahepatic cholangiocarcinoma. Ann Surg Oncol 2019;26(6):1841–50.

25. Zhang X-F, Bagante F, Chakedis J, et al. Perioperative and long-term outcome for intrahepatic cholangiocarcinoma: Impact of major versus minor hepatectomy. J Gastrointest Surg 2017;21(11):1841–50.

26. Spolverato G, Kim Y, Alexandrescu S, et al. Is hepatic resection for large or multi-focal intrahepatic cholangiocarcinoma justified? results from a multi-institutional collaboration. Ann Surg Oncol 2014;22(7):2218–25.

27. Petrowsky H, Hong JC. Current surgical management of hilar and intrahepatic cholangiocarcinoma: the role of resec- tion and orthotopic liver transplantation. Transplant Proc 2009;41:4023–35.

28. Spolverato G, Vitale A, Cucchetti A, et al. Can hepatic resection provide a long-term cure for patients with intrahepatic cholangiocarcinoma? Cancer 2015; 121(22):3998–4006.

29. Becker NS, Rodriguez JA, Barshes NR, et al. Outcomes analysis for 280 patients with cholangiocarcinoma treated with liver transplantation over an 18-year period. J Gastrointest Surg 2007;12(1):117–22.

30. McMillan RR, Javle M, Kodali S, et al. Survival following liver transplantation for locally advanced, unresectable intrahepatic cholangiocarcinoma. Am J Trans-plant 2022;22(3):823–32.

31. Bowlus CL, Arrivé L, Bergquist A, et al. Aasld practice guidance on primary scle-rosing cholangitis and Cholangiocarcinoma. Hepatology 2022;77(2):659–702.

32. Panayotova G, Lunsford KE, Latt NL, et al. Expanding indications for liver trans-plantation in the era of liver transplant oncology. World J Gastrointest Surg 2021; 13(5):392–405.

33. Sapisochin G, de Lope CR, Gastaca M, et al. Intrahepatic cholangiocarcinoma or mixed hepatocellular-cholangiocarcinoma in patients undergoing liver transplan-tation. Ann Surg 2014;259(5):944–52.

34. Sapisochin G, Facciuto M, Rubbia-Brandt L, et al. Liver transplantation for "very early" intrahepatic cholangiocarcinoma: International Retrospective study sup-porting a prospective assessment. Hepatology 2016;64(4):1178–88.

35. Facciuto ME, Singh MK, Lubezky N, et al. Tumors with intrahepatic bile duct dif-ferentiation in cirrhosis. Transplantation 2015;99(1):151–7.

36. De Martin E, Rayar M, Golse N, et al. Analysis of liver resection versus liver trans-plantation on outcome of small intrahepatic cholangiocarcinoma and combined hepatocellular-cholangiocarcinoma in the setting of cirrhosis. Liver Transplant 2020;26(6):785–98.

37. Lunsford KE, Javle M, Heyne K, et al. Liver transplantation for locally advanced intrahepatic cholangiocarcinoma treated with neoadjuvant therapy: a prospective case-series [published correction appears in Lancet Gastroenterol Hepatol. 2018 Jun;3(6):e3]. Lancet Gastroenterol Hepatol 2018;3(5):337–48.

38. Moeini A, Sia D, Bardeesy N, et al. Molecular pathogenesis and targeted thera-pies for intrahepatic cholangiocarcinoma. Clin Cancer Res 2016;22(2):291–300.

39. Ye Y, Zhou L, Xie X, et al. Interaction of B7-H1 on intrahepatic cholangiocarci-noma cells with PD-1 on tumor-infiltrating T cells as a mechanism of immune evasion. J Surg Oncol 2009;100(6):500–4.

Liver Transplantation for Colorectal Liver Metastases

Emily J. Schepers, MD*, Stephen J. Hartman, MD,
Jenna N. Whitrock, MD, Ralph C. Quillin III, MD

KEYWORDS

- Colorectal metastases • Liver transplantation • Nonresectable metastases
- Colon cancer • Transplant oncology

KEY POINTS

- Liver transplantation improves overall survival for nonresectable colorectal liver metastases (CRLM) compared to chemotherapy.
- The main limitation to transplant for CRLM is organ availability.
- Ongoing efforts are evaluating optimal patient selection and perioperative management of unresectable CRLM.
- Transplant oncology is a modern field emerging as a promising alternative to palliative chemotherapy for unresectable metastatic disease.

INTRODUCTION
Incidence and Epidemiology

Colorectal cancer (CRC) is the third most common malignancy diagnosed among adults in the United States with more than 150,000 new cases diagnosed in 2022.[1,2] It affects nearly 1 million patients worldwide and is currently the second leading cause of cancer death.[3,4] Epidemiologic studies identified male sex and age as the most important non-modifiable risk factors for CRC; however, recent studies are showing rising incidence in patients less than 55 years of age.[5,6] At the time of diagnosis, approximately 20% of patients will have metastatic disease or synchronous metastases.[7,8] The most common sites for metastasis include the liver (colorectal liver metastases [CRLM]), accounting for approximately 80% of metastasis.[9,10] Overall, up to 50% of patients will develop liver metastases during their disease course. Survival for metastatic CRC (mCRC) is dismal without treatment, with a median survival of 6 to 12 months.[5] Liver resection of CRLM can achieve 5-year survival rates approaching 50%; however, relapse remains high, occurring in 75% of patients.[4,5,11]

Division of Transplantation, Department of Surgery, University of Cincinnati College of Medicine, 231 Albert Sabin Way, Cincinnati, OH 45267-0558, USA
* Corresponding author. University of Cincinnati, 231 Albert Sabin Way, Cincinnati, OH 45267-0558.
E-mail address: schepeey@ucmail.uc.edu

Surg Clin N Am 104 (2024) 227–242
https://doi.org/10.1016/j.suc.2023.08.003
0039-6109/24/© 2023 Elsevier Inc. All rights reserved.

Diagnosis and Staging

CRC classically presents in 3 ways: routine screening colonoscopy; symptoms and laboratory findings such as weight loss, fatigue, anemia, rectal bleeding, or altered bowel habits; or emergently with bowel perforation or obstruction.[12,13] Clinical symptoms are often based on the location of the primary tumor with right-sided tumors presenting with vague or generalized findings, such as fatigue and anemia.[5,14,15] In contrast, left-sided tumors often present with altered bowel habits such as constipation, narrow caliber stool, or rectal bleeding.[14] Meta-analyses of clinical trials for mCRC have shown that right-sided tumors are associated with significantly worse progression-free survival (PFS) and overall survival (OS).[16] For this reason, the primary tumor location has been included as a variable impacting survival in patients with mCRC.

Diagnosis and staging of CRC include pathologic confirmation of primary tumor and screening for metastatic disease, including contrast-enhanced computed tomography of the chest, abdomen, and pelvis. In addition, serum carcinoembryonic antigen (CEA) levels should be obtained as an important tool for surveillance after surgical resection.[12] The American Joint Committee on Cancer (AJCC) and the Union for International Cancer Control recommend the tumor, nodes, metastases staging system (**Table 1**). Risk of metastasis increases with stage: less than 10% stage I, 10% to 20% stage II; 25% to 50% stage III.[8,15,17] Due to the significant difference in OS in patients with stage IV disease, the AJCC seventh edition in 2010 changed stage IV disease to subcategories IVA (metastasis to one site) and IVB (metastasis to more than one site).[7] For further evaluation of the metastatic disease, additional imaging including PET/CT scan as well as MRI of the liver should be considered.

Molecular Subtypes of Colorectal Cancer

Management of metastatic CRC has evolved significantly in the past several years in part due to the development of targeted biological and immunotherapy agents.[16] Current recommendations for diagnosis of CRC include molecular analysis of the primary tumor to evaluate tumor gene status for *RAS* and *BRAF* mutations, HER2 amplifications, and determination of tumor deficiency of mismatch repair or presence of microsatellite instability (MSI).[18,19] CRC is one of the first solid tumors to be molecularly characterized.[18] Based on transcriptomic analysis, the consensus molecular subtypes (CMS) were identified with 4 different classifications including CMS1 (MSI immune), CMS2 (canonical), CMS3 (metabolic), and CMS4 (mesenchymal).[18,20] These classifications have been found to correlate with clinical outcomes; in addition, these will guide treatment strategies. For instance, CMS4 mesenchymal tumors have an increased incidence of relapse, and CMS1 MSI immune tumors have poor prognosis in the metastatic setting.[20]

Furthermore, there are several genetic mutations that have been established as prognostic biomarkers and are being used as therapeutic targets with immunotherapy.[21] For instance, the use of epidermal growth factor receptor (EGFR) inhibitors, such as cetuximab or panitumumab, for management of *RAS* and *BRAF* wildtype mCRC.[22] *RAS* mutations are found in more than 50% of tumors.[18] Although seen in a smaller proportion of cases (up to 8%), *BRAF* mutations are associated with poorer prognosis. Similarly, *HER2* overexpression is associated with resistance to EGFR monoclonal antibodies in the refractory setting, but also a positive predictive marker for response to HER2-targeted agents in mCRC. There are numerous ongoing phase II/III trials utilizing targeted agents against these biomarkers with the intention to improve survival in mCRC. As we understand more about tumor biology, we will improve our patient selection as well as improve systemic treatment options to improve OS.

Table 1
Tumor, node, metastasis staging of colorectal cancer

Primary Tumor Staging

T0	No evidence of primary tumor
Tis	Carcinoma in situ
T1	Tumor invades submucosa
T2	Tumor invades the muscularis propria
T3	Tumor invades through muscularis propria into the pericolonic tissue
T4a	Tumor penetrates to the surface of the visceral peritoneum (serosa)
T4b	Tumor invades and/or is adherent to the other organs or structures

Regional lymph node staging

N0	No regional lymph node metastases
N1a	Metastasis in 1 regional lymph node
N1b	Metastasis in 2–3 regional lymph nodes
N1c	Tumor deposits in subserosa, mesentery, or nonperitonealized pericolic or perirectal tissues without regional nodal metastases
N2a	Metastases in 4–6 regional lymph nodes
N2b	Metastases in 7 or more regional lymph nodes

Distant metastases staging

M0	No distant metastases
M1a	Metastasis confined to 1 organ or site
M1b	Metastasis in more than 1 organ/site or the peritoneum

Stage	T	N	M
0	Tis	N0	M0
I	T1-2	N0	M0
IIA	T3	N0	M0
IIB	T4a	N0	M0
IIC	T4b	N0	M0
IIIA	T1-2	N1-N1c	M0
	T1	N2a	M0
IIIB	T3-4a	N1-N1c	M0
	T2-3	N2a	M0
	T1-2	N2b	M0
IIIC	T4a	N2a	M0
	T3-4a	N2b	M0
	T4b	N1-2	M0
IVA	Any T	Any N	M1a
IVB	Any T	Any N	M1b

Abbreviations: M, distant metastases staging; N, regional lymph node staging; T, primary tumor staging.

Adapted from Amin MB, Edge S, Greene F, Byrd DR, Brookland RK, Washington MK, Gershenwald JE, Compton CC, Hess KR, et al. (Eds.). AJCC Cancer Staging Manual (8th edition). Springer International Publishing: American Joint Commission on Cancer; 2017.

Synchronous Verses Metachronous Colorectal Cancer Liver Metastases

Synchronous colorectal metastases are distant metastases present at time of diagnosis, although some variability in the definition exists.[23,24] As expected, synchronous CRLM have worse prognosis, with reduced OS compared to metachronous

CRLM.[23,25] In a cohort study of 26,813 patients, they found the incidence of metachronous liver metastases decreased from 1976 to 2018. In contrast, the incidence of synchronous metastases has remained stable since 2000.[24] Survival of patients with synchronous liver metastases at 1, 3, and 5 years was 41.8%, 13.1%, and 6.2%, respectively, compared to survival of patients with metachronous liver metastases at 1, 3, and 5 years of 49.9%, 22.3%, and 13.2%. There are 3 key approaches to the management of synchronous CRLM: staged resection with the primary-first approach, the liver-first approach, and simultaneous resection of the primary and the liver disease.[23,26] In general, there appear to be better outcomes for simultaneous resection; however, the difference in patient populations limits the ability for an unbiased comparison. Currently, the practice is center-specific and patient-specific with further study needed to delineate selection criteria.

CURRENT GUIDELINES FOR MANAGEMENT OF METASTATIC COLORECTAL CANCER

Surgery is the cornerstone of curative-intent treatment regardless of staging with increasing number of available therapies aimed at long-term disease control and possible cure for mCRC.[5] Hepatic resection of isolated liver metastases is shown to have survival advantages over complete resection of liver metastases resulting in 10-year and 20-year survival rates of 23% and 18%, respectively.[27] Unfortunately, recurrence rates remain high in the remnant liver, which has prompted ongoing studies comparing perioperative and adjuvant treatment strategies to improve outcomes in these patients.[28]

Hepatectomy

Indications for curative-intent treatment of CRLM have expanded in recent years with approximately 25% of patients eligible for resection.[29] The definition of operable metastases has changed over time. Fong and colleagues established a clinical risk score to estimate recurrence based on clinical features of the metastatic disease and improve patient selection for invasive surgical procedures in the late 1990s.[27] These included 5 features: nodal status of the primary, disease-free interval from diagnosis of the primary tumor to liver metastases less than 12 months, number of tumors greater than 1, preoperative CEA level greater than 200 ng/ml, and size of the largest tumor greater than 5 cm (**Table 2**). The current approach to liver resection focuses on the technical ability to achieve an R0 resection with sufficient future liver remnant (FLR).[11,29] FLR is an estimate of the remaining liver volume after resection with established criteria for acceptable FLR based on patient's current hepatic function.[30]

Systemic Chemotherapy

Adjuvant chemotherapy is routinely given for advanced CRC to improve disease-free survival (DFS) and OS.[31] There are numerous studies evaluating systemic

Table 2	
Clinical risk scores for tumor recurrence after liver resection and transplantation	
Fong Clinical Risk Scores (Resection)	**Oslo Score (Transplant)**
Node-positive primary	Size >5.5 cm
Disease-free < 12 mo	Disease-free < 2 y
>1 tumor	No disease progression
Size > 5 cm	
Carcinoembryonic antigen > 200 ng/mL	

chemotherapy for advanced CRC, beyond the scope of this review; however, the overarching goals are either to improve DFS/OS in patients with resectable mCRC or attempt to downstage unresectable disease. For initially resectable mCRC, phase III trials have failed to show a statistically significant survival benefit comparing combined chemotherapy and surgery versus surgery-alone. Additionally, the approach to systemic chemotherapy, either given perioperatively or in the adjuvant setting, remains controversial. Portier and colleagues conducted a phase III randomized control trial (RCT) comparing combination surgery with adjuvant fluorouracil to surgery-alone, they found improved outcomes with chemotherapy; however, these results were not statistically significant.[4,32,33] EORTC (European Organisation for Research and Treatment of Cancer) 40983 was an RCT comparing perioperative chemotherapy with FOLFOX (leucovorin, fluorouracil , and oxaliplatin) to surgery-alone.[4] FOLFOX, a combination chemotherapy regimen including leucovorin, fluorouracil, and oxaliplatin, had previously shown survival benefit in patients with CRLM.[34] There was no statistically significant difference in OS; however, there was a modest improvement in PFS at 3 years, 35.1% versus 28.1% (hazard ratio 0.79 [0.62–1.02]; $P = .058$). These trials demonstrate patients able to tolerate both chemotherapy and surgery have a survival benefit, with a major limitation being lack of statistical significance due to underpowering of the studies. Current National Comprehensive Cancer Network guidelines recommend neoadjuvant FOLFOX in oxaliplatin-naïve patients with resectable CRLM.[16] Further research is needed to evaluate the benefits of perioperative verses adjuvant chemotherapy as well as optimal treatment regimen.

The management of borderline resectable disease has also advanced with multidisciplinary approach and increasing alternative treatment options. Currently there are 2 basic approaches, including downstaging disease or expansion of the FLR. Both options will allow for surgical resection. OLIVIA is a clinical trial that randomized initially unresectable CRLM to FOLFOX verses FOLFOX plus irinotecan (FOLFOXIRI) and bevacizumab. The results demonstrated a higher rate of R0 resection and PFS in the FOLFOXIRI cohort.[35] Another challenge in resection for CRLM is an insufficient size of predicted FLR after resection. There are several strategies utilized to increase the FLR including 2-stage hepatectomy with either portal vein embolization (PVE) or portal vein ligation (PVL).[11] An alternative strategy is the procedure known as associating liver partition and portal ligation for staged hepatectomy or ALPPS.[36] This strategy achieves rapid growth of the FLR compared to PVE or PVL, but the utility of this procedure remains controversial due to increase perioperative complications.

ALTERNATIVE TREATMENT APPROACHES

In addition to surgery and systemic therapies for management of mCRC, local ablative techniques can serve as adjunct treatments for CRLM.[37] Radiofrequency ablation is still the preferred local ablative therapy for the liver; for larger lesions and those close to vascular structures, microwave ablation or stereotactic radiotherapy are alternative options.

LIVER TRANSPLANTATION

Despite efforts to increase the number of resectable cases of CRLM, approximately 75% of CRLM remain unresectable and therefore are offered chemotherapy and palliative care with a dismal prognosis.[11] For unresectable CRLM, the OS has doubled from 12 to 24 months with the start of first-line chemotherapy in the last decade; however, oncological treatment alone is not curative and 5-year survival remains around 10%.[11]

The first attempts at treating CRLM with liver transplantation (LT) began in the 1980s.[10] The largest single-center experience with LT was at the Medical University of Vienna which transplanted 25 patients between 1982 and 1994.[38] They had a 30-day mortality rate of ~30%; with 1-year, 3-year, and 5-year OS of 76%, 32%, and 12%, respectively. There were an additional 58 cases of LT for CRLM in the European Liver Transplant Registry performed between 1977 and 1995.[39] They had similar survival rates with 1-year, 3-year, and 5-year survival of 73%, 36%, and 18%, respectively. Notably, this cohort also experienced a 44% graft loss in the absence of tumor recurrence. Initial attempts to utilize LT for CRLM were unsuccessful due to cancer-specific reasons, including poor patient selection resulting in poor OS and high rates of relapse, as well as inexperience with LT resulting in the high perioperative mortality and graft loss.[6] In addition, there were no standardized immunosuppression protocols with limited options available at that point in time.

As perioperative transplant survival and technique has improved, LT has emerged as a standard treatment approach for both primary and metastatic unresectable malignancies in the liver.[40–42] Similar to LT for CRLM, initial utilization of LT for hepatocellular carcinoma (HCC) was slow due to poor outcomes; however, after the Milan criteria were developed and brought into practice in the 1990s, HCC has become one of the major indications for LT.[11] Cholangiocarcinoma, another primary liver malignancy derived from the biliary system, and metastatic neuroendocrine tumors are also using LT in select cases.[43,44] The success of these experiences has advanced the field of transplant oncology and led to the resurgence of LT as a potential curative treatment strategy for unresectable liver malignancies. Patient selection, a cornerstone of any cancer treatment, remains the most important factor in improving survival after LT as established by the Milan criteria for HCC.

Clinical Trials of Liver Transplantation for Colorectal Liver Metastases

Due to the improving outcomes after LT for other cancers, renewed interest for LT of unresectable CRLM resurged in 2006.[10] The University of Oslo performed a pilot study that demonstrated a survival benefit for patients who underwent LT compared with chemotherapy alone for unresectable CRLM.[45] The Secondary Cancer I (SECA-I) study enrolled 21 patients who underwent deceased donor LT.[46] The study included patients who had undergone an R0 resection of their primary disease, received 6 weeks of chemotherapy, and did not have evidence of extrahepatic disease. There were no standardized preoperative or adjuvant chemotherapy protocols and every patient received sirolimus for immunosuppression. They reported DFS (1-year 35%; 3-year 0%; 5-year NA) and OS (1-year 95%; 3-year 68%; 5-year 60%). The median time to recurrence was 6 months (range 2–24 months). Notably, the 12 patients with relapsed disease that did not include the liver were alive at the end of the study period.

Despite the high recurrence rates, this ground-breaking study demonstrated LT for CRLM was associated with nearly 30% improvement in survival compared to the standard of care. Four factors were independently associated with survival and risk of recurrence after LT, which were referred to as the "Oslo criteria": (1) maximal hepatic tumor diameter greater than 5.5 cm, (2) time from primary cancer surgery less than 2 years, (3) CEA greater than 80ug/L, and (4) progressive disease at time of LT (see **Table 2**). This study established several important factors: first that OS was improved with LT compared to palliative care with chemotherapy, and unresectable CRLM had the potential for curative-intent treatment.

Coinciding with this first prospective trial, 2 retrospective studies were published that demonstrated a survival benefit after LT for CRLM. Toso and colleagues reviewed the outcomes of 12 patients who underwent LT for CRLM between 1995 and 2015 and found 5-year OS of 50%.[47] Dueland and colleagues performed a retrospective study comparing DFS and OS from patients in SECA study to PFS and OS in a similar cohort of liver-only mCRC from the NORDIC-VII trial.[48] The NORDIC-VII study was a multi-center, phase III trial with 3 arms designed to evaluate the OS in patients treated with either cetuximab plus continuous or intermittent fluorouracil, folinic acid, and oxaliplatin (Nordic FLOX) versus FLOX alone in the first-line treatment of mCRC.[49,50] The DFS/PFS were similar between the 2 cohorts; however, the OS was significantly improved in the patients managed with LT for CRLM.

Following SECA-I, a phase II prospective trial was developed with stricter inclusion criteria to determine if there was a survival benefit and difference in the quality of life (QoL) for LT compared to chemotherapy for unresectable CRLM in 2012.[51] The SECA-II study (NCT01479608) enrolled 25 participants with Oslo scores ranging from 0 to 2, which correlated with low-risk disease and at least 10% response to chemotherapy. The DFS was 53% and 35% at 1 and 3 years, respectively, with OS of 100%, 73%, and 73% at 1, 2, and 4 years. Relapse affecting only the lungs occurred in 40% of cases, with liver relapse occurring in 6.6% of cases.

An additional arm of the SECA-II study, arm D, was established to extend inclusion criteria for both recipient and donors. They enrolled 10 participants who had worse tumor biology, measured by the Oslo Score and the Fong Clinical Risk Score (FCRS), and included patients with resectable pulmonary metastases. The participants had a shorter median time from primary surgery to relapse, 16.5 months, increased number of metastases (median number of 20, range 1–45), and size of metastases (median 5.9 cm, range 1.5–9.4 cm). As expected, the outcomes were poorer with median DFS of 4 months and OS of 18 months.

Predicting post-transplant survival and recurrence in patients with mCRC is still uncertain. The clinical risk scores, including the FCRS and the Oslo Score, and PET metabolic tumor volume (MTV) liver uptake values utilized in the trials were not consistent with outcomes observed in SECA-I and II. PET MTV is a volumetric measure estimating the total tumor burden as an imaging-based tool to predict clinical outcomes.[52] For instance, FCRSs in arm D of SECA-II were similar to SECA-I; however, patients with Oslo scores of 1 to 2 had significantly shorter OS than patients with similar Oslo scores in SECA-I, suggesting additional determining factors. Additional selection criteria need to be taken into account including tumor location, histologic differentiation, and lymph node status of the primary tumor to optimize the outcomes.[53] At the conclusion of these studies, LT for CRLM demonstrated significant improvement in OS compared to palliative chemotherapy; however, these were both nonrandomized, low accrual studies. This has led to the modern era of LT for unresectable CRLM.

MODERN ERA OF LIVER TRANSPLANTATION FOR COLORECTAL LIVER METASTASES

There are now several multicenter RCTs worldwide evaluating the survival benefit of LT over standard of care (**Table 3**). In 2016, SECA III (NCT03494946) and TRANSMET (Liver Transplantation in Patients with Unresectable Colorectal Liver Metastases Treated by Chemotherapy) (NCT0259748) began enrolling into phase III RCTs. TRANSMET was the first clinical trial outside of Norway. Three additional trials have opened, SOULMATE (The Swedish Study of Liver Transplantation for Non-resectable Colorectal Cancer Metastases) (NCT04161092) in Sweden, COLT (Improving Outcome of Selected Patients with Non-resectable Hepatic Metastases from Colo-rectal Cancer With Liver Transplantation) (NCT03803436) in Italy, and TRASMETIR (Liver Transplantation in Patients With Unresectable Colorectal Liver Metastases) (NCT04616495) in Spain. All except for COLT, are phase III RCT with

Table 3
Active clinical trials comparing outcomes for liver transplantation for colorectal liver metastases

Study	Location	Study Start Date	Study Type	Inclusion Criteria	Exclusion Criteria	Target Accrual	Study Interventions	Primary Outcomes	Secondary Outcomes
SECA III (NCT03494946)	Norway	December 2016	Phase III RCT	No extrahepatic metastases or local relapse except resectable lung lesion (<15 mm); disease progression on first-line chemotherapy	Prior resection of local relapse or extrahepatic metastasis within 2 y; presence of CNS or bone disease; extrahepatic extension involving diaphragm; size >10 cm; 3 negative prognostic factors (CEA>80, <2 y from diagnosis, diameter of largest lesion >5.5 cm)	30	(A) Liver transplant or (B) Chemotherapy with other treatment options including TACE and SIRT	2-y OS	
TRANSMET (NCT02597348)	France/ Belgium	February 2016	Phase III RCT	DFS >1 y; ≧3 mo chemotherapy; <2 lines of chemotherapy for metastatic disease; CEA <80ug/L or decrease >50% of highest CEA; no extrahepatic disease	Non-standard of care for primary disease; prior extrahepatic disease or local relapse	95	(A) Liver transplantation with ECD or (B) standard of care	5-y OS	3-y OS; DFS; recurrence rates at 3-y and 5-y; QoL questionnaires

Trial	Country	Date	Study type	Inclusion criteria	Exclusion criteria	n	Intervention	Primary endpoint	Secondary endpoints
SOULMATE (NCT04161092)	Sweden	December 2020	Phase III RCT	DFS >1 y; no extrahepatic disease; >2 y DFS from prior local or extrahepatic relapse; nonPD with >2 mo chemotherapy	BRAF mutation; MSI-high; size >10 cm, PD	45	(A) Liver transplantation with ECD or (B) Standard of care	5-y OS	2-y OS; median OS; 5-y PFS; hepatic PFS; extrahepatic recurrence-free survival; QoL questionnaires; Health economic evaluation (Estimation of quality adjusted life year)
COLT (NCT03803436)	Italy	January 2019	Phase II, prospective, non-randomized	Metachronous disease; >4 mo without disease progression on first-line chemotherapy with ≦ 2 lines chemotherapy	RAS or BRAF mutations; hereditary CRC syndromes including FAP and Lynch syndrome; prior extrahepatic metastatic disease or local relapse; extra-peritoneal cancers (rectum)	22	Liver transplant: compared OS to matched COLT-eligible population in a phase III RCT on triple chemotherapy	5-y OS	5-y PFS; Complication rate
TRASMETIR (NCT04616495)	Spain	September 2021	Phase III RCT	No extrahepatic disease; disease response to ≦ 2 lines chemotherapy; ≧ 1 y from diagnosis to listing	BRAF mutation; size >5 cm; CEA >80 ng/mL (at time of enrollment on waitlist); no neoadjuvant chemotherapy	30	(A) Liver transplantation with ECD or (B) Standard of care	5-y OS	1-y, 3-y, and 5-y DFS and QoL

Abbreviations: CEA, carcinoembryonic antigen; CNS, central nervous system; CRC, colorectal cancer; DFS, disease-free survival; ECD, extended criteria donor; FAP, familial adenomatous polyposis; MSI, microsatellite instability; OS, overall survival; PD, progress disease; PFS, progression-free survival; QoL, quality of life; RCT, randomized control trial; SIRT, selective internal radiation therapy; TACE, trans-arterial chemoembolization.

participants randomized to LT or standard of care. The COLT trial is a phase II study comparing outcomes of LT to a COLT-eligible matched cohort in another open phase III trial for chemotherapy with anti-EGFR. Inclusion criteria include standard of care treatment and R0 resection of primary disease, no evidence of extrahepatic disease, and require non-progressive disease on several months of first-line or second-line chemotherapy. Exclusion criteria changed between the initial trials and the more recent studies. Current studies exclude patients with RAS and BRAF mutations in primary tumors. In addition, another aim of the SOULMATE trial is to evaluate the use of extended criteria donors (ECDs).[54] Unlike Norway, most of the world has an already limited donor pool with high waitlist mortality. Outcomes for ECDs are not well established, and demonstrating a lack of inferiority could mitigate the burden of an additional indication for LT.

Outside of clinical trials, there are an increasing number of individual institutions using LT for CRLM. Selection criteria are variable and institution-specific. For this reason, the International Hepato-Pancreato-Biliary Association published consensus guidelines in 2021 for LT of unresectable CRLM.[55] The current guidelines include (1) no evidence of extrahepatic disease, (2) primary tumor meets established molecular criteria, including BRAF wildtype, and (3) a trial of chemotherapy with appropriate response to first-line or second-line treatment. At any time point, if progressive disease excludes its eligibility for LT, they transition to palliative therapy.

In the United States, LT for unresectable CRLM is limited to a few high-performance centers with a non-standardized, institution-specific treatment algorithm for patient selection and management of unresectable CRLM. Despite the lack of consensus, there has been a tenfold increase in the number of LT for unresectable CRLM between 2017 and 2022.[56–58] A retrospective study published in early 2023 reported the outcomes for individuals listed for transplant on the UNOS (United Network for Organ Sharing) database during the study period.[57] There were a total of 64 patients listed; 46 received a transplant, 10 remained on the list at the end of the study, and 8 had been removed for unknown reasons. The cumulative DFS and OS at 1 and 3 years were 75.1% and 53.7%, and 89% and 60.4%, respectively. Compared to other trials, donor characteristics were significantly different in the United States with a larger number of patients undergoing living donor liver transplant (LDLT), with living donor recipients having lower Model for End-Stage Liver Disease (MELD) scores, shorter waitlist time, and improved OS compared to deceased-donor transplants. An important takeaway from this study is the need for established standardized practice among centers and development of a national registry to better understand the outcomes for LT of CRLM.

LIMITATIONS TO LIVER TRANSPLANTATION FOR COLORECTAL LIVER METASTASES

An important consideration as the indications for LT continue to expand is the limited availability of grafts. In the United States, 1 in 6 patients listed will die prior to transplant, and the current allocation system shifts available grafts to higher MELD scores, with no exception points for CRLM.[59] Strategies to overcome this include optimizing graft survival, expanding the donor pool, and utilizing LDLTs. Current studies described earlier demonstrate similar graft survival between LT for CRLM compared to other indications. LDLT and ECDs are being evaluated to expand access to grafts for LT for CRLM. In the SECA-II study, there were 10 grafts that met the ECD criteria, median survival was 16 months, and only 1 patient with greater than 80% steatosis required re-transplantation after 43 days. The SOULMATE trial will provide further information on the impact of these grafts on patient outcomes. In addition, novel perfusion strategies such as hypothermic oxygenated machine perfusion are miti-gating the risk of biliary complications, a major limitation of donation after circulatory death, with long-term potential to extend the restrictive time criteria for these do-nors.[60] In addition to expanding the deceased donors, LDLT is an option for patients who fit the criteria and have donors available. A prospective trial performed at 3 US transplant centers, evaluated the outcomes of patients undergoing LDLT for unresect-able CRLM.[61] Ten out of the 12 patients that met the criteria for LT for unresectable CRLM underwent LDLT. The cohort of patients was extensively pre-treated, including a combination of prolonged intensive chemotherapy, liver resection, hepatic artery infusion chemotherapy, and tumor ablation. The median follow-up was 1.5 years, with disease and OS similar to the Norwegian studies. This study provides initial evi-dence supporting LDLT for unresectable CRLM in highly selective patients with favor-able tumor biology, low MELD, and high-performance status.

Finally, there are several non-traditional transplant strategies in the early clinical tri-als. RAPID (Resection and Partial Liver Segment 2/3 Transplantation with Delayed To-tal Hepatectomy) (NCT02215889) is an ongoing phase I/II trial with a two-stage approach to transplant and resection, similar in concept to the ALPPS procedure. First described by Line and colleagues in 2015, this procedure involves the surgical resec-tion of the left lateral segment with orthotopic transplant of small partial grafts.[62,63] Completion hepatectomy of the native liver is performed after sufficient growth of the donor segments. The LIVER-T(W)O-HEAL (Living Donor Liver Transplantation with Two-Stage Hepatectomy for Patients with Isolated, Irresectable Colorectal Liver Metastases) (NCT03488953) trial is currently enrolling participants to evaluate the out-comes using living-donor grafts for the RAPID procedure. In addition to 3-year PFS/OS, these studies are evaluating the time from LT to completion hepatectomy and the percentage of patients that undergo both procedures. Donor availability is critical and appropriate ethical consideration is essential as the field evolves and LT becomes routine in the treatment of unresectable CRLM.

RECURRENCE AFTER LIVER RESECTION VERSUS TRANSPLANTATION

Recurrence after curative-intent surgery and chemotherapy occurs in 26.6% of all stages of CRC.[64] After surgery for CRLM, the overall recurrence rates are 50% to 70%.[65] Approximately half of the relapse occurs within the remnant liver. Re-resection, or curative-intent treatment results in 5-year survival of 50%. Trends and patterns of recurrence after LT are continuing to evolve; however, prospective trials have demonstrated a shift in the pattern of recurrence. In SECA II, median time to recurrence was 6 months. Lung-only relapse occurred in 40% of cases, with liver relapse occurring in 6.6% of cases. The 5-year survival with lung-only relapse was 72% with either surgical resection or chemotherapy.[66]

The observed high rates of recurrence after hepatectomy raise the concern for the presence of occult disease in the liver remnant despite extensive pretreatment and absence of radiographic evidence of the disease.[67] Our ability to detect residual dis-ease is restricted to preoperative multimodal imaging and use of intraoperative ultra-sound. In a recent study, Chavez-Villa and colleagues evaluated 14 total hepatectomy specimens for occult disease.[67] There were several key findings in their study, including the presence of viable tumor despite aggressive pretreatment and "com-plete response" on multimodal imaging. Additional studies are needed; however, these findings raise important questions about the sensitivity of our current imaging guidelines to characterize active disease in heavily pretreated patients and the true ability to downstage disease for anatomic resection. As LT for CRLM becomes more routine in practice, there will likely be a time when the therapeutic benefit of aggressive chemotherapy and surgery versus LT will have to be addressed. Despite significant improvements in OS, metastatic cancer is rarely cured; instead, the paradigm is shifting to the management of a chronic disease, which includes minimizing toxicity and focusing on overall QoL for patients.

SUMMARY

Transplant oncology is an emerging field that will continue to expand our utilization of LT for primary and secondary liver malignancies. Though limited in patient size, recent data has demonstrated that there is a dramatic survival benefit with LT for CRLM; however, standardized guidelines and recommendations are urgently needed. As we extend the definition of resectable disease surgically, we will need to define appropriate criteria for establishing survival benefits for both liver resection and transplant. In addition, a multidisciplinary approach will be essential for the management of LT for CRLM.

CLINICS CARE POINTS

- Liver resection of CRLM have 50% 5-year OS, unresectable disease has 10% 5-year OS, trials have demostrated up to 60% 5-year OS after liver transplant in appropriately selected patients.
- Recurrence after curative-intent surgery is 26.6% of all stages of CRC, with high rates of liver recurrence after resection, another benefit of LT was the observed decreased in liver recurrence after transplant.

DISCLOSURE

The authors have nothing to disclose.

REFERENCES

1. Cancer Stat Facts: Colorectal Cancer: National Cancer Institute Surveillance, Epidemiology, and End Results Program; (updated 2022. Available at: https://seer.cancer.gov/statfacts/html/colorect.html. Accessed April 12, 2023.
2. Patrlj L, Tuorto S, Fong Y. Combined blunt-clamp dissection and LigaSure ligation for hepatic parenchyma dissection: postcoagulation technique. J Am Coll Surg 2010;210(1):39–44.
3. Wolf AM, Fontham ET, Church TR, et al. Colorectal cancer screening for average-risk adults: 2018 guideline update from the American Cancer Society. CA: a cancer journal for clinicians 2018;68(4):250–81.
4. Nordlinger B, Sorbye H, Glimelius B, et al. Perioperative chemotherapy with FOLFOX4 and surgery versus surgery alone for resectable liver metastases from colorectal cancer (EORTC Intergroup trial 40983): a randomised controlled trial. Lancet 2008;371(9617):1007–16.
5. Dekker E, Tanis P, Vleugels J, et al. Colorectal cancer. Lancet [Internet] 2019; 394(10207):1467–80.
6. Gorgen A, Muaddi H, Zhang W, et al. The new era of transplant oncology: liver transplantation for nonresectable colorectal cancer liver metastases. Canadian Journal of Gastroenterology and Hepatology 2018;2018.

7. Chakedis J, Schmidt CR. Surgical treatment of metastatic colorectal cancer. Surgical Oncology Clinics 2018;27(2):377–99.
8. Biller LH, Schrag D. Diagnosis and Treatment of Metastatic Colorectal Cancer. JAMA 2021;325(7).
9. Riihimäki M, Hemminki A, Sundquist J, et al. Patterns of metastasis in colon and rectal cancer. Sci Rep 2016;6(1):1–9.
10. Ros J, Salva F, Dopazo C, et al. Liver transplantation in metastatic colorectal cancer: are we ready for it? Br J Cancer 2023;1–10.
11. Hagness M. Liver transplantation in treatment of colorectal liver metastases. Hepatic oncology 2015;2(2):181–90.
12. Mahmoud NN. Colorectal cancer: preoperative evaluation and staging. Surgical Oncology Clinics 2022;31(2):127–41.
13. National Cancer Institute Surveillance, Epidemiology, and End Results Program. 2021 Available at: https://seer.cancer.gov/statfacts/html/colorect.html. Accessed April 27, 2023.
14. Moreno CC, Mittal PK, Sullivan PS, et al. Colorectal cancer initial diagnosis: screening colonoscopy, diagnostic colonoscopy, or emergent surgery, and tumor stage and size at initial presentation. Clin Colorectal Cancer 2016;15(1):67–73.
15. Ulanja MB, Rishi M, Beutler BD, et al. Colon cancer sidedness, presentation, and survival at different stages. Journal of oncology 2019;2019.
16. Sandhu J, Lavingia V, Fakih M. Systemic treatment for metastatic colorectal cancer in the era of precision medicine. J Surg Oncol 2019;119(5):564–82.
17. National Cancer Institute website. Available at: https://seer.cancer.gov/archive/csr/1975_2016/. Accessed April 12, 2023.
18. Dienstmann R, Salazar R, Tabernero J. Molecular subtypes and the evolution of treatment decisions in metastatic colorectal cancer. American Society of Clinical Oncology Educational Book 2018;38:231–8.
19. Messersmith WA. NCCN guidelines updates: management of metastatic colorectal cancer. J Natl Compr Cancer Netw 2019;17(55):599–601.
20. Guinney J, Dienstmann R, Wang X, et al. The consensus molecular subtypes of colorectal cancer. Nature medicine 2015;21(11):1350–6.
21. Dariya B, Aliya S, Merchant N, et al. Colorectal cancer biology, diagnosis, and therapeutic approaches. Critical Reviews™ in Oncogenesis 2020;25(2).
22. Martinelli E, Ciardiello D, Martini G, et al. Implementing anti-epidermal growth factor receptor (EGFR) therapy in metastatic colorectal cancer: challenges and future perspectives. Ann Oncol 2020;31(1):30–40.
23. Adam R, de Gramont A, Figueras J, et al. Managing synchronous liver metastases from colorectal cancer: a multidisciplinary international consensus. Cancer Treat Rev 2015;41(9):729–41.
24. Reboux N, Jooste V, Goungounga J, et al. Incidence and Survival in Synchronous and Metachronous Liver Metastases From Colorectal Cancer. JAMA Netw Open 2022;5(10):e2236666–.
25. Miller G, Biernacki P, Kemeny NE, et al. Outcomes after resection of synchronous or metachronous hepatic and pulmonary colorectal metastases. J Am Coll Surg 2007;205(2):231–8.
26. Kasai S, Ashida R, Sugiura T, et al. Long-term outcomes of staged liver resection for synchronous liver metastases from colorectal cancer and the clinical impact of early recurrence: A single-center retrospective cohort study. Ann Gastroenterol Surg 2022;7(2):318–25.

27. Fong Y, Fortner J, Sun RL, et al. Clinical score for predicting recurrence after hepatic resection for metastatic colorectal cancer: analysis of 1001 consecutive cases. Ann Surg 1999;230(3):309–18 [discussion: 18-21].

28. Riesco-Martinez MC, Modrego A, Espinosa-Olarte P, et al. Perioperative Chemotherapy for Liver Metastasis of Colorectal Cancer: Lessons Learned and Future Perspectives. Curr Treat Options Oncol 2022;23(9):1320–37.

29. Engstrand J, Nilsson H, Strömberg C, et al. Colorectal cancer liver metastases - a population-based study on incidence, management and survival. BMC Cancer 2018;18(1):78.

30. Pawlik TM, Scoggins CR, Zorzi D, et al. Effect of surgical margin status on survival and site of recurrence after hepatic resection for colorectal metastases. Annals of surgery 2005;241(5):715.

31. Hari DM, Leung AM, Lee J-H, et al. AJCC Cancer Staging Manual 7th edition criteria for colon cancer: do the complex modifications improve prognostic assessment? J Am Coll Surg 2013;217(2):181–90.

32. Khoo E, O'Neill S, Brown E, et al. Systematic review of systemic adjuvant, neoadjuvant and perioperative chemotherapy for resectable colorectal-liver metastases. Hpb 2016;18(6):485–93.

33. Portier G, Elias D, Bouche O, et al. Multicenter randomized trial of adjuvant fluorouracil and folinic acid compared with surgery alone after resection of colorectal liver metastases: FFCD ACHBTH AURC 9002 trial. J Clin Oncol 2006;24(31): 4976–82.

34. de Gramont Ad, Figer A, Seymour M, et al. Leucovorin and fluorouracil with or without oxaliplatin as first-line treatment in advanced colorectal cancer. J Clin Oncol 2000;18(16):2938–47.

35. Gruenberger T, Bridgewater J, Chau I, et al. Bevacizumab plus mFOLFOX-6 or FOLFOXIRI in patients with initially unresectable liver metastases from colorectal cancer: the OLIVIA multinational randomised phase II trial. Ann Oncol 2015; 26(4):702–8.

36. Schadde E, Ardiles V, Slankamenac K, et al. ALPPS offers a better chance of complete resection in patients with primarily unresectable liver tumors compared with conventional-staged hepatectomies: results of a multicenter analysis. World J Surg 2014;38:1510–9.

37. Abdel-Rahman O, Cheung WY. Integrating systemic therapies into the multimodality treatment of resectable colorectal liver metastases. Gastroenterology Research and Practice 2018;2018.

38. Muhlbacher F. Is orthotopic liver transplantation a feasible treatment for secondary cancer of the liver? Transpl Proc 1991;23:1567–8.

39. Foss A, Adam R, Dueland S. Liver transplantation for colorectal liver metastases: revisiting the concept. Transpl Int 2010;23(7):679–85.

40. Le Treut YP, Grégoire E, Klempnauer J, et al. Liver transplantation for neuroendocrine tumors in Europe—results and trends in patient selection: a 213-case European liver transplant registry study. Annals of surgery 2013;257(5): 807–15.

41. Murad SD, Kim WR, Harnois DM, et al. Efficacy of neoadjuvant chemoradiation, followed by liver transplantation, for perihilar cholangiocarcinoma at 12 US centers. Gastroenterology 2012;143(1):88, 98. e3.

42. Masuoka HC, Rosen CB. Transplantation for cholangiocarcinoma. Clin Liver Dis 2011;15(4):699–715.

43. RizviS K. Cholangiocarcinoma - evolving concepts andtherapeuticstrategies. Nat Rev Clin Oncol 2018;15:95.

44. Barbier L, Neuzillet C, Dokmak S, et al. Liver transplantation for metastatic neuro-endocrine tumors. Hepatic Oncology 2014;1(4):409–21.

45. Line P-D, Dueland S. Liver transplantation for secondary liver tumours: The difficult balance between survival and recurrence. J Hepatol 2020;73(6):1557–62.

46. Hagness M, Foss A, Line P-D, et al. Liver transplantation for nonresectable liver metastases from colorectal cancer. Annals of surgery 2013;257(5):800–6.

47. Toso C, Marques HP, Andres A, et al. Liver transplantation for colorectal liver metastasis: Survival without recurrence can be achieved. Liver Transplant 2017;23(8):1073–6.

48. Dueland S, Guren TK, Hagness M, et al. Chemotherapy or liver transplantation for nonresectable liver metastases from colorectal cancer? Annals of surgery 2015;261(5):956–60.

49. Guren TK, Thomsen M, Kure EH, et al. Cetuximab in treatment of metastatic colorectal cancer: final survival analyses and extended RAS data from the NORDIC-VII study. British journal of cancer 2017;116(10):1271–8.

50. Tveit KM, Guren T, Glimelius B, et al. Phase III trial of cetuximab with continuous or intermittent fluorouracil, leucovorin, and oxaliplatin (Nordic FLOX) versus FLOX alone in first-line treatment of metastatic colorectal cancer: the NORDIC-VII study. J Clin Oncol 2012;30(15):1755–62.

51. Dueland S, Syversveen T, Solheim JM, et al. Survival Following Liver Transplantation for Patients With Nonresectable Liver-only Colorectal Metastases. Ann Surg 2020;271(2).

52. Rahmim A, Bak-Fredslund KP, Ashrafinia S, et al. Prognostic modeling for patients with colorectal liver metastases incorporating FDG PET radiomic features. European journal of radiology 2019;113:101–9.

53. Smedman TM, Line PD, Hagness M, et al. Liver transplantation for unresectable colorectal liver metastases in patients and donors with extended criteria (SECA-II arm D study). BJS open 2020;4(3):467–77.

54. Reivell V, Hagman H, Haux J, et al. SOULMATE: the Swedish study of liver transplantation for isolated colorectal cancer liver metastases not suitable for operation or ablation, compared to best established treatment-a randomized controlled multicenter trial. Trials 2022;23(1):831.

55. Bonney GK, Chew CA, Lodge P, et al. Liver transplantation for non-resectable colorectal liver metastases: the International Hepato-Pancreato-Biliary Association consensus guidelines. The Lancet Gastroenterology & Hepatology 2021;6(11):933–46.

56. Zingg SW, Shah SA. Where are We with Liver Transplant for Unresectable Colorectal Metastases? Its Early, but Some Initial Insights are Evident. Ann Surg Oncol 2023;1–2.

57. Sasaki K, Ruffolo LI, Kim MH, et al. The current state of liver transplantation for colorectal liver metastases in the United States: a call for standardized reporting. Ann Surg Oncol 2023;1–9.

58. Whitrock JN, Hartman SJ, Shah SA. Transplant for colorectal cancer liver metastases. Surgery 2023;174(1):106–7.

59. Ishaque T, Massie AB, Bowring MG, et al. Liver transplantation and waitlist mortality for HCC and non-HCC candidates following the 2015 HCC exception policy change. Am J Transplant 2019;19(2):564–72.

60. van Rijn R, Schurink IJ, de Vries Y, et al. Hypothermic Machine Perfusion in Liver Transplantation — A Randomized Trial. N Engl J Med 2021;384(15):1391–401.

61. Hernandez-Alejandro R, Ruffolo LI, Sasaki K, et al. Recipient and Donor Outcomes After Living-Donor Liver Transplant for Unresectable Colorectal Liver Metastases. JAMA Surgery 2022;157(6):524–30.
62. Line P-D, Hagness M, Berstad AE, et al. A novel concept for partial liver transplantation in nonresectable colorectal liver metastases: the RAPID concept. Annals of surgery 2015;262(1):e5–9.
63. Nadalin S, Settmacher U, Rauchfuß F, et al. RAPID procedure for colorectal cancer liver metastasis. Int J Surg 2020;82:93–6.
64. Schellenberg AE, Moravan V, Christian F. A competing risk analysis of colorectal cancer recurrence after curative surgery. BMC Gastroenterol 2022;22(1):95.
65. Buisman FE, Galjart B, Van der Stok EP, et al. Recurrence patterns after resection of colorectal liver metastasis are modified by perioperative systemic chemotherapy. World J Surg 2020;44:876–86.
66. Lanari J, Dueland S, Line P-D. Liver transplantation for colorectal liver metastasis. Current Transplantation Reports 2020;7:311–6.
67. Chávez-Villa M, Ruffolo LI, Al-Judaibi BM, et al. The high incidence of occult carcinoma in total hepatectomy specimens of patients treated for unresectable colorectal liver metastases with liver transplant. Ann Surg 2023;10:1097.

Moving?

Make sure your subscription moves with you!

To notify us of your new address, find your **Clinics Account Number** (located on your mailing label above your name), and contact customer service at:

Email: journalscustomerservice-usa@elsevier.com

800-654-2452 (subscribers in the U.S. & Canada)
314-447-8871 (subscribers outside of the U.S. & Canada)

Fax number: 314-447-8029

Elsevier Health Sciences Division
Subscription Customer Service
3251 Riverport Lane
Maryland Heights, MO 63043

*To ensure uninterrupted delivery of your subscription, please notify us at least 4 weeks in advance of move.

Printed and bound by CPI Group (UK) Ltd, Croydon, CR0 4YY

03/10/2024

01040469-0007